TOPICS IN CANCER SURVIVORSHIP

Edited by **Ravinder Mohan**

Topics in Cancer Survivorship
Edited by Ravinder Mohan

Published by InTech
Janeza Trdine 9, 51000 Rijeka, Croatia

Publishing Process Manager Masa Vidovic

Technical Editor Teodora Smiljanic

Cover Designer InTech Design Team

Additional hard copies can be obtained from orders@intechopen.com

Topics in Cancer Survivorship, Edited by Ravinder Mohan
p. cm.
ISBN 978-953-307-894-6

For EU product safety concerns:
IN TECH d.o.o., Prolaz Marije Krucifikse Kozulić 3, 51000 Rijeka, Croatia,
info@intechopen.com or visit our website at intechopen.com.

Meet the editor

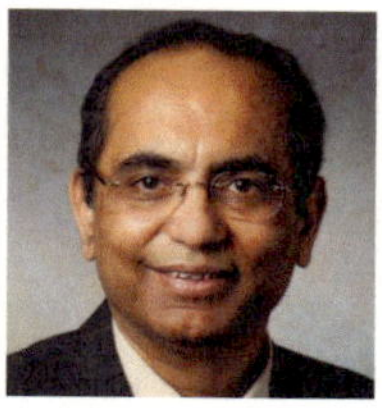

Dr Ravinder Mohan, MD, PhD teaches and practices family medicine in Virginia and also works as a hospitalist physician. He became interested in research on health-related quality of life in Belgium, where he followed clinical outcomes in heart surgery patients. He later used similar methods in Virginia, to evaluate the quality of life of patients who had knee arthritis, and subsequently of patients before and after treatment of localized prostate cancer. Dr. Mohan's research has been published in over 35 high-impact factor peer-reviewed journals and he has also contributed to chapters in five books.

Contents

Preface

"You have cancer," these words almost always cause devastation in the lives of their recipients. Feelings of uncertainty and loss of control over one's life are common reactions. Over time, cancer patients face several challenges that disrupt their quality of life. Examples include: making sense of complex medical information; making difficult treatment decisions; dealing with treatment side effects; living with the fear of recurrence; and for some, facing the possibility of impending death. Thus, in addition to prolonging survival, a key goal of cancer care is to minimize the impact of the disease and treatment on patients' functioning and well-being.

Cancer survivors are all those patients who have ever been diagnosed with cancer. The term "survivor" connotes that patients have been through a harrowing experience. Newly-diagnosed patients are included because this experience begins with the moment of diagnosis. From that time quality of life is almost constantly at peril because of uncertainties and side effects associated with diagnostic and treatment procedures, chronic pain, frequent hospitalizations, disfigurement, depression, and bodily dysfunctions. The spectrum of threats is wide, and so is the potential to address these threats.

In this book, authors present a variety of interventions ranging from the effect of cancer and its treatment on physical appearance and function, expectations regarding survival, mood, sexuality, fertility, and immune function, and describe lifestyle interventions to mitigate these effects and solutions for specific symptoms such as alopecia and lymphedema.

Assoc. Prof. Dr. Ravinder Mohan
Full-time Clinical Faculty,
Department of Family and Community Medicine,
Eastern Virginia Medical School, Norfolk, Virginia,
USA

1

Living With and Beyond Cancer: New Challenges

Neel Bhuva, Sonia P. Li and Jane Maher
Mount Vernon Cancer Centre, Northwood, Middlesex, UK

1. Introduction

'An illness in stages, a very long flight of steps that led assuredly to death, but whose every step represented a unique apprenticeship. It was a disease that gave death time to live and its victims time to die, time to discover time, and in the end to discover life.' Hervé Guilbert

The incidence of cancer is increasing with most current published statistics suggesting that approximately 300,000 new cases are being diagnosed annually in the UK. 1 in 3 will develop cancer during their lifetime. However, despite the incidence of cancer rising by almost 25% in the last 30 years, mortality rates have fallen by almost 20% in the same time period. In the UK, the overall cancer mortality rate in 2008 stood at just over 150,000 (Cancer Research UK, 2010). At present it is thought that two million people have cancer in the UK and as survival rates continue on an upward trend, this figure will only continue to rise (Table 1, Figures 1 and 2). This means that more and more people are living with or beyond a diagnosis of cancer especially with improving cure rates. Cancer is no longer a death sentence for an increasing number of patients.

	UK	%	ENGLAND
Total	2,000,000	100	1,670,000
Male	800,000	40	670,000
Female	1,200,000	60	1,000,000
Age			
0-17	16,000	0.8	13,000
18-64	774,000	38.7	645,000
65+	1,210,000	60.5	1,010,000
Breast	550,000	28	460,000
Colorectal	250,000	12	210,000
Prostate	215,000	11	180,000
Lung	65,000	3	54,000
Other	920,000	46	766,000

Kings College London, MacMillan Cancer Support and National Cancer Intelligence Network,Cancer Prevalence in the UK, 2008

Table 1. Number of people living in the UK and England who have had a cancer diagnosis

Relative five-year estimates based on survival probabilities observed during 2000-2001, by sex and site, England and Wales

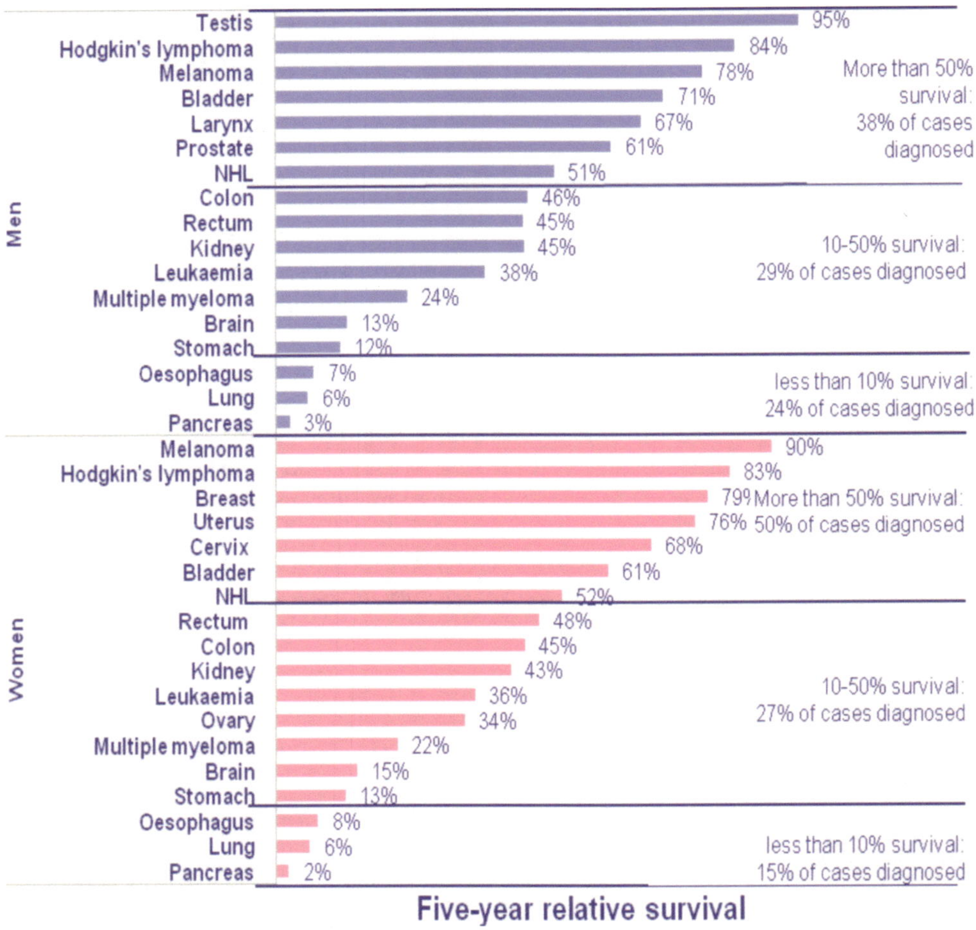

[1]Cancer Research UK, Cancer Stats
[2]Coleman MP et al. Trends and socioeconomic inequalities in cancer survival in England and Wales up to 2001.Br J Cancer, 2004. 90(7): 1367-73

Fig. 1. Relative 5-year survival rates[1,2]

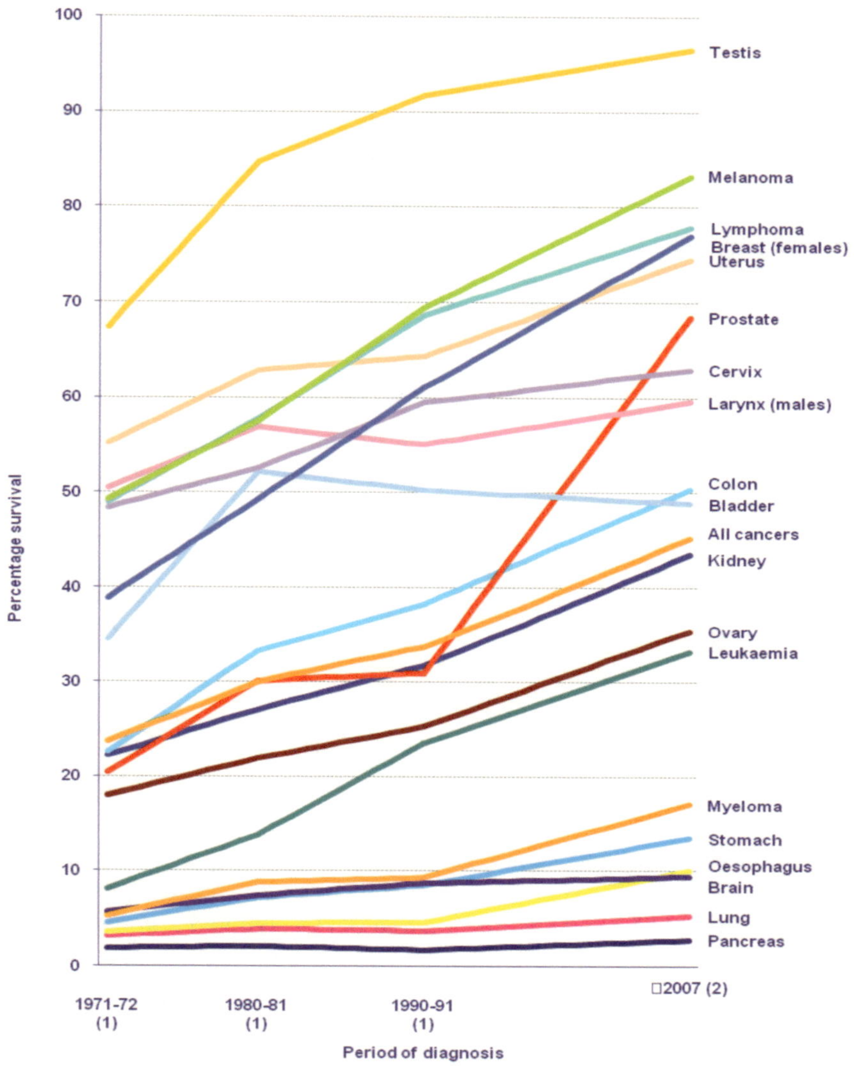

(1) 1971-1991 Cohort Analysis - actual survival, (2) 2007 Hybrid Analysis - predicted survival
1Coleman MP et al. Research commissioned by Cancer Research UK, 2010

Fig. 2. Ten year relative survival (%), adults (15-99 years), selected cancers, England and Wales: survival trends for selected cancers 1971-2007

In fact, survival is increasing and we extrapolate that by 2030 the number of cancer survivors will rise to 4 million (Armes et al., 2009). For the most part, these individuals remain well and healthy but a small number will experience changes to their well-being. As more people live with cancer the proportion of this latter group will go up as well. Cross-sectional studies of populations with chronic illnesses reveal similar health and wellness profiles to populations in whom cancer is present but not active (Birgisson et al., 2008) This suggests that we are living long enough to develop conditions related to the treatment as well as the cancer itself and that we must focus on the quality of survival after different treatments.

A quarter of cancer patients will experience long-term effects that compromise their quality of life. These effects may manifest up to 10 years later and range from minor ailments in the majority to complex and debilitating problems for an unlucky few. Treatments now used to cure patients may no longer be considered ideal when treatment related adverse effects are taken into account and although most will be able to cope with minor conditions, a substantial minority will not. As a result, we must recognise and address the needs of these individuals. Early detection of symptoms, appropriate management and patient education are all key aspects to this. As curative approaches to different cancers become increasingly widespread, the focus needs to be more on quality of survival and reducing the disability associated with them. This is our challenge for the future.

At present it is estimated that almost half a million cancer survivors in the UK suffer from a chronic treatment related condition which impacts their quality of life. In the United States, a National Health Interview study (Hewitt et al., 2003) compared 5,000 cancer survivors with 90,000 people without any history of cancer. It found that cancer survivors were more likely to report being in poor health both psychologically and physically. As we move forward, this will translate into a huge burden on our health resources, especially in the primary care setting. These findings are mirrored by results of similar studies in the UK which have also highlighted the financial impact on cancer patients as a result of no longer being able to work or who are subject to extra costs incurred due to their treatment and/or long-term disability (Fobair, 2007; Macmillan Cancer Support, 2006; Yabroff et al., 2007). It is important therefore, that measures are put in place now to minimise this.

2. Addressing the late effects of cancer treatment

2.1 Definition of late effects

There is currently no agreed definition for the late effects of treatment with some differentiating between long term effects (those occurring during treatment and persisting after completion) and late effects (toxicities not apparent during primary treatment but manifesting some time later). However, the internationally accepted classification of adverse effects of treatment, the Common Toxicities Common Adverse Effects criteria (CTCAE) does not distinguish "acute" and "late" effects.

In response to this, the National Cancer Survivorship Initiative Late Effects workstream has proposed the following definition that "late effects are the long-term consequences of cancer and its treatment, including those which appear during, or soon after treatment, as well as those which appear months or years later".

These effects include:

- Heart (e.g. heart failure following anthracyclines and herceptin)
- Lungs (e.g. radiotherapy, bleomycin)
- Kidneys (e.g. cisplatin)
- Gastrointestinal tract (eg pelvic radiotherapy)
- Musculoskeletal system (eg amputations)
- Lymphatic system (eg lymphoedema)
- Brain (eg impact on cognition following chemotherapy or radiotherapy)
- Peripheral nerves (eg neuropathy related to platinum based drugs)
- Endocrine system (eg growth, fertility, thyroid deficiency, early menopause)
- Sexual interest and function

- Genitourinary system (e.g. following pelvic radiotherapy)
- Second cancers (e.g. breast cancer following radiotherapy for Hodgkin's disease)
- Emotional impact of long-term and late effects of cancer and its treatment.

2.2 Treatment related late effects

Surgery, chemotherapy and radiotherapy all have consequences, which may become apparent immediately or after several years. These include urinary, bowel and sexual dysfunction, neuropathy, cardiovascular and endocrine abnormalities. Those treated as children are at greater risk of complex and inter-related issues arising after a substantial period of time with the risk of a second malignancy becoming an increasingly real threat.

Surgery and radiotherapy can result in significant ongoing co-morbidities. For those patients, for example, who underwent bowel resections, gastrointestinal sequelae of treatment can be severe and most often manifest as loose stool and incontinence. Pelvic radiotherapy has led to increasing cure rates of many cancers but the incidence of long term gastrointestinal problems is even higher (Flentje & Guckenberger, 2006) than with surgery including problems such as urgency, flatulence, abdominal pain and intermittent or regular soiling. Studies report that only a third of patients report normal or good bowel function (Lundby et al., 2005; Marijnen et al., 2005). Despite this, only few gastroenterologists feel adequately trained to deal with such side effects of treatment.

Management of long-term gastrointestinal effects is poorly represented in the literature with little research in the field. Such problems are often very embarrassing to patients and therefore under-reported. Patients may feel that nothing can be done and physicians may not encourage patients to discuss these issues due to their minimal experience in dealing with them (Andreyev et al., 2003a, Andreyev et al., 2003b; Putta & Andreyev, 2005). Such patients inevitably withdraw from social interaction from fear of uncontrollable symptoms (Faithfull, 1995). It is not just bowel related difficulties that these patients face but also urological and sexual dysfunction. Furthermore, fractures, neurological issues and thrombo-embolic phenomena are also seen, although less frequently. 17,000 patients a year are treated with radiotherapy to the pelvis with almost 80,000 survivors of this treatment in the UK. Almost half of these individuals feel that sequelae of treatment has had an impact on their quality of life with 27,000 describing this impact as moderate to severe. These figures are probably an underestimation, particularly as follow-up times for most studies preclude the true magnitude of late effects. Furthermore, few patients freely admit to diarrhoea or incontinence unless directly asked and therefore questionnaires may be too insensitive and not reproducible. The British Society of Gastroenterology is due to publish guidelines on the management of treatment-related late effects this year.

The formation of RAGE (Radiotherapy Action Group Exposure) campaign was to address and improve conditions for patients with breast cancer who experienced late radiation injury as a consequence of radiotherapy at a time when there were no national standards in the United Kingdom. Although radiation damage is relatively rare, serious injuries such as those to the brachial plexus nerves causing weakness of the ipsilateral shoulder, arm and hand and vascular compromise have been reported. Less serious consequences such as rib fractures and skin discoloration may also arise. However, with many women now alive more than a decade after their diagnosis, the consequences of treatment of radiotherapy are becoming an increasing reality and a burden. Macmillan Cancer Support UK have focused on six main areas in response to RAGE (Hanley & Staley, 2006).

1. The development of a national register of consequences of treatment.
2. The improvement of communication between primary and secondary care.
3. Increasing the support to patients by providing information and assistance to patients in understanding the potential changes in their own health after treatment and on when to seek help.
4. The development of easily accessible pathways to access multidisciplinary specialist expertise to patients with late side-effects.
5. The development of an expert patient program for chronic treatment related conditions.
6. The development of innovative commissioning models to help patients get the care they need.

It is not just surgery and radiotherapy that have consequences. Chemotherapy is toxic and mutagenic, causing short-term multi-organ toxicity and increasing the risk of secondary malignancy. Two of the biggest hurdles women with breast cancer face after treatment is the fatigue associated with the cumulative effect of months of treatment and the after-effects of chemotherapy, together with mild cognitive impairment such as memory deficits, often termed "chemobrain" (Tannock et al., 2004). Furthermore, ongoing treatments in patients with breast cancer such as endocrine therapies which are often continued for at least five years, can affect recovery, leaving patients with physical problems such as fatigue, hot flushes, weight gain, joint pains and muscle aches. Tamoxifen can cause endometrial hyperplasia and increase the risk of endometrial malignancy. Osteoporosis and arthalgia are potential adverse effects that can arise from the use of aromatase inhibitors. Although hospital based follow-up systems have been developed to help monitor and detect any late toxicities, it may actually be more effective to educate patients to recognize problems. It is also important that adaptive strategies are discussed with patients in order to help them cope with these side-effects.

2.3 Complex treatment related late effects

A small proportion will suffer from severe or complex problems associated with treatment requiring specialist input. Some of these could be avoided through the prompt recognition and correct management of symptoms thereby avoiding the potential distressing complications resulting from inappropriate procedures. Occasionally, there may be people with unexpected effects associated with treatments which may require a national process of recall, reassessment and commissioning of new services. An example of this is in the group of young patients who received "Mantle" field radiotherapy for Hodgkin's lymphoma which was subsequently associated with a high incidence of breast cancer. There are challenges both in identifying which patients should be recalled as well as how to link them to appropriate specialist multidisciplinary management.

2.4 Secondary malignancies

Secondary malignancies can develop as a consequence of primary treatment, in particular, for patients who received treatment for a childhood cancer. Treatment for Hodgkin's lymphoma is associated with secondary leukaemia and breast cancer. Secondary malignancies are the sixth most common cancer in the USA (after skin, breast, prostate, bowel and lung cancers) and a cancer survivor has twice the risk of a comparable individual without cancer of developing another primary. This makes it all the more important to educate patients and GPs about potential warning signs of another malignancy.

3. Surviving cancer

Mullan (1985) in his seminal paper "Seasons of Survival" describes the evolving process of surviving cancer as beginning from diagnosis and involving the following 3 phases (Mullan, 1985):

- Acute Survival: the first year, recovery from the diagnosis and treatment.
- Extended Survival: five years after treatment.
- Permanent Survival: the long term.

The **acute phase** is particularly difficult with a multitude of physical and psychosocial issues that patients may face. The organic side effects of treatment are the first hurdle but with the completion of treatment, a whole host of unexpected emotions such as uncertainty, fear of recurrence and abandonment may surface (Pelusi, 1997). There are huge psychological hurdles that patients may need to deal with; a sustained mortal threat, unrelenting personal and domestic turmoil, long difficult medical treatments and a prolonged uncertainty about the future. At this point, patients may find that they need to face up to the realities from being an ill person to being a survivor, from feeling time is unlimited to a having finite lifespan and from being fully able to living with a disfigurement or disability. Returning to work can be a huge physical and mental challenge. Patients' view of themselves may have changed and side effects of treatment such as mood changes and hot flushes may make social interaction difficult (Charmaz, 1983; Wyatt 1996). Hospitals form a protective bubble, having become a familiar and comfortable place in which patients often feel a sense of togetherness and reassurance. The sudden foray into the world outside can therefore be lonely and unpredictable. As time passes, most begin to feel a sense of security return and find that their health becomes more predictable. However a significant proportion, approximately 20-30%, will still suffer from continuing distress (Absolom, 2009; Foster, 2009) and will require increasing support in the community. Predictors of persistent, moderate and severe problems with daily living may include a high level of unmet physical needs, fear of recurrence, stress of looking after a family and increasing imposition on their health by unrelated co-morbidities or iatrogenic interventions.

Extended survival is the period where active hospital based surveillance is the mainstay of follow-up. However, these first five years after treatment has ended also represent the period of highest recurrence risk. Reduced levels of activity and less acute symptomatology may persist which over time could erode into the ability to enjoy life and maintain relationships. For example, menopausal symptoms are experienced by 70% of patients treated for breast cancer and can persist for several years impacting severely on quality of life (Carpenter & Andrykowski, 1999; Fenlon et al., 2009; Hunter et al., 2004; Walker et al., 2007). An online survey found that over 30% of breast cancer survivors stopped adjuvant aromatase inhibitor therapy due to their side effects (Zivian & Salgado, 2007). Long term sexual difficulties are also a challenge, with loss of libido, decreased orgasm and physical difficulties (retrograde ejaculation and impotence in men on GHRH antagonists, dyspareunia in women on endocrine therapy). Such issues are often considered taboo or difficult to discuss with medical professionals. Many more women are being diagnosed at a younger age due to screening programmes and therefore wish to maintain fertility. Access to fertility preserving facilities is variable and simply potentiates an already sensitive issue (Amir & Ramati, 2002; Bloom et al., 2004; Broeckel et al., 2002).

Permanent survival refers to treatment related problems that emerge years or decades after the initial diagnosis. This is most apparent in children, a group in whom, as cancer treatment has become more successful, has an increasing number of survivors developing treatment related sequelae such as premature ischaemic heart disease and dyslipidemia after radiation to the heart. Ominously, a similar pattern is developing in adults also. Survivors of breast cancer who were given radiotherapy at a relatively young age are now demonstrating an increased incidence of cardiac problems with age. Despite evidence suggesting that these patients are also at a significantly higher risk of recurrence of a second primary later on in life, many are not receiving more intense screening than the normal population.

4. Responding to the changing cancer story: Focus on the future

In the past and even in the present, cancer services continue to focus predominantly on the acute recovery phase with little emphasis on a five or even ten-year support plan. The first year after treatment is merely the 'tip of the iceberg' and it is crucial that our approach to treating cancer is more visionary and holistic, viewing cancer as a chronic illness rather than an acute condition.

A recent UK survey concluded that at present, follow-up is primarily a check for signs of recurrence or spread (Theis et al., 2010), and checking for recurrence is perceived by the patient as the most important reason for engaging in follow-up. Several studies are currently underway exploring different follow-up methods. What is clear, particularly in the case of colorectal cancer, is that more intense follow-up in the first two years does improve survival, as evidenced by five out of six recent systematic reviews (Figueredo et al., 2003; Richard & Mcleod, 1997; Rosen et al., 1998, Tjandra & Chan, 2007). However, what is not clear is which aspects of follow-up are associated with this. Within the NHS in the UK, consensus meetings have concluded that many follow-up appointments are not required and for many, the common cancers signs of recurrence are as easily and reliably detectable by the patients as they are by expensive surveillance investigations. As long as there is a robust method of feedback to the clinician, i.e. through a specialist nurse, unnecessary appointments can be avoided thus releasing resources and achieving a system, which is more geared to focus on assessment of the cancer, rehabilitation and dealing with the emotional, psychosocial and financial burdens of patients. We need a more bespoke service tailored to the needs of the individual person rather than a 'one size fits all' approach.

The English National Cancer Survivorship Initiative (NCSI) aims to address this issue and provides a vision for better care and support for cancer survivors in the UK. It highlights the importance of recognition and self-management of ongoing problems and raises awareness of the longer-term consequences of cancer (DH, Macmillan Cancer Support & NHS Improvement, 2010). The NCSI is a partnership between Macmillan Cancer Support and the Department of Health and sets out five key shifts in its Vision document of January 2010, outlining ways to assess need, plan care and support cancer survivors to recognise and manage ongoing problems:

- A cultural shift with greater focus on recovery, health and well-being after cancer treatment.
- A shift towards personalized assessment, information provision and care planning.
- A shift towards support for self management.
- A shift from a single model of clinical follow-up to tailored support that enables early recognition and preparation for both the signs of further disease and the longer-term consequences of treatment.
- A shift towards using Patient Reported Outcome Measures as well as clinical measures.

This should raise awareness and allow intervention to help deal with the longer term consequences of cancer treatment, including the recognition that survivors of cancer have particular risks in relation to unhealthy lifestyles. Some long term cancer survivors express a preference for hospital-based services including telephone based services and those who have experience of such services are generally very positive about them. Furthermore, as part of the National Cancer Survivorship Initiative, different ways to deliver after cancer treatment care such as "end of treatment care packages" including information about "what to expect", written care plans, description of symptoms indicating a need for tests, coping strategies and a variety of educational interventions are being investigated and these will be reported in 2011-12 to aid in the commissioning of new pathways.

If change is to be successfully implemented it will require coordination of services and teamwork between secondary care, primary care and the patients themselves. The transitions between the three phases of survivorship according to Mullan's model have been dubbed as 'teachable moments' (Denmark-Wahnefried et al., 20045). These are seen to be opportunities for giving information on health surveillance and healthy living. Cancer survivors are receptive to any initiatives that will improve their health, but many are not aware that lifestyle changes are especially important for them, given that they are at an increased risk of chronic illnesses and further malignant disease. Not only do we need to equip patients to know what symptoms to look for and when they require to be seen by a medical professional, but we must also unlock these gateways in order that they may benefit from programmes supporting lifestyle change, such as smoking cessation, weight loss and exercise.

Primary care will also need to play an increasingly important role. General practitioner should no longer see cancer in simple terms i.e. 'cured and back to normal' or 'incurable and terminal'. Many general practitioner have not received any training or education about the long-term consequences of cancer and its treatment and therefore may not always make the connection between a symptom or series of symptoms and past cancer treatment. Furthermore, in some cases, they may not view it as their responsibility to identify and manage these consequences. Progressive, complex problems related to rare conditions and/or obsolete treatments may often go unrecognised. Symptoms of all patients with a cancer history should be considered as possibly relating to that cancer. Furthermore, practices must employ up-to-date and accurate recording of patients so that previous cytotoxic or radiation treatments are highlighted on computer systems. Visual alerts can bring an individual's cancer diagnosis to the forefront of the primary care physician's mind during a consultation. The flow of information between oncologist and GP is vital with one of the mandates of the NCSI specifically addressing how this can be improved. GPs also need to be educated on being pro-active in asking about physical symptoms, such as those with heart disease, as well as providing and facilitating psychological support. It is crucial that GPs and patients are given access to freely available information regarding the long term sequelae of oncological treatments, and those patients identified as being at higher risk are more closely monitored and receive appropriate lifestyle advice.

5. Transition

The landscape of cancer treatment is changing. In today's world we do not just treat cancer - we live with it. In tomorrow's world we will survive it.

'Survival machines which can simulate (i.e.imagine) the future are one jump ahead of survival machines who can learn only by trial and error…'
Richard Dawkins

6. References

(2010) In: *Cancer Research UK,* Accessed 21 June 2010, www.info.cancerresearchuk.org/cancerstats/types/cervix/incidence. Http://info.cancerresearchuk.org/cancerstats/types/breast/survival/index.htm#depr

Absolom, K. et al. (2009). Follow-up care for cancer survivors: views of the younger adult. *British Journal of Cancer,* Vol.101, No.4, pp. 561-567

Amir, M. & Ramati ,A. (2002). Post-traumatic symptoms, emotional distress and quality of life in long-term survivors of breast cancer: a preliminary research. *Journal Anxiety Disorder,* Vol.16, pp. 195-206

Andreyev, H.J.N. et al. (2003). GI symptoms developing after pelvic radiotherapy require gastronenterological review but is this happening in the UK? *Clin Oncol,* Vol.15, No.2, S12 (abstract)

Andreyev, H. et al. (2003). GI symptoms developing after pelvic radiotherapy require gastroenterological review. *Gut* Vol.52, supplement 1, A90

Armes, J. et al. (2009). Patients' supportive care needs beyond the end of treatment: aprospective and longitudinal survey. *Clin Oncol,* Vol.27, No.36, pp. 6172-6179.

Birgisson, H. et al., (2008). Late gastrointestinal disorders after recal cancer surgery with and without pre-operative radiation therapy. *British Journal of Surgery,* 2008, Vol.95, No.2, pp. 206-213.

Bloom, J.R. et al. (2004). Then and now: quality of life of young breast cancer survivors.*Psycho-Oncology,* Vol.13, pp. 147-160

Broeckel, J.A., et al. (2002). Sexual functioning in long-term breast cancer survivors treated with adjuvant chemotherapy. *Breast Cancer Research and Treatment,* Vol.75, pp. 241-248

Carpenter, J.S. & Andrykowski, M.A. (1999). Menopausal symptoms in breast cancer survivors. *Oncology Nursing Forum,* Vol.26, No.8, pp. 1311-1317

Charmaz, K. (1983). Loss of self: a fundamental form of suffering in the chronically ill. *Sociology of Health& Illness,* Vol.5, No.2, pp.168-95

Demark-Wahnefried, W. et al. (2005). Riding the crest of the teachable moment: promoting long-term health after the diagnosis of cancer. *Clin Oncol,* Vol.23, No.24, pp. 5814-5830

DH, Macmillan Cancer Support and NHS Improvement. The National Cancer Survivorship Initiative Vision 2010. Available from http://www.dh.gov.uk/publications

Faithfull, S. (1995). 'Just grin and bear it and hope that it will go away': coping with urinary symptoms from pelvic radiotherapy. *Eur J Cancer Care,* Vol.4, No.4, pp. 158-165

Fenlon, D.R. et al. (2009). Menopausal hot flushes after breast cancer. *Eur J of Cancer Care,* Vol.18, No.2, pp. 140-148

Figueredo, A. et al. (2003). Follow-up of patients with curatively resected colorectal cancer: a practice guideline. *BMC Cancer*, Vol. 3, pp. 26

Fobair, P. (2007). Oncology social work for survivors. *Cancer Survivorship Today andTomorrow*. Ed Patricia Ganz pub Springer pp. 114-121

Foster, C. et al. (2009). Psychosocial implications of living five years or more following a cancer diagnosis. A systematic review of the research evidence. *Eur J. of Cancer Care*, Vol.18, pp. 223-247

Guckenberger, M. & Flentje, M. (2006). Late small bowel toxicity after adjuvant treatment for rectal cancer. *Int J Colorectal Dis*, Vol. 21, pp. 209-220

Hunter, M.S. et al. (2004). Menopausal symptoms in women with breast cancer: prevalence and treatment preferences. *Psycho-Oncology*, Vol.13, No.11, pp. 769-778

Lange, M.M. et al. (2007). Risk factors for faecal incontinence after rectal cancer treatment. *Br Journal of Surgery*, Vol.94, Ch.10, pp. 1278-1284

Lundby, L. et al. (2005). Long term anorectal dysfunction after postoperative radiotherapy for rectal cancer. *Dis Colon Rectum*, Vol.48, Ch.7, pp. 1343-1352

Macmillan Cancer Support. *Cancer Costs 2006*. www.macmillan.org.uk

Marijnen, C.A. et al. (2005). Impact of short term preoperative radiotherapy on health related quality of life and sexual functioning in primary rectal cancer: report of a multi-center randomized trial. *Clin Oncol*, Vol.23, Ch.9, pp. 1847-1858

Mullan, R. (1985) Seasons of survival: reflections of a physician with cancer. *NEJM*, Vol.313, pp. 270-273

Pelusi, J. (1997). The lived Experience of Surviving Breast Cancer. *Oncology Nursing Forum*, Vol. 24, No.8, pp.1343-1353

Putta, S. & Andreyev, H.J.N. (2005). Faecal incontinence - a late side effect of pelvic radiotherapy. *Clin Oncol*, Vol.7, Ch.6, pp. 469-477

Richard, C.S. & Mcleod, R.S. (1997). Follow-up of patients after resection for colorectal cancer: a position paper of the Canadian Society of Surgical Oncology and the Canadian Society of Colon and Rectal Surgeons. *Can J Surg*, Vol.40, pp. 90-100

Rosen, M. et al. (1998). Follow-up of colorectal cancer: a meta-analysis. *Dis Colon Rectum* Vol.41, pp. 1116-1126

Tannock, I.F. et al. (2004). Cognitive impairment associated with chemotherapy for cancer: areport of a workshop. *Clin Oncol*, Vol.22, No.11, pp. 2233-2239

Theis, V.S. et al. (2010). Chronic Radiation Enteritis. Clin Oncol, Vol.22, pp. 70-83

Tjandra, J.J. & Chan, M.K.Y. (2007). Follow-up after curative resection of colorectal cancer: a meta-analysis. *Dis Colon Rectum*, available from http://www.springerlink.com/content/r95uqr6x328u7130/

Walker, G., et al. (2007). Ear acupuncture for hot flushes--the perceptions of women with breast cancer. *Complement Ther Clin Pract*, Vol.13, No.4, pp. 250-257

Wyatt, G. & Friedman, L.L. (1996). Long term female cancer survivors: quality of life issues and clinical implications. *Cancer Nursing*, Vol. 19, pp. 1-7

Yabroff, K.R. et al,. (2007). Patient time costs associated with cancer care. *JNCI* , Vol.99, No.1, pp. 14-23

Zivian, M. & Salgado, B. (2007). Side effects revealed: Women's experiences with Aromatase Inhibitors. *Breast Cancer Action,* San Francisco

2

Body Image and Cancer

Hanne Konradsen
Gentofte University Hospital,
Denmark

1. Introduction

Human beings have always been interested in their appearance. Most of us make active efforts to influence the way we look: we exercise, we lose or put on weight, we use make-up and dye our hair, we dress in certain ways, and some of us even have surgery to change parts of the body with which we are dissatisfied. Changes in appearance are sometimes desired, and sometimes not. According to Giddens, the body is easily changeable and reflects our identity (Giddens 1991). Individuals therefore have the ability to change their bodies, if they so wish. The healthy body symbolises a healthy society, while the sick or imperfect body represents a sick society. In advertising, good-looking models are often used, as it is expected that this will cause us to buy the product they are advertising (Rumsey N. & Harcourt D. 2005). Visual appearance is sometimes also linked with inner values. Most societies have their own traditional links; in Western society, for example, red hair is associated with a hot temper, and a link has been found between appearance and the chance of being convicted in court through false consensus (Miyake & Zuckerman 1993). Stereotypical conceptions of links between visual appearance and a person's inner qualities have also been experienced by patients (Rumsey N. 2003). Plough Hansen has, for example, described how women with chemotherapy-induced hair loss experienced this as a loss of womanhood, associated with sickness and death, and therefore used wigs and make-up to control and minimize the effects of the changed appearance (Hansen H.P. 2007). Jutel and Buetow argue that outer appearance and a tendency to focus on first impressions may imply a tendency for health care professionals to use this as an indicator of health, with the risk that this could harm medical practice (Jutel & Buetow 2007). However, although there is an emphasis on visual appearance in our society, such norms as "true beauty comes from within", "do not judge a book by its cover" or "beauty lies in the eye of the beholder" are often more acceptable. People do not generally wish to be regarded as being overly concerned about their appearance, or as someone who judges others on their appearance. This makes it difficult for patients to talk about issues of appearance. It might therefore also seem a contradiction that many smokers continue to smoke rather than risk gaining an extra five kilos, even though the health risk from smoking is many times greater than that of a small amount of extra weight. Similarly, young amateur bodybuilders risk taking anabolic steroids in order to increase their muscle mass, even though this affects their bodies in many ways, and may involve the risk of impotence. In a study of patients attending a cancer rehabilitation centre, it was found that the lack of communication about appearance was experienced as a socially-accepted norm, supported by the taboo on speaking out about cancer (Rasmussen, Hansen, & Elverdam 2009).

Visual appearance affects first impressions when two people meet. In addition, another determinant is how those impressions are understood and socially returned. It has for example been shown that people who undergo facial changes experience social encounters in ways that are different from others, with behaviour or rules of social conduct that differ from the norm, e.g. greater standing distance (Rumsey N., Bull R., & Gahagan D. 1982), staring and comments, or differences expressed in "silent language" such as body movements and gestures (Macgregor F.C. 1990). This is an example of how reactions are determined, not only by the actual physically changed appearance, but also by social interaction between people. In patients who have undergone a changed appearance after surgery for head, neck or eye cancer, this was described in their first year post-operatively as "interactional integration" (Konradsen H. 2010). The integration of disfigurement was affected not only by the attitudes of the patients themselves, but equally by their social interaction with the surrounding society, also described as the movement from becoming disfigured, to being a disfigured person, to becoming a person with a disfigurement.

One of the first philosophers to talk about the body was Plato, who lived from 427 – 347 BC. He regarded the body and mind as two separate entities, and this dualistic view of body and mind still underlies much of our health care today. Others have criticised this approach. The anthropologists Scheper-Huges and Lock (Scheper-Hughes & Lock 1987), for example, view the body on three levels: the individual body, the social body and the political body. According to them, society socialises us and our bodies, and our bodies therefore represent our ability to live up to these norms. This puts a great deal of pressure on those who fall ill.

In the early 1990s, Bob Price developed the "Body Image Care Model" (Price 1990). This model focuses on how we experience our bodies, and our reaction to how others regard us. The model describes our body image as influenced by three dimensions: body ideal, body reality and body appearance (Figure 1)

Subsequently, other people have developed other models. Professor Robert Newell, for example, has developed the "fear-avoidance model" (Newell 1999). His model can help to evaluate body image-related concerns and provide possible suggestions for intervention. (Figure 2).

In healthcare research, the use of the concept of body image began in the nineteen-sixties, and was at first mainly related to social psychology, with the main emphasis on eating disorders. Most research at that time focused on how the disturbed body image or body ideal was perceived by the person herself: the fact that you did not see yourself as others saw you. This way of looking at body image-related concerns is for example reflected in the NANDA classifications (Ackly & Ladwig 2008). Here, disturbed body image is defined as "confusion in the mental picture of one's physical self". More recently, the concept of body image has received wider clinical application. Today, we know that bodily changes, and related body image concerns, occur independently of medical diagnosis. Most diseases cause bodily changes, whether they are temporary, recurrent or chronic. These changes may be visible or invisible, physical or psychological, and may interfere in various ways with our everyday lives. Such bodily changes are not merely objective visible changes, but are also subjective, and are linked to the ways in which we see our bodies, the world and our relationships with others. Health-related quality of life studies have explored this and have shown how changed appearance in relation to illness is an important issue, for example in cases of HIV and AIDS (Huang et al. 2006b; Huang et al. 2006a), as well as obstetrics (Hawighorst-Knapstein et al. 2004). It is also important irrespective of patients' age, gender, social situation or ethnicity (Cash T.F. & Pruzinsky T. 2002).

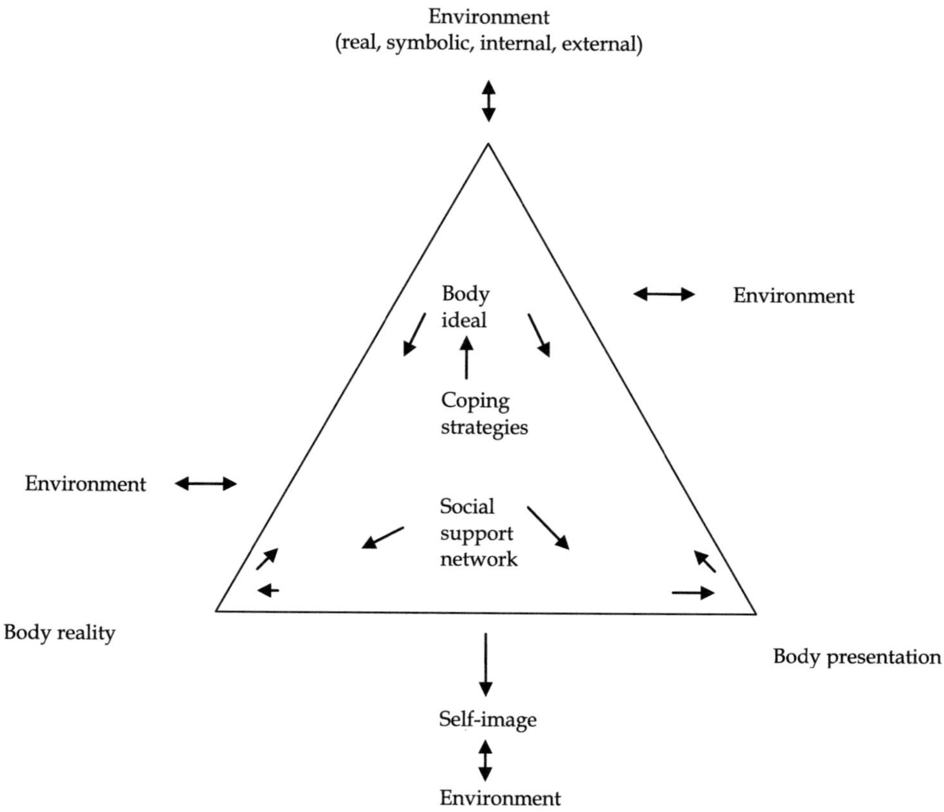

Fig. 1. The body-image care model. Arrows indicate direction, influence or interaction. (Price 1990)

Facial disfigurement as a result of surgical treatment for head, neck or eye cancer, for example, poses a great challenge to the person experiencing it. The face is a major contributor to what is labelled "first impressions", and it expresses a great deal of our personality (Bar M., Neta M., & Linz H. 2006;Hess U., Adams R.B., & Kleck R.E. 2009;Naumann L.P. et al. 2009). Changes in the face cannot be hidden, and are therefore often more difficult for patients to deal with than changes elsewhere in the body (Dropkin M.J. 1999). According to Callahan, facial disfigurement poses a challenge, in that the patient must deal with both a changed appearance and an altered sense of self (Callahan C. 2004). Facial disfigurement is associated with a high degree of psychosocial problems and a lower self-reported quality of life. The problems occur irrespective of the patient's age or the extent of the disfigurement (Blood G.W. et al. 1995;Tebble N.J., Thomas D.W., & Price P. 2004), and include anxiety, depression and social isolation (D`Antonio L. et al. 1998;Rumsey N. 2003;Rumsey N. et al. 2004) Marks 2000, Tebble 2006). Close family members or partners may also be affected (Drabe N. et al. 2008;Krouse H.J. et al. 2004;Verdonck-de Leeuw I.M. et al. 2007;Vickery L.E.Latchford G. et al. 2003). In relation to quality of life, socio-cultural factors seem to matter more than physical dysfunction (Morton R.P. 2003). In 1983, Dropkin (Dropkin M.J. et al. 1983) found no differences in the evaluation of men's and women's degree of disfigurement after identical surgical treatment, whereas Lockhart found such differences in 1999, and based the explanation of the results on a generally increased focus in society on "the perfect female body" (Lockhart J.S. 1999).

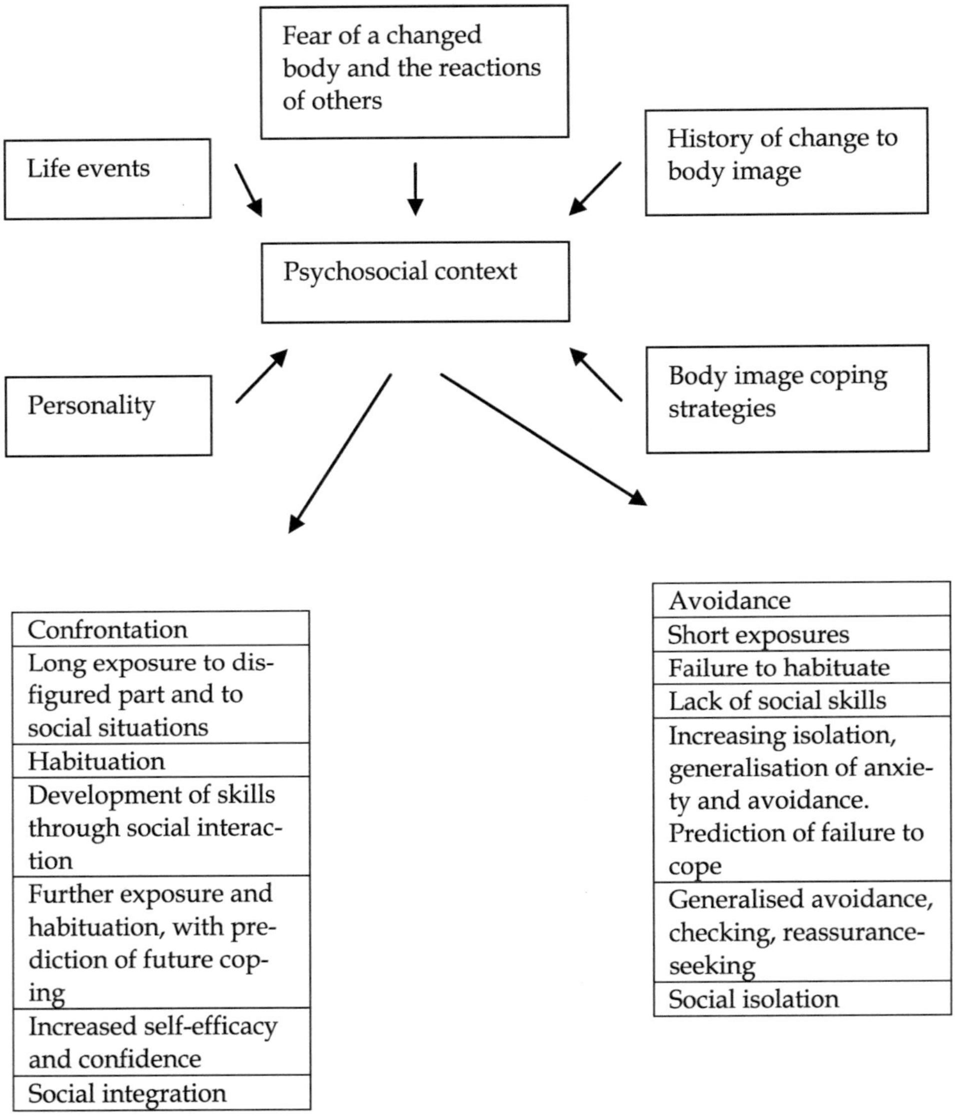

Fig. 2. A fear-avoidance model of psychosocial difficulties following disfigurement. (Newell 1999).

When we encounter illness our attention is directed towards the body, a mechanism Leder calls "the dysappearing body" (Leder D. 1990). When our body is changing, or not functioning as we expect, our attention is drawn towards it. Others have found that the experience of bodily change is influenced by various underlying self-schemas (Thompson A. & Kent G. 2001), the degree to which people have a negative view of themselves (Moss T. & Carr T. 2004), or social self-efficacy (Hagedoorn & Molleman 2006).

Cancer, i.e. the disease itself, its treatment and side effects, significantly interferes with the body. There are bodily changes associated with the specific cancer site, but in addition to this, many cancer patients also struggle with symptoms such as tiredness, pain, etc. Due to the seriousness of the disease, psychosocial concerns are also of great importance and influence the way in which the body is perceived.

In general, body image is a multidimensional concept which is used in many different ways. In 2002, White wrote that "much of the literature on body image and cancer is observational, atheoretical, and anecdotal. Though more empirical research has recently emerged, it is often of poor quality, resulting in inconsistent findings" (Cash T.F. & Pruzinsky T. 2002). This is still partly true, but body image as a research subject has been attracting increasing attention.

2. What we know

In the following, the literature relating to body image and cancer is briefly reviewed. What do we know about body image in relation to cancer patients? And what are the benefits and limitations of the research?

The research studies examined date from 1997 to 2010. As the aim is to understand how issues and concerns relating to bodily changes are experienced by adults, only studies which employed a qualitative approach have been examined. In order to obtain an overview, all of the studies were arranged according to the Matrix Method (Garrad J. 2011). The research includes studies of adult women, men, both men and women, and families. The medical diagnoses included breast cancer, gynaecological cancer, head and neck cancer, testicular cancer and colorectal cancer. A few also included persons with a mixture of different diagnoses. This indicates that the research has mainly concentrated on diagnoses for which treatment most often results in a visibly changed body.

2.1 Body image and gender

Overall, most of our knowledge about body image and cancer is related to the diagnosis of breast cancer, and thereby relates specifically to women. Breast cancer has been described as associated with the fear of losing one's attractiveness and desirability (Elmir et al. 2010), and has been seen as a threat to intimate relationships (Ashing-Giwa et al. 2006) and as challenging a person's female identity (Piot-Ziegler et al. 2010). Studies focusing on men are rare. A few studies have been undertaken of testicular cancer, e.g. (Chapple & McPherson 2004), and of male breast cancer (Pituskin et al. 2007). Even fewer studies have been undertaken of how the cancer experience relates to body image when gay or lesbian patients are involved; one example is a study by Katz (Katz 2009). In relation to body image concerns, it seems that the emphasis is on gender as a sexual component, and little is known about how women and men experience bodily changes in relation to cancer diseases that are not related to a person's specific gender.

2.2 Body image as a static or changing problem

Problems relating to body image are often described as a static issue, clearly associated in time with the period after cancer treatment. A few studies have examined changes in body image pre- and post treatment, e.g. Adamsen's study of how young athletes regain their bodily control and identity through exercise, and Bredin's study of women with breast cancer, and how they experienced their body image in combination with therapeutic massage (Adamsen et al. 2009; Bredin 1999). Body image problems are also often presented as being static post-treatment. In general, the findings give a picture of BI-related concerns at a specific point in time. We know that adjustment to other chronic diseases must be viewed over a substantial period of time if they are to be fully understood. Adjustment is the psychosocial adaptation to a life change, as expressed in the Nursing Outcome Classification (Johnson M., Maas M., & Moorhead S. 2000), so if body image is regarded as a chronic or stable situation, this approach could prove fruitful. In the case of multiple sclerosis, for example, patients diagnosed at least five years previously stated that it was a process that "one can learn to live with" in time (Irvine H. et al. 2009). For patients adjusting to lower-limb amputation, it has been found to be a question of developing an altered sense of self and identity over the months and years following the amputation (Horgan O. & MacLachlan M. 2004). In an article, Morse describes findings from a study of patients who survived traumatic injury, covering their experiences from the initial impact of the surgery until recovery (Morse J.M. & O'Brian B. 1995). She describes a four-stage process of vigilance, disruption, enduring the self, and striving to regain the self. In the final stage, the participants learned to redefine the self as a disabled person by accepting the consequences and reformulating their expectations. Learning to see oneself as a disabled person is also one of the end-points in a qualitative meta-analysis of the individual's responses to acute or chronic illness or injury (Morse J.M. 1997).

The elucidation and exploration of body image is also seen as a static problem, in that only a few studies describe the late effects of cancer and how these are experienced. Frid found that lower limb lymphedema exerts a considerable influence on the psychosocial situation of cancer patients in palliative care (Frid et al. 2006). There are very few studies that examine how a patient's body image concerns change over time. One example is the study by Roing on the experiences of patients with oral cancer of their illness and treatment (Roing, Hirsch, & Holmstrom 2007). The study found that the need of patients for support increased during treatment, and it was suggested that this need might be greatest at the conclusion of radiotherapy, when the patients returned home. This is an example of how the degree and extent of patient concerns can be greatest at the time of discharge, rather than, as is often thought, at the time of admission to hospital. Another way of elucidating change in body image over time is described by Frith in a study of chemotherapy-induced hair loss among patients treated for breast cancer (Frith, Harcourt, & Fussell 2007). Here it was shown that the women made use of the anticipation of altered appearance as a form of anticipatory coping.

A more detailed picture is required of interventions targeted at specific problems relating to body image; how do the problems change over time, and when is the most appropriate time for intervention?

2.3 Context-related or universal

In most of the studies, context is very sparsely elucidated. In some studies the cultural aspect is described, examining such issues as religious approaches in newly-diagnosed Iranian women coping with breast cancer (Taleghani, Yekta, & Nasrabadi 2006), how spiritual belief is part of the cancer belief among Asian American women with breast cancer (Tam et al. 2003), or how culture and the role of the woman in Lebanese families creates a foundation for various coping strategies among women with breast cancer (Doumit et al. 2010). Another study described women from a low-income socio-economic group with early-stage breast cancer and their various styles of decision-making (McVea, Minier, & Johnson Palensky 2001). While it is plausible that body image-related concerns could have a universal inner structure, it is also plausible that body image-related concerns could be highly culturally dependent. The latter is suggested by a study of Jewish/Middle Eastern cancer patients from Israel, where religious belief systems, amongst other things, can influence how patients deal with existential concerns (including body image-related concerns) (Blinderman & Cherny 2005). It seems evident that body image-related concerns are not only dependent on how an individual experiences her own body. The surrounding society and the people with whom one interacts also have a substantial influence - an influence that is often overlooked in research.

2.4 Multiple effects

Body image is very often described as a concept that relates to the visible, objective signs of changed appearance: the absence of a breast or hair, deterioration in muscle function, or a change in bodily functions such as amenorrhoea or loss of control over bodily functions.

When body image is addressed in a study's results, the terms in which it described are often powerful, such as identity-changing, hopelessness, fear, poor self-esteem, frustration and so on. The concept of body image itself is rarely defined, and is most often used without a theoretical basis. One of the few studies to actually define the term body image as it used is Jenks et al (Jenks, Morin, & Tomaselli 1997), who state that the definition of body image they employ is based on the individual's own perception of the physical appearance and physical functions of the body.

However, as with any other concept in research, the use of the body image concept is strongly linked to how the concept is defined. This may be exemplified by examining three different studies.

In 1983, Dropkin developed a visual scale to measure the perception of the severity of visible disfigurement and dysfunction following head and neck cancer surgery (Dropkin et al. 1983). Evaluations were made by measuring how nurses assessed a certain disfiguring surgical procedure. The study argues that quantitative measurement of the grade of disfigurement could be used to foresee the course of a patient's rehabilitation. This thus implies that the way in which others perceive a person with a disfigurement is an important factor in the rehabilitation process.

Later, Newell developed his fear-avoidance model of psychosocial difficulties following disfigurement (Newell 1999). This model suggests that the problems experienced by patients with disfigurement could be compared to those experienced by patients with phobias. It therefore recommends cognitive behavioural therapy. The model thus implies that a person's own perception of himself or herself and their own way of behaving are important factors.

The third study is from 2006; here Furness argues that social support and a person's ability to cope with challenging situations are important (Furness P.J. et al. 2006). This study implies that social interaction and a person's own psychological resources are important factors.

These three studies present different theoretical perspectives on the psychosocial issues relating to disfigurement. These theoretical views contribute to determining how one might regard, elucidate and examine these problems, how data is collected and analysed, and where to look for data. Determining and describing the theoretical view of the concept of body image thus seems to be important in order to assess the results of the study. Doing so could potentially strengthen the whole body of knowledge within this clinical area and improve the possibilities for developing adequate and effective interventions which will target the patients' problems.

2.5 Relationships

One major theme that emerges in connection with how patients with body image-related concerns relate to health care professionals is that of lack of support. In head, neck and eye cancer, for example, this is described by Konradsen (Konradsen, Kirkevold, & Zoffmann 2009) as an issue that is silenced in the communication between patient, relatives and professionals. In a study of patients surgically treated for laryngeal cancer, it was found that for a period of three years, the most difficult areas of psychosocial adaptation were work and family relationships (Ramirés M.J. et al. 2003), while in patients with orofacial injury, it was found that the perception of a diminished level of social support was associated with a higher risk of post-traumatic stress (Lui A., Glynn S., & Shetty V. 2009). Others have found that patients' family members also go through a process of adjustment, from being concerned about the survival of the patient to becoming concerned with how disfigurement might affect the patient socially (Bonanno A. et al. 2010).

It seems that for cancer patients, body image-associated issues relate to some of the basic and fundamental structures of a person's identity, and thereby also to social interaction in a broad sense. For patients with colorectal cancer, the experience of having to deal with a stoma is described as a loss of adulthood (Rozmovits & Ziebland 2004), which also influences their sense of dignity, independency and sexual confidence.

3. Future research

With the exception of one study's additional use of journal narrative, the research has exclusively employed individual interviews or focus group interviews for data collection. These are data collection methods which are well established in qualitative research, and are capable of collecting valuable data. However, a wider range of data collection methods might enrich the body of knowledge in the field of body image.

A closer look at changing body ideals in the surrounding society of patients might also be beneficial. How does the changing body ideal among both women and men influence the experience of bodily change? If more is learned about this, it might be possible to develop better patient trajectories.

All of the studies included an adult population, but few included old people. As an example, it has been shown that body image is important when older women are making treatment decisions about breast cancer, and that treatment outcomes influenced body image two years after treatment (Figueiredo et al. 2004). It might therefore be of great interest to examine the impact on body image of experiencing cancer either as an older person, or how this changes (or does not change) in the course of a lifetime. Collecting this knowledge and obtaining an overview might help the health care system to improve both the overall and the individual quality of treatment and care.

4. Interventions

Measuring body image implies a wide range of challenges. The definition of the term 'body image' reflects what is being measured. One proposal for a means of measuring body image, specifically in relation to cancer patients, has been advanced by Hopwood (Hopwood et al. 2001). The scale focuses on how body image is experienced by the patients themselves. It is a valuable scale, but it may omit the contribution of relatives and society generally to the way in which patients experience their own body image. The scale can provide valuable knowledge about the extent of body image concerns among cancer patients. It has for example been used to describe how half of a multi-ethnic population of women in the USA diagnosed with breast cancer experienced two or more body image problems during the early months after diagnosis (Fobair et al. 2006). Another scale is Dropkin's disfigurement/dysfunction scale, which measures how others view the extent of a patient's disfigurement. This is also important, and has been used to show how body image reintegration is critical to subsequent quality of life after head and neck cancer surgery (Dropkin M.J. 1999).

Qualitative studies are important when developing intervention studies targeted at the psychosocial problems experienced by cancer patients in relation to body image. In many areas there is a lack of effective intervention methods. In relation to head and neck cancer, for example, reviews have shown that no intervention method has so far been successful (Semple et al. 2004). Another example is in relation to gynaecological cancer patients; in this context there is only weak evidence to suggest an effect from cognitive behavioural interventions for body image-related concerns (Hersch et al. 2009). Overall, Bessell concluded in a review of the effectiveness of psychosocial interventions targeting individuals with visible disfigurement unrelated to diagnosis that none of the studies demonstrated adequate clinical effectiveness in the interventions (Bessell & Moss 2007).

Qualitative studies have the potential to direct the researcher's attention to possible elements of future interventions. Studies using grounded theory as a research method have for example demonstrated this in other contexts, such as diabetes care (Zoffmann & Lauritzen 2006). To demonstrate how this can be viewed, a case is presented elucidating how a longitudinal study of patients with facial disfigurement as a result of surgical treatment for head, neck or eye cancer could point to possible elements of future interventions (Konradsen H. 2010).

In the study, the researcher met and interviewed the participating patients several times during the first postoperative year. Grounded theory analysis of the early patient-nurse interaction during hospitalisation revealed that disfigurement in this context was silenced, and this situation continued. The researcher, on the other hand, brought up disfigurement as a central theme in every interview. The fact that the researcher became a familiar person who accompanied the patients throughout their trajectory also meant that the researcher knew the patient's history and was aware of his or her concerns. While hospitalised, the patients met various nurses, albeit a limited number, whereas during outpatient treatment they met a different nurse at almost every visit. In contrast to this, the researcher was the same person throughout the entire process.

Throughout the study, there were numerous signs of the patients' willingness to participate, e.g. repeatedly devoting their spare time to talking to the researcher, inviting the researcher to their homes and serving coffee and cake, wishing to continue talking after the interview was completed, and so on. Regardless of not being asked about the benefits of participation in the study, six of the twelve patients spontaneously stated that they had benefited from this. The positive effects were related to the patients' feeling that there was someone who

was willing to listen to their story, the feeling of being able to look to the future with some confidence, and a sense of being able to exert some kind of influence over how to tackle the possible obstacles the patient would meet in the future.
The positive effects of participation in the study indicate and help to point out various possible effective components of interventions, which future intervention studies may subsequently evaluate. Examples are shown in table 1.

- Setting the issue on the agenda
- Regular meetings for patients and their significant others with a nurse at the hospital
- Emotional intimacy between nurse and patient
- Establish a relationship between nurse and patient
- Promote trust between the patient and the nurse to talk about any issue the patient wishes
- Encourage patients to tell their stories
- Give patients the time needed for reflection
- Explicitly ask the patients questions about disfigurement
- Ask open questions in order for the nurse to understand the patient's experiences and in order for the nurse to help the patient to understand own experiences
- Develop specific communication skills among nurses in order to redirect communication from the area of general practicalities and physical needs to patient-specific psychosocial needs
- Organise the entire patient trajectory towards higher nurse-patient continuity

Table 1. Possible elements in interventions targeting psychosocial concerns related to body image

5. References

Ackly, B. & Ladwig, G. 2008, *Nursing diagnosis handbook. An evidence-based guide to planning care.* Mosby Elsevier.

Adamsen, L., Andersen, C., Midtgaard, J., Moller, T., Quist, M., & Rorth, M. 2009, "Struggling with cancer and treatment: young athletes recapture body control and identity through exercise: qualitative findings from a supervised group exercise program in cancer patients of mixed gender undergoing chemotherapy", *Scand.J Med Sci.Sports*, vol. 19, no. 1, pp. 55-66.

Ashing-Giwa, K. T., Padilla, G. V., Bohorquez, D. E., Tejero, J. S., & Garcia, M. 2006, "Understanding the breast cancer experience of Latina women", *J Psychosoc.Oncol.*, vol. 24, no. 3, pp. 19-52.

Bar M., Neta M., & Linz H. 2006, "Very first impressions", *Emotion*, vol. 6, no. 2, pp. 269-278.

Bessell, A. & Moss, T. P. 2007, "Evaluating the effectiveness of psychosocial interventions for individuals with visible differences: a systematic review of the empirical literature", *Body Image*, vol. 4, no. 3, pp. 227-238.

Blinderman, C. D. & Cherny, N. I. 2005, "Existential issues do not necessarily result in existential suffering: lessons from cancer patients in Israel", *Palliat.Med*, vol. 19, no. 5, pp. 371-380.

Blood G.W., Blood S., Raimondi S.C., & Dineen M. 1995, "A comparison of older and younger individuals living after the surgical treatment of laryngeal cancer", *Journal of Rehabilitation*, vol. 61, no. 4, pp. 41-45.

Bonanno A., Esmaeli B., Fingeret M.C., Nelson D.V., & Weber R.S. 2010, "Social challenges of cancer patients with orbitofacial disfigurement", *Ophthalmic Plastic and Reconstructive Surgery*, vol. 26, no. 1, pp. 18-22.

Bredin, M. 1999, "Mastectomy, body image and therapeutic massage: a qualitative study of women's experience", *J Adv.Nurs*, vol. 29, no. 5, pp. 1113-1120.

Callahan C. 2004, "Facial disfigurement and sense of self in head and neck cancer", *Social Work in Health Care*, vol. 40, no. 2, pp. 73-87.

Cash T.F. & Pruzinsky T. 2002, *Body image. A handbook of theory, research and clinical practice* The Guilford Press, New York.

Chapple, A. & McPherson, A. 2004, "The decision to have a prosthesis: A qualitative study of men with testicular cancer", *Psycho-Oncology*, vol. 13, no. 9, pp. 654-664.

Doumit, M. A., Huijer, H. A., Kelley, J. H., El, S. N., & Nassar, N. 2010, "Coping with breast cancer: a phenomenological study", *Cancer Nurs*, vol. 33, no. 2, p. E33-E39.

Drabe N., Zwahlen D., Büchi S., Moergeli H., Zwahlen R.A., & Jenewein J. 2008, "Psychiatric morbidity and quality of life in wives of men with long-term head and neck cancer", *Psycho-Oncology*, vol. 17, pp. 199-204.

Dropkin M.J. 1999, "Body image and quality of life after head and neck cancer surgery", *Cancer Practice*, vol. 7, no. 6, pp. 309-313.

Dropkin M.J., Malgady R.G., Scott D.W., Oberst M.T., & Strong E.W. 1983, "Scaling of disfigurement and dysfunction in postoperative head and neck patients", *Head and Neck*, vol. 6, no. 559, p. 570.

Dropkin, M. J., Malgady, R. G., Scott, D. W., Oberst, M. T., & Strong, E. W. 1983, "Scaling of disfigurement and dysfunction in postoperative head and neck patients", *Head and Neck Surgery*, vol. 6, no. 1, pp. 559-570.

D`Antonio L., Long S., Zimmerman G., Peterman A., Petti G., & Chonkich G. 1998, "Relationship between quality of life and depression in patients with head and neck cancer", *Laryngoscope*, vol. 108, no. 6, pp. 806-811.

Elmir, R., Jackson, D., Beale, B., & Schmied, V. 2010, "Against all odds: Australian women's experiences of recovery from breast cancer", *J Clin.Nurs*, vol. 19, no. 17-18, pp. 2531-2538.

Figueiredo, M. I., Cullen, J., Hwang, Y. T., Rowland, J. H., & Mandelblatt, J. S. 2004, "Breast cancer treatment in older women: does getting what you want improve your long-term body image and mental health?", *J Clin.Oncol.*, vol. 22, no. 19, pp. 4002-4009.

Fobair, P., Stewart, S. L., Chang, S., D'Onofrio, C., Banks, P. J., & Bloom, J. R. 2006, "Body image and sexual problems in young women with breast cancer", *Psycho-Oncology*, vol. 15, no. 7, pp. 579-594.

Frid, M., Strang, P., Friedrichsen, M. J., & Johansson, K. 2006, "Lower limb lymphedema: experiences and perceptions of cancer patients in the late palliative stage", *J Palliat.Care*, vol. 22, no. 1, pp. 5-11.

Frith, H., Harcourt, D., & Fussell, A. 2007, "Anticipating an altered appearance: women undergoing chemotherapy treatment for breast cancer", *Eur.J Oncol.Nurs*, vol. 11, no. 5, pp. 385-391.

Furness P.J., Garrud, P., Faulder, A., & Swift, J. 2006, "Coming to terms: a grounded theory of adaptation to facial surgery in adulthood", *J.Health Psychol.*, vol. 11, no. 3, pp. 453-466.

Garrad J. 2011, *Health sciences litterature review made easy: The matrix method* Sudbury.

Giddens, A. 1991, *Modernity and self-identity. Self and society in the late modern age* Polity Press, Cambridge.

Hagedoorn, M. & Molleman, E. 2006, "Facial disfigurement in patients with head and neck cancer: the role of social self-efficacy", *Health Psychol*, vol. 25, no. 5, pp. 643-647.

Hansen H.P. 2007, "Hair loss induced by chemotherapy: An anthrpological study of women, cancer and rehabilitation", *Anthropology and Medicine*, vol. 14, no. 1, pp. 15-26.

Hawighorst-Knapstein, S., Fusshoeller, C., Franz, C., Trautmann, K., Schmidt, M., Pilch, H., Schoenefuss, G., Knapstein, P. G., Koelbl, H., Kelleher, D. K., & Vaupel, P. 2004, "The impact of treatment for genital cancer on quality of life and body image--results of a prospective longitudinal 10-year study", *Gynecologic Oncology*, vol. 94, no. 2, pp. 398-403.

Hersch, J., Juraskova, I., Price, M., & Mullan, B. 2009, "Psychosocial interventions and quality of life in gynaecological cancer patients: a systematic review", *Psycho-Oncology*, vol. 18, no. 8, pp. 795-810.

Hess U., Adams R.B., & Kleck R.E. 2009, "The face is not an empty canvas: how facial expressions interact with facial appearance", *Philosophical Transactions of the Royal Society of London.Series B: Biological Sciences*, vol. 364, pp. 3497-3504.

Hopwood, P., Fletcher, I., Lee, A., & Al, G. S. 2001, "A body image scale for use with cancer patients", *Eur.J Cancer*, vol. 37, no. 2, pp. 189-197.

Horgan O. & MacLachlan M. 2004, "Psychosocial adjustment to lower-limb amputation: a review", *Disability and Rehabilitation*, vol. 26, no. 14/15, pp. 837-850.

Huang, J. S., Harrity, S., Lee, D., Becerra, K., Santos, R., & Mathews, W. C. 2006a, "Body image in women with HIV: a cross-sectional evaluation", *AIDS Res Ther.*, vol. 3, p. 17.

Huang, J. S., Lee, D., Becerra, K., Santos, R., Barber, E., & Mathews, W. C. 2006b, "Body image in men with HIV", *AIDS Patient Care STDS.*, vol. 20, no. 10, pp. 668-677.

Irvine H., Davidson C., Hoy K., & Lowe-Strong A. 2009, "Psychosocial adjustment to multiple sclerosis: exploration of identity redefinition", *Disability and Rehabilitation*, vol. 31, no. 8, pp. 599-606.

Jenks, J. M., Morin, K. H., & Tomaselli, N. 1997, "The influence of ostomy surgery on body image in patients with cancer", *Appl.Nurs Res*, vol. 10, no. 4, pp. 174-180.

Johnson M., Maas M., & Moorhead S. 2000, *Nursing outcomes classification (NOC)*, second edicition edn, Mosby, Inc., St. Louise, Missouri.

Jutel, A. & Buetow, S. 2007, "A picture of health? Unmasking the role of appearance in health", *Perspect.Biol.Med*, vol. 50, no. 3, pp. 421-434.

Katz, A. 2009, "Gay and lesbian patients with cancer", *Oncol.Nurs Forum*, vol. 36, no. 2, pp. 203-207.

Konradsen H. 2010, *From silent problem to interactional integration. A qualitative longitudinal study of patients with facial disfigurement.*, PhD Dissertation edn, Faculty of Health Science, Aarhus University, Aarhus.

Konradsen, H., Kirkevold, M., & Zoffmann, V. 2009, "Surgical facial cancer treatment: the silencing of disfigurement in nurse-patient interactions", *J Adv.Nurs*, vol. 65, no. 11, pp. 2409-2418.

Krouse H.J., Rudy S., Vallerand A.H., Hickey M.M., Klein M.N., Kagan S.H., & Walizer E.M. 2004, "Impact of thracheostomy or laryngectomy on spousal and caregiver relationships", *ORL-Head and Neck Nursing*, vol. 21, no. 1, pp. 10-25.

Leder D. 1990, *The absent body* University of Chicago Press, Chicago.

Lockhart J.S. 1999, "Nurses´ perception of head and neck oncology patients after surgery: Serverity of facial disfigurement and patient gender", *ORL-Head and Neck Nursing*, vol. 17, no. 4, pp. 12-25.

Lui A., Glynn S., & Shetty V. 2009, "The interplay of perceived socail support and posttraumatic psychological distress folllowing orofacial injury", *Journal of Nervous and Mental Disease*, vol. 197, no. 9, pp. 639-645.

Macgregor F.C. 1990, "Facial disfigurement: Problems and management of social interaction and implications for mental health", *Aesthetic Plastic Surgery*, vol. 14, pp. 249-257.

McVea, K. L., Minier, W. C., & Johnson Palensky, J. E. 2001, "Low-income women with early-stage breast cancer: physician and patient decision-making styles", *Psycho-Oncology*, vol. 10, no. 2, pp. 137-146.

Miyake, K. & Zuckerman, M. 1993, "Beyond personality impressions: effects of physical and vocal attractiveness on false consensus, social comparison, affiliation, and assumed and perceived similarity", *J Pers*, vol. 61, no. 3, pp. 411-437.

Morse J.M. 1997, "Responding to threats to integrity of self", *Advances in Nursing Science*, vol. 19, no. 4, pp. 21-36.

Morse J.M. & O'Brian B. 1995, "Preserving self: from victim, to patient, to disabled person", *Journal of Advanced Nursing*, vol. 21, pp. 886-896.

Morton R.P. 2003, "Studies in the quality of life of head and neck cancer patients: Results of a two-year langitudinal study and a comparative cross-sectional cross-cultural survey", *Laryngoscope*, vol. 113, pp. 1091-1103.

Moss T. & Carr T. 2004, "Understanding adjustment to disfigurement: The role of self-concept", *Psychol-Health*, vol. 19, no. 6, pp. 737-748.

Naumann L.P., Vazire S., Rentfrow P.J., & Gosling S.D. 2009, "Personality judgments based on physical appearance", *Pers Soc Psychol Bull*, vol. 35, no. 12, pp. 1661-1671.

Newell, R. J. 1999, "Altered body image: a fear-avoidance model of psycho-social difficulties following disfigurement", *J Adv.Nurs*, vol. 30, no. 5, pp. 1230-1238.

Piot-Ziegler, C., Sassi, M. L., Raffoul, W., & Delaloye, J. F. 2010, "Mastectomy, body deconstruction, and impact on identity: a qualitative study", *Br.J Health Psychol*, vol. 15, no. Pt 3, pp. 479-510.

Pituskin, E., Williams, B., Heather-Jane, A., & Martin-McDonal, K. 2007, "Experiences of men with breast cancer: a qualitative study", *JMHG*, vol. 4, no. 1, pp. 44-51.

Price, B. 1990, "A model for body-image care", *J Adv.Nurs*, vol. 15, no. 5, pp. 585-593.

Ramirés M.J., Ferriol E.E., Doménech F.G., Llatas M.C., Suárez-Varela M.M., & Martinez R.L. 2003, "Psychosocial adjustment in patients surgically treated for laryngeal cancer", *Otolaryngology - Head and Neck Surgery*, vol. 129, no. 1, pp. 92-97.

Rasmussen, D. M., Hansen, H. P., & Elverdam, B. 2009, "How cancer survivors experience their changed body encountering others", *European Journal of Oncology Nursing.*

Roing, M., Hirsch, J. M., & Holmstrom, I. 2007, "The uncanny mouth - a phenomenological approach to oral cancer", *Patient Education and Counseling,* vol. 67, no. 3, pp. 301-306.

Rozmovits, L. & Ziebland, S. 2004, "Expressions of loss of adulthood in the narratives of people with colorectal cancer", *Qual.Health Res,* vol. 14, no. 2, pp. 187-203.

Rumsey N. 2003, "Exploring the psychosocial concerns of outpatients with disfigureing conditions", *Journal of Wound Care,* vol. 12, no. 7, pp. 247-252.

Rumsey N., Bull R., & Gahagan D. 1982, "The effect of facial disfigurement on the proxemic behaviour of the general public", *Journal of Applied Social Psychology,* vol. 12, pp. 137-150.

Rumsey N., Clarke A., White P., Wyn-Williams M., & Garlick W. 2004, "Altered body image: Appearance-related concerns of people with visible disfigurement", *Journal of Advanced Nursing,* vol. 48, no. 5, pp. 443-453.

Rumsey N. & Harcourt D. 2005, *The psychology of appearance* Open University Press, Berkshire.

Scheper-Hughes, N. & Lock, M. 1987, "The Mindful Body: A prolegomenon to future work in medical anthropology", *Medical Anthropology Quarterly,* vol. 1, pp. 6-41.

Semple, C. J., Sullivan, K., Dunwoody, L., & Kernohan, W. G. 2004, "Psychosocial interventions for patients with head and neck cancer: past, present, and future", *Cancer Nurs,* vol. 27, no. 6, pp. 434-441.

Taleghani, F., Yekta, Z. P., & Nasrabadi, A. N. 2006, "Coping with breast cancer in newly diagnosed Iranian women", *J Adv.Nurs,* vol. 54, no. 3, pp. 265-272.

Tam, A. K., Padilla, G., Tejero, J., & Kagawa-Singer, M. 2003, "Understanding the breast cancer experience of Asian American women", *Psycho-Oncology,* vol. 12, no. 1, pp. 38-58.

Tebble N.J., Thomas D.W., & Price P. 2004, "Anxiety and self-consciousness in patients with minor facial lacerations", *Journal of Advanced Nursing,* vol. 47, no. 4, pp. 417-426.

Thompson A. & Kent G. 2001, "Adjustment to disfigurement: Processes involved in dealing with being visibly different", *Clinical Psychology Review,* vol. 21, no. 5, pp. 663-682.

Verdonck-de Leeuw I.M., Eerenstein S.E., Van der Linden M.H., Kuik D.J., Bree R., & Leemans C.R. 2007, "Distress in spouses and patients after treatment for head and neck cancer", *Laryngoscope,* vol. 117, pp. 238-241.

Vickery L.E.Latchford G., Hewison J., Bellew M., & Feber T. 2003, "The impact of head and neck cancer and facial disfigurement on the quality of life of patients and their partners", *Head and Neck,* vol. 25, pp. 289-296.

Zoffmann, V. & Lauritzen, T. 2006, "Guided self-determination improves life skills with type 1 diabetes and A1C in randomized controlled trial", *Patient Education and Counseling,* vol. 64, no. 1-3, pp. 78-86.

3

Changes in Body Image in Women with Early Stage Breast Cancer

Brenda L. Den Oudsten, Alida F.W. Van der Steeg,
Jan A. Roukema and Jolanda De Vries
*Tilburg University, St. Elisabeth Hospital,
Emma Children's Hospital AMC & VU University Medical Centre,
The Netherlands*

1. Introduction

Worldwide, breast cancer is the predominant form of malignancy in women (Hortobagyi *et al.*, 2005). However, when diagnosed in an early stage, women have a good chance to survive for a longer period of time. Therefore, it is important to focus on the impact of breast cancer and its treatment on long-term psychosocial outcomes. In recent years, quality of life (QOL) has become a primary endpoint in oncology (Movsas, 2003, Sprangers, 2002). Body image is an important aspect of QOL, especially in breast cancer patients (Avis *et al.*, 2005), because of the mutilating effect surgical treatment may have. Body image is a component of the self-concept of a woman, which includes feeling attractive and feminine (Fobair *et al.*, 2006). Body image is defined in different ways, but typically conceived as a multidimensional construct, consisting of perceptual, attitudinal, and behavioral aspects.(Jolly *et al.*, , Sarwer and Cash, 2008) Body image evaluation (e.g., satisfaction or dissatisfaction) and body image investment (i.e., the psychological importance of one's appearance to his or her sense of self or self-worth) are the most central body image dimensions.(Sarwer and Cash, 2008) Patients experience a body image problem when a marked discrepancy exists between the actual or perceived appearance or function of a discrete bodily attribute(s) and an individual's expressed ideal regarding this bodily attribute(s).(White, 2000) A positive body image is related to patients' ability to cope with cancer (Pikler and Winterowd, 2003). In this study, the focus will be on the dimension of body image evaluation.

Women with breast cancer often experience a decrease in satisfaction with body image after surgery, irrespective of type of surgical treatment (Brandberg *et al.*, 2008, Ganz *et al.*, 1992, Kraus, 1999, Lindop and Cannon, 2001). There is no consensus whether the type of surgery received is related to dissatisfaction with body image after surgery. Some studies found that women receiving MTC report lower scores on body image compared with women receiving BCT (Anagnostopoulos and Myrgianni, 2009, Engel *et al.*, 2004, Ganz *et al.*, 1992, Janni *et al.*, 2001, Janz *et al.*, 2005, Kenny *et al.*, 2000, Schou *et al.*, 2005). However, a number of studies did not find type of surgery to be a relevant factor in satisfaction with body image (Fobair *et al.*, 2006, Goldberg *et al.*, 1992, Schover *et al.*, 1995, Wolberg *et al.*, 1989). Furthermore, previous research was also inconsistent regarding adjuvant therapy. Although most studies showed that chemotherapy (Fehlauer *et al.*, 2005, Joly *et al.*, 2000), hormone therapy (Ganz *et al.*, 1998), and radiotherapy (Fehlauer *et al.*, 2005, Hopwood *et al.*) did not negatively affect body image, Schover et al. (Schover *et al.*, 1995) concluded that chemotherapy did have a negative impact on body image, while hormonal and radiation therapy did not.

Women's perception about their bodies may be influenced by the length of time since treatment. In general, most studies found that body image improved over time (Hopwood *et al.*), for MTC and BCT (Ganz *et al.*, 1992, King *et al.*, 2000). However, in a more recent study, it was found that most body image scores were quite stable, especially for MTC patients. Only BCT patients felt more attractive and feminine after two years (Engel *et al.*, 2004). Information about the effect of surgery across time is lacking and few studies measured body image before diagnosis making it impossible to know the effect of treatment on patients' body image. Therefore, the first aim of this prospective follow-up study was to examine changes in body image across one year, starting before diagnosis and comparing women with benign breast problems (BBP group) with women with breast cancer (MTC and BCT).

The impact of disease and treatment on general QOL seems to vary with age, marital status, and educational level, with younger women and women with lower levels of education reporting lower QOL scores when patients received chemotherapy (Janz *et al.*, 2005, King *et al.*, 2000). Two studies reported a strong relationship between age and body image (Al-Ghazal *et al.*, 1999, King *et al.*, 2000, Yeo *et al.*, 2004). The largest negative impact of MTC on body image was found amongst young, married women (King *et al.*, 2000, Yeo *et al.*, 2004). In contrast, other studies did not find differences in scores on body image between younger and older women (Engel *et al.*, 2004, Hartl *et al.*, , Kenny *et al.*, 2000, Zimmermann *et al.*, 2009).

Body image is not only influenced by life events such as having breast cancer, but also by culture, socio-economic status, and personality (Diener *et al.*, 2003). The personality traits extraversion (the disposition towards cheerfulness, sociability, and high activity) and neuroticism (the tendency to experience distressing emotions, such as fear, guilt, and frustration) may have an effect on QOL (Diener *et al.*, 2003). Only one study examined these characteristics and found that neuroticism was acting as a vulnerability factor for anxiety and/or depressive symptoms one year after breast cancer surgery (Millar *et al.*, 2005). Besides, Costa et al. (Costa *et al.*, 1992) found that neuroticism was correlated with a negative body image and extraversion was correlated with a positive body image. However, there is a lack of prospective data on possible relationships between psychological, clinical, and demographic factors and body image (Hartl *et al.*, 2003, Zimmermann *et al.*, 2009). Therefore, the second aim of this prospective study was to examine the effects of personality, sociodemographic factors, and type of surgery on body image in breast cancer patients at different time points after treatment over a one-year period. In contrast with previous studies on satisfaction with body image in breast cancer patients, this study examined which factors from a combination of factors (age, marital status, educational level, work status, disease stage, type of surgery, chemotherapy, radiotherapy, hormone therapy, neuroticism, extraversion, agreeableness, openness to experiences, conscientiousness) predicted body image. It is hypothesized that body image problems arise from surgery and are most commonly experienced following MTC. In addition, body image problems are a function of personality (i.e., neuroticism).

2. Methods

2.1 Participants

Women with a palpable lump in the breast or an abnormality on a screening mammography were referred by their general practitioner to the outpatient clinic of the St. Elisabeth Hospital (Tilburg), the Maasland Hospital (Sittard; since August 2004), or the Jeroen Bosch Hospital (Den Bosch; since January 2006) in the Netherlands between September 2002 and September 2007. Women were included if they had an abnormality in the breast, were able to read, speak and write Dutch, and were 18 years or older. Women who had a history of abnormalities in the breast, benign or malignant, or had a breast tumor that was too large (>5 centimeter) for BCT, were excluded from the study. After written informed consent and before the first appointment with the surgeon, the participating women completed a set of questionnaires. Thus, women completed the first set of questionnaires when the diagnosis was still unknown. After this baseline measurement (Time-1), a set of questionnaires was also completed one (Time-2), three (Time-3), six (Time-4), and 12 months (Time-5) after diagnosis (BBP) and/or surgical treatment (BC). The breast cancer group consisted of 219 patients; the women with benign breast problems (BBP group) consisted of 381 patients (See Figure 1). Non-participants (57.8 ± 10.1 yrs) were older than participants (55.0 ± 10.4 yrs; $p=.001$) in the study. They did not differ on other sociodemographic (i.e., living with a partner, having children, educational level) or clinical characteristics (i.e., disease stage, type of surgery, adjuvant therapy). The length of the questionnaires and the amount of stress the women experienced during the diagnostic period were the reasons for not participating in the study. This study was approved by the local ethics committee.

2.2 Questionnaires

All women completed questionnaires on personality factors (only at baseline) and the WHOQOL-100 Body Image and Appearance facet (all time points). The BC group also completed the EORTC-QLQ-BR23 Body image subscale from Time-2 onwards. Both instruments were chosen since both subscales complement each other, i.e., the Body and Appearance facet covers more general concerns (satisfaction with they way the body looks, acceptance of bodily appearance, and inhibition by own looks), while the Body image subscale covers feelings of low attractiveness and femininity as a result of cancer or treatment.

The Neuroticism-Extraversion-Openness Five Factor Inventory (NEO-FFI) (Costa and McCrae, 1992, Hoekstra *et al.*, 1996) was developed to study an individual's personality by testing the five domains of the Five Factor or Big Five Model: neuroticism (i.e., the tendency to experience distressing emotions, such as fear, guilt, and frustration), extraversion (i.e., the disposition towards cheerfulness, sociability, and high activity), openness (i.e., the tendency to have a receptive orientation towards varied experiences and ideas), agreeableness (i.e., the inclination towards interpersonal trust and consideration of others) and conscientiousness (i.e., the tendency towards persistence, sense of duty, organizing, planning, and self-discipline). This self-report questionnaire consists of 60 statements. Each statement is rated on a 5-point scale ranging from 1 (*strongly disagree*) to 5 (*strongly agree*), resulting in dimension scores ranging from 12 to 60. The psychometric properties are acceptable to good.(Costa and McCrae, 1992)

The World Health Organization Quality of Life assessment instrument-100 (WHOQOL-100) (De Vries and Van Heck, 1997, WHOQOL Group, 1998) is a cross-culturally developed generic multi-dimensional quality of life measure. This questionnaire consists of 100 items that are divided in 24 facets covering four domains (Physical health, Psychological health, Social Relationships, and Environment) and an Overall Quality of Life and General Health facet. Each facet is measured with four items using 5-point Likert scales. In the present study, only the facet Body Image and Appearance was used. The facet body image consists of four items, for instance 'Are you able to accept your bodily appearance?' A high facet score indicates good body image (score range: 4 - 20). The reliability and validity are adequate and sensitivity is high. (De Vries and Van Heck, 1997, Den Oudsten *et al.*, 2009b, O'Carroll *et al.*, 2000) The Cronbach's alpha coefficients of the facet Body Image and Appearance in this study were .85 (BCT group), .87 (BBP group), and .88 (MTC group).

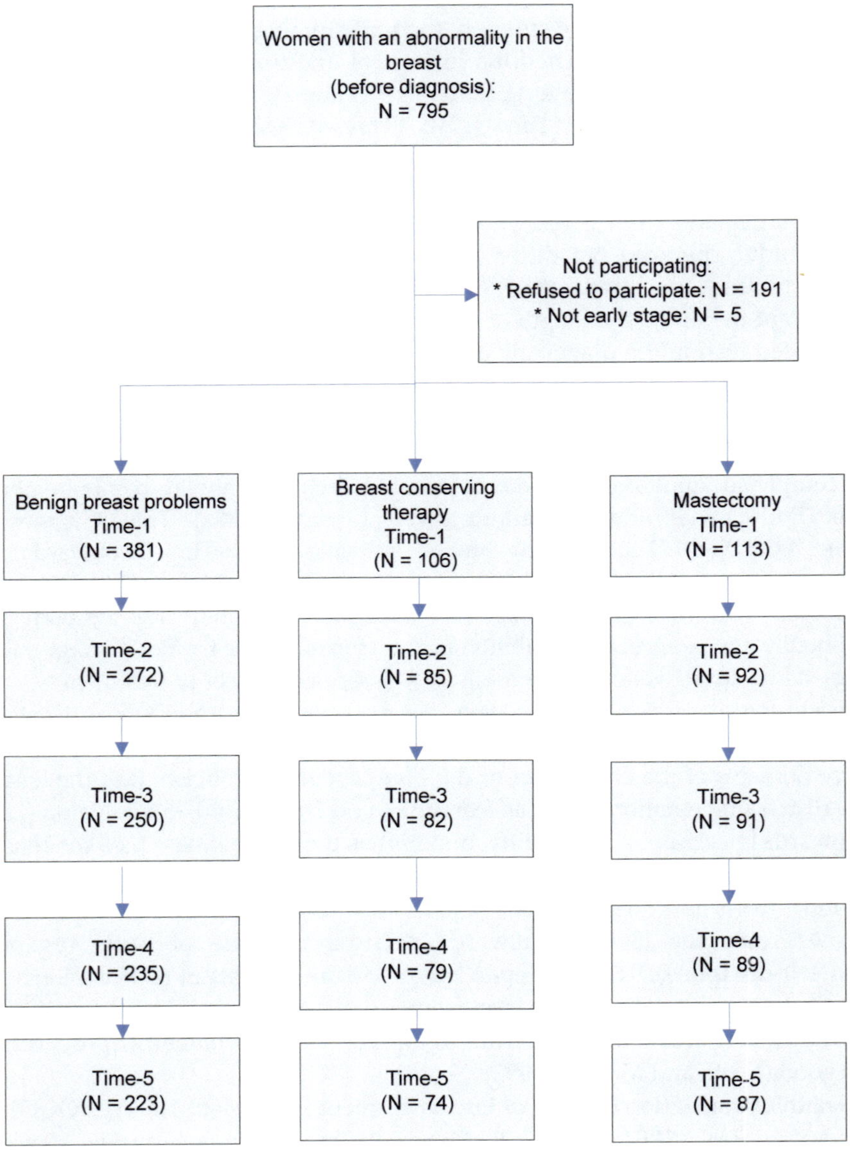

Fig. 1. Flow chart

The EORTC QLQ-BR23 is a 23-item disease-specific questionnaire measuring health status in breast cancer patients. The BR-23 is a supplementary module of the EORTC QLQ C30, which covers the physical, personal, cognitive, emotional, and social domains.(Montazeri *et al.*, 2000, Sprangers *et al.*, 1996) The EORTC QLQ BR-23 incorporates two functional scales (Body Image and Sexual Functioning) and three symptom scales (Arm Symptoms, Breast Symptoms, and Systematic Therapy Side Effects). The remaining items assess sexual enjoyment and being upset by hair loss. The reliability and validity are adequate(Montazeri *et al.*, 2000, Sprangers *et al.*, 1996, Yun *et al.*, 2004). In this study, only the scale Body Image was used. The Body Image scale consists of four items, for instance 'Did you feel less feminine as a consequence of your illness or treatment?' This scale was linearly transformed (score range 0-100). A higher score represent higher levels of functioning. The reliability and validity of this scale is adequate.(Sprangers *et al.*, 1996, Yun *et al.*, 2004) The Cronbach's alpha coefficients of the Body Image scale in this study were .87 (BCT group) and .89 (MTC group).

Patients were asked to respond to a number of questions concerning age, marital status, having children, and years of education. Marital status was dichotomized in two categories, i.e. being involved in a relationship or not being involved in a relationship.

Data concerning diagnosis, type of surgical treatment (BCT or MTC), disease stage, and type of adjuvant treatment (chemotherapy, hormone therapy, and radiotherapy) were obtained from the medical records of the included patients.

2.3 Statistical procedures

Student t-tests and chi-square tests were used to examine differences between participants and non-participants and women who had undergone BCT and MTC. General linear model for repeated measures was used to examine if scores on Body Image changed over time, if scores on Body Image were different for (women with a benign diagnosis,) women who undergone BCT or MTC, and if the pattern of Body Image scores over time was different for BCT and MTC. Subsequently, multivariate analysis of covariance (MANCOVA) with repeated measures was performed to adjust for the effect of potential confounders on the relationship between body image and group (benign breast problems, MTC, BCT). Radiotherapy and disease stage were selected as covariates based on statistical differences between treatment groups on baseline characteristics. Post-hoc paired samples t-tests were conducted to determine differences in body image for group separately. Linear regression analyses were performed to examine which, and to what extent, sociodemographic, clinical, and personality variables predicted the scores on body image (WHOQOL-100, EORTC QLQ-BR23). For the time points, one, three, six, and 12 months after surgery, a hierarchical multiple regression analysis (method: enter) was conducted. As a first step, aiming at minimizing the number of independent variables in the final regression analysis, separate preliminary regression analyses were performed with sociodemographic (age, marital status, educational level, work status), clinical (disease stage, type of surgery, chemotherapy, radiotherapy, and hormone therapy), psychological (body image at baseline), and personality factors (neuroticism, extraversion, agreeableness, openness to experiences, conscientiousness) as independent variables. Subsequently, significant predictors ($p<.05$) were entered in the final regression analysis. Chemotherapy, radiotherapy, and hormone therapy were not entered at Time-2 as a factor, since women with breast cancer did not yet received adjuvant therapy at that time. Mean and standard deviations are provided as ($M \pm SD$). SPSS 17.0 was used for all calculations.

3. Results

The sociodemographic, clinical, and psychological characteristics of women who received BCT or MTC and the women who had a benign breast problem are summarized in Table 1.

	BBP (n = 381)	BCT (n = 106)	MTC (n = 113)	p-value
Demographics				
Age at diagnosis, yrs	52.9 ± 10.4	58.4 ± 8.5	58.5 ± 9.7	.91
No partner	50 (13.1%)	14 (13.2%)	21 (18.6%)	.29
No children	57 (14.9%	14 (13.2%)	14 (12.4%)	.77
Educational level				
0-9 years	123 (32.1%)	38 (35.8%)	43 (38.1%)	.84
10-14 years	171 (44.6%)	46 (43.4%)	47 (41.6%)	
> 14 years	72 (18.8%)	19 (17.9%)	17 (15.0%)	
Clinical values				
Disease stage	-			
Stage 0		8 (7.5%)	17 (15.5%)	<.0001
Stage I		60 (56.6%)	32 (28.3%)	
Stage IIa		33 (31.1%)	34 (30.1%)	
Stage IIb		5 (4.7%)	30 (26.5%)	
Adjuvant therapy[1]				
Chemotherapy	-	20 (18.9%)	41 (36.3%)	.01
Radiotherapy	-	96 (90.6%)	20 (17.7%)	<.0001
Hormone therapy	-	32 (30.2%)	52 (46.0%)	.02
Psychological				
Body image WHOQOL[2] [range: 4-20]	16.0 ± 3.3	16.6 ± 2.8	16.5 ± 3.1	.81
Neuroticism [range: 12-60]	31.1 ± 6.9	30.7 ± 7.5	29.4 ± 7.1	.23
Extraversion [range: 12-60]	40.1 ± 5.8	40.6 ± 5.7	41.9 ± 5.4	.09
Openess to experience [range: 12-60]	36.7 ± 5.4	36.2 ± 6.6	35.0 ± 4.9	.20
Agreeableness [range: 12-60]	43.7 ± 4.2	43.7 ± 4.2	43.3 ± 4.2	.44
Conscientiousness [range: 12-60]	45.4 ± 4.9	45.9 ± 5.6	45.9 ± 5.2	.96

Note: [1] more than one treatment possible; [2] higher scores on body image indicate higher quality of life
Abbreviations: BBP: Benign Breast Problems; BCT: Breast-Conserving Therapy; MTC = mastectomy

Table 1. Patient characteristics

Patients who underwent MTC were more often treated with chemotherapy and hormone therapy, compared to patients who received BCT ($p < .05$). As expected, based on standard treatment, women with BCT were more often treated with radiotherapy ($p < .0001$) and differed regarding disease stage ($p < .0001$). No other differences between the surgical groups were found with regard to other sociodemographic, clinical, and psychological variables.
Figure 2 shows the change in scores on WHOQOL-facet Body Image. Body Image changed significantly over time [$F(4,239) = 3.0$; $p = .020$], after correcting for potential confounders. Furthermore, an interaction effect was found for time by surgical treatment, indicating that the pattern of change over time in Body Image is different for women with MTC, women with BCT, and women with BBP [$F(8,480) = 2.8$; $p = .004$]. From Time-1 to Time-2, women with MTC reported a significant deterioration in their Body Image ($p = .035$), while women with BCT and BBP were stable. Although their Body Image improved in time, they had significantly lower scores at Time-5 when compared to Time-1 ($p = .004$). Radiotherapy and disease stage did not interact with Body Image ($p > .05$). Overall, women with BBP and women with BCT and MTC did not score differently on Body Image, except at Time-2 ($p < .036$).

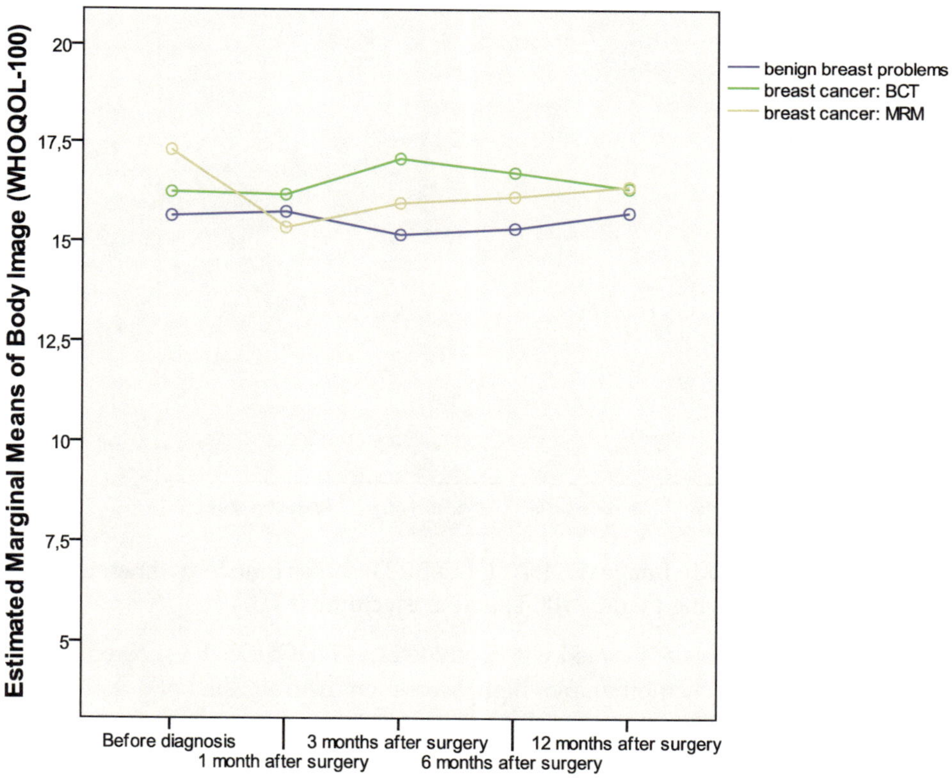

Fig. 2. Mean scores on Body Image and Appearance (WHOQOL-100) across time for women who undergonebreast-conserving therapy (BCT) and mastectomy (MTC) and women with a benign diagnosis

Figure 3 shows the change in scores on EORTC QLQ BR-23 subscale Body Image. In the adjusted analysis, Body Image improved significantly over time when correcting for potential confounders [F(3,93) = 2.8; p =.043]. Scores on Time-4 (85.2 ± 20.3), and Time-5 (86.4 ± 18.4) were statistically higher compared with the scores on Time-2 (79.7 ± 23.1; ps<.05). On average, women with BCT and MTC scored differently on Body Image, i.e. women with BCT scored significantly higher on Body Image [F(1,95) = 7.4; p =.008]. However, no interaction effect was found, indicating that the pattern of change over time in Body Image was not significantly different for both groups (p =.348). Radiotherapy and disease stage did not interact with Body Image (p >.05).

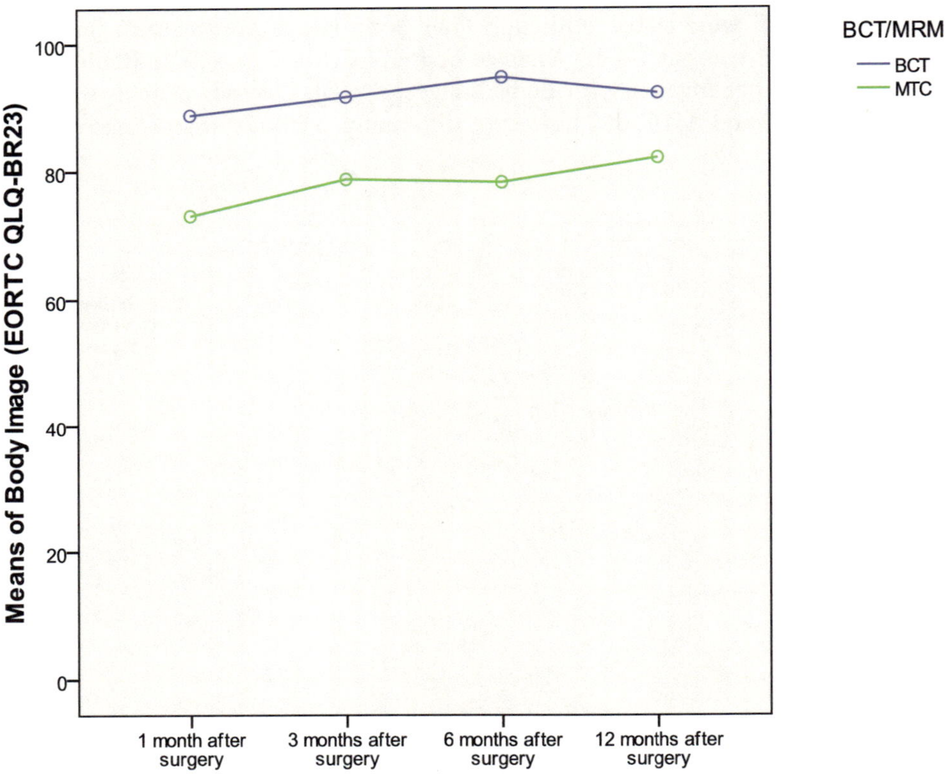

Fig. 3. Mean scores on Body Image (EORTC QLQ-BR23) across time for women who undergone breastconserving therapy (BCT) and mastectomy (MTC)

Table 2 shows those factors associated with Body Image (WHOQOL-100) scores across time. Being older, receiving chemotherapy, high scores on neuroticism, and low scores on agreeableness were significantly associated with lower Body Image scores at all time points. The regression models at different time points explained 26% to 32% of the variance. Table 3 shows those factors associated with Body Image (EORTC QLQ BR23) scores across time. High scores on neuroticism were significantly associated with lower Body Image scores at all time points. The regression models at different time points explained 16% to 30% of the variance. Chemotherapy, radiotherapy, and hormone therapy were not entered in the regression analysis at Time-2 and Time-3, since women not received this treatment yet.

Timepoint	Factor	β-value	R^2	Adjusted R^2	p-value
Time-2*	Age	.31	.34	.32	<.0001
	BCT/MTC	-.21			.005
	Neuroticism	-.31			<.0001
	Agreeableness	.20			.011
Time-3*	Age	.35	.27	.26	<.0001
	Disease stage	-.25			.001
	Neuroticism	-.29			<.0001
Time-4	Age	.18	.29	.26	.024
	Educational level	.08			.328
	Chemotherapy	-.28			.001
	Neuroticism	-.23			.006
	Agreeableness	.24			.003
Time-5	Age	.22	.30	.28	.006
	Chemotherapy	-.16			.038
	Neuroticism	-.30			<.0001
	Agreeableness	.26			.001

Note: *chemotherapy was not entered at Time-2 and Time-3 as a factor, since women with breast cancer had not yet received chemotherapy

Table 2. Final results of hierarchical multiple regression analysis with body image (WHOQOL-100) as the dependent variable, for one (Time-2), three (Time-3), six (Time-4), and 12 months after surgery (Time-5)

4. Discussion

Body image is an important aspect of QOL in women with breast cancer. For years, it was hypothesized that MTC contributed to some extent to the development of psychological problems of women with breast cancer. It was intuitively thought that BCT would remove some of the stress because of its less mutilating effect compared to MTC.(Meyer and Aspegren, 1989) Until now, body image was mostly studied in cross-sectional designs. Therefore, this prospective study examined the impact of surgical treatment, personality, and sociodemographic factors on body image during a follow-up period of one year after primary surgical treatment. In addition, this study examined if scores on body image were lower in women who received MTC compared to women who underwent BCT or women with benign breast problems. In general, a temporary decrease was found in body image scores due to treatment. Although we found that scores of women with MTC were lower compared with women with benign breast problems and women with BCT, the results were only significant at one month after surgery. Type of surgical treatment predicted body image at one month (WHOQOL-100; EORTC QLQ-BR23), three months (EORTC QLQ-BR23), and six months after surgical treatment (EORTC QLQ-BR23). Most studies found BCT to be superior with regard to scores on body image, which is in line with our study. (Avis *et al.*, 2004, Ganz *et al.*, 2002, Hartl *et al.*, 2003, King *et al.*, 2000, Schou *et al.*, 2005, Yeo *et al.*, 2004) BCT patients were more satisfied with their appearance than patients who received MTC. (Engel *et al.*, 2004, Janni *et al.*, 2001)

Timepoint	Factor	β-value	R^2	Adjusted R^2	p-value
Time-2*	BCT/MTC	-.29	.18	.16	.001
	Neuroticism	-.24			.008
	Agreeableness	.16			.079
Time-3*	Age	.26	.33	.31	<.0001
	BCT/MTC	-.30			<.0001
	Neuroticism	-.43			<.0001
	Conscientiousness	-.29			<.0001
Time-4	Age	.28	.34	.30	.001
	Educational level	.07			.400
	BCT/MTC	-.21			.007
	Chemotherapy	-.16			.044
	Neuroticism	-.32			<.0001
	Agreeableness	.19			.024
	Conscientiousness	-.22			.007
Time-5	Age	.22	.23	.20	.006
	Neuroticism	-.25			.004
	Agreeableness	.27			.002
	Conscientiousness	-.29			.001

Note: *chemotherapy was not entered at Time-2 and Time-3 as a factor, since women with breast cancer had not yet received chemotherapy

Table 3. Final results of hierarchical multiple regression analysis with body image (EORTC-QLQ BR23) as the dependent variable, for one (Time-2), three (Time-3), six (Time-4), and 12 months after surgery (Time-5)

Studies in this field show a wide variation with regard to the methodological aspects. First, different instruments were used to assess body image. There is a wide variation in body image scales, and they are composed of different items. For example, some instruments contain items assessing satisfaction with body image, as the breast specific module from the European Organization for Research and Treatment of Cancer (EORTC QLQ-BR23)(Fehlauer et al., 2005, Janz et al., 2005), or with the Cancer Rehabilitation Evaluation System (CARES). (Avis et al., 2004, Ganz et al., 1992) Others constructed their own scale or added questions to general questionnaires to measure body image.(Engel et al., 2004, Hartl et al., 2003, Janni et al., 2001, King et al., 2000) In this study, a generic QOL instrument (WHOQOL-100) and a disease-specific health status instrument (EORTC QLQ BR-23) were used. The results based on both instruments indicated that body image scores changed significantly over time, irrespective of diagnosis/treatment. However, this effect was partly explained by the differences in scores between the baseline measure and the first follow-up measure (WHOQOL-100), when body image scores dropped considerably in the MTC group. Body image scores measured with the EORTC-QLQ BR23 also improved significantly; but, this measure could not register the drop in body image scores between Time-1 and Time-2, since it can only be assessed in a cancer population. In our study, the baseline assessment was before diagnosis. (Engel et al., 2004) Our findings are in line with other studies. For instance, Ganz et al. (Ganz et al., 1992) reported an improvement in body image one year after surgery in both surgical groups, just as Bloom et al. (Bloom et al., 2004) did between baseline (soon after diagnosis) and five year follow-up. In our study, body image scores completely returned to baseline values, except for the body image scores of women with MTC. It is possible that a study in which a longer follow-up is taken, body image will further improve.

Older women were more satisfied with their bodies, which is in line with the majority of other studies in this field. (Al-Ghazal *et al.*, 1999, Fehlauer *et al.*, 2005, Janz *et al.*, 2005, Kenny *et al.*, 2000, King *et al.*, 2000) However, it should be noted that the results on the direction of the relationship between age and body image in the literature is inconsistent. That is, several studies did not find differences in body image scores between age groups(Engel *et al.*, 2004, Schou *et al.*, 2005) or found that body image issues may be particularly salient for younger women(Avis *et al.*, 2005). Since older women are often excluded from clinical studies, future studies should examine the psychosocial concerns in this age group.

Adjuvant therapies, like radiotherapy and hormone therapy were not strongly related to body image. Chemotherapy predicted scores on body image at all time points included. From the few studies that are available on this topic, women who received chemotherapy reported lower scores on body image (Janz *et al.*, 2005, Schover *et al.*, 1995), probably due to the loss of hair that is accompanied by this type of treatment.

Personality characteristics (neuroticism and agreeableness) played an important role in predicting outcome in this study. Neuroticism contributed in a negative way to scores on body image at all follow-up measures, after controlling for all other variables. This result is consistent with other research on personality in breast cancer, in which patients, who experienced high levels of chronic stress one year after treatment for breast cancer, were characterized by higher levels of neuroticism. (Millar *et al.*, 2005) In other studies, this trait also in part explained the variance in depressive symptoms after breast cancer surgery (Den Oudsten *et al.*, 2009a, Golden-Kreutz and Andersen, 2004), as well as of poor adjustment to mastectomy. (Morris *et al.*, 1977)

After discussing the results of the study, certain limitations and strengths should be acknowledged. Strength of the underlying study is the baseline measurement, before the diagnosis is known. At the same time, this is also a weakness, because women are probably scared and nervous because an abnormality has been seen on the mammography (i.e., only applies for those women who had a screening mammography) or that a lump (whether it is benign or malign) is in the breast. However, in this study the BBP group showed stable scores regarding body image. The optimal moment for the baseline measurement would be before visiting the doctor or taking a mammography, and then it is probably of better prospective value. The one-year follow-up period is another advantage of this study, because body image is a concept that probably changes over time when a woman is confronted with a threat to her body image. Moreover, this study included also a control group consisting of women with benign breast problems. Few studies have included a comparison group. (Andrykowski *et al.*, 1996) Finally, the data was collected in several hospitals in the Netherlands, which may facilitation generalization in women with breast cancer. Studies, like the current one, often show relatively high attrition(Arving *et al.*, 2008). Our study had 73.5% of the women with early stage BC in the study at one-year after surgical treatment. This may have influenced our results. However, women with breast cancer who dropped out of the study did not differ from women remaining in the study, except for age with women staying in the study being significantly younger. A limitation of this study is that a specific body image scale would have been appropriate, for instance Body Image Scale(Hopwood *et al.*, 2001). In addition to the EORTC QLQ BR23 items on body image, this scale includes also items on change in self-consciousness with appearance, less sexually attractive, less feminine, dissatisfaction with appearance when dressed, dissatisfaction with scars, body feeling less whole, and avoidance of people because of appearance. These topics were not assessed in our study. However, it should be noted that the women with BBP could not have been assessed on body image.

More longitudinal studies need to focus on body image, whether body image in the MTC group will eventually return to baseline values (i.e., before the breast cancer diagnosis), but also examine the associations with self-esteem, sexual functioning, and quality of life. In addition, studies should also include elderly women. Moreover, it is also reasonable to take women's partners into account, since patients and partners coping with cancer will exchange experiences and influencing each others acceptation process. (Manne and Badr, 2008, 2009) Recently, Zimmerman et al. (Zimmermann *et al.*, 2009) have shown that dyadic factors are important. They found that women's depressive symptoms, women's age and men's marital satisfaction predicted women's body image, explaining 24% of the variance. Given the importance of the marital relationship in adaptation, a greater understanding of this dyadic process may aid in the development of psychosocial interventions for couples adapting to breast cancer who may be at risk for distress.

5. Conclusion

In conclusion, results from this study confirm previous findings that breast cancer temporarily affects satisfaction with body image in a negative way. Results are more obvious for women who underwent MTC, than for women who have had BCT. Older women seemed to have more problems with body image after surgery. Overall, it is important for women facing breast cancer to get assistance in adjusting to alterations in body image. (Kraus, 1999) Personality factors that influence these changes should be taken into account.

6. References

Al-Ghazal, S. K., Blamey, R. W., Stewart, J. & Morgan, A. A. (1999). The cosmetic outcome in early breast cancer treated with breast conservation. *Eur J Surg Oncol* 25, 566-70.

Anagnostopoulos, F. & Myrgianni, S. (2009). Body image of Greek breast cancer patients treated with mastectomy or breast conserving surgery. *J Clin Psychol Med Settings* 16, 311-21.

Andrykowski, M. A., Curran, S. L., Studts, J. L., Cunningham, L., Carpenter, J. S., McGrath, P. C., Sloan, D. A. & Kenady, D. E. (1996). Psychosocial adjustment and quality of life in women with breast cancer and benign breast problems: a controlled comparison. *J Clin Epidemiol* 49, 827-34.

Arving, C., Glimelius, B. & Brandberg, Y. (2008). Four weeks of daily assessments of anxiety, depression and activity compared to a point assessment with the Hospital Anxiety and Depression Scale. *Qual Life Res* 17, 95-104.

Avis, N. E., Crawford, S. & Manuel, J. (2004). Psychosocial problems among younger women with breast cancer. *Psycho-oncology* 13, 295-308.

Avis, N. E., Crawford, S. & Manuel, J. (2005). Quality of life among younger women with breast cancer. *J Clin Oncol* 23, 3322-30.

Bloom, J. R., Stewart, S. L., Chang, S. & Banks, P. J. (2004). Then and now: quality of life of young breast cancer survivors. *Psycho-oncology* 13, 147-60.

Brandberg, Y., Sandelin, K., Erikson, S., Jurell, G., Liljegren, A., Lindblom, A., Linden, A., von Wachenfeldt, A., Wickman, M. & Arver, B. (2008). Psychological reactions, quality of life, and body image after bilateral prophylactic mastectomy in women at high risk for breast cancer: a prospective 1-year follow-up study. *J Clin Oncol* 26, 3943-9.

Costa, P. T., Jr., Fagan, P. J., Piedmont, R. L., Ponticas, Y. & Wise, T. N. (1992). The five-factor model of personality and sexual functioning in outpatient men and women. *Psychiatr Med* 10, 199-215.

Costa, P. T. & McCrae, R. R. (1992). *Revised NEO Personality Inventory (NEO-PI-R) and NEO Five Factor Inventory (NEO-FFI) professional manual.* Psychological Assessment Resources Inc.: Odessa, FL.

De Vries, J. & Van Heck, G. L. (1997). The World Health Organization Quality of Life assessment instrument (WHOQOL-100): validation study with the Dutch version. *Eur J Psychol Assess* 13, 164-178.

Den Oudsten, B. L., Van Heck, G. L., Van der Steeg, A. F., Roukema, J. A. & De Vries, J. (2009a). Predictors of depressive symptoms 12 months after surgical treatment of early-stage breast cancer. *Psychooncology* 18, 1230-7.

Den Oudsten, B. L., Van Heck, G. L., Van der Steeg, A. F., Roukema, J. A. & De Vries, J. (2009b). The WHOQOL-100 has good psychometric properties in breast cancer patients. *J Clin Epidemiol* 62, 195-205.

Diener, E., Oishi, S. & Lucas, R. E. (2003). Personality, culture, and subjective well-being: emotional and cognitive evaluations of life. *Annu Rev Psychol* 54, 403-25.

Engel, J., Kerr, J., Schlesinger-Raab, A., Sauer, H. & Holzel, D. (2004). Quality of life following breast-conserving therapy or mastectomy: results of a 5-year prospective study. *Breast J* 10, 223-31.

Fehlauer, F., Tribius, S., Mehnert, A. & Rades, D. (2005). Health-related quality of life in long term breast cancer survivors treated with breast conserving therapy: impact of age at therapy. *Breast Cancer Res Treat* 92, 217-22.

Fobair, P., Stewart, S. L., Chang, S., D'Onofrio, C., Banks, P. J. & Bloom, J. R. (2006). Body image and sexual problems in young women with breast cancer. *Psycho-oncology* 15, 579-94.

Ganz, P. A., Desmond, K. A., Leedham, B., Rowland, J. H., Meyerowitz, B. E. & Belin, T. R. (2002). Quality of life in long-term, disease-free survivors of breast cancer: a follow-up study. *J Natl Cancer Inst* 94, 39-49.

Ganz, P. A., Rowland, J. H., Desmond, K., Meyerowitz, B. E. & Wyatt, G. E. (1998). Life after breast cancer: understanding women's health-related quality of life and sexual functioning. *J Clin Oncol* 16, 501-14.

Ganz, P. A., Schag, A. C., Lee, J. J., Polinsky, M. L. & Tan, S. J. (1992). Breast conservation versus mastectomy. Is there a difference in psychological adjustment or quality of life in the year after surgery? *Cancer* 69, 1729-38.

Goldberg, J. A., Scott, R. N., Davidson, P. M., Murray, G. D., Stallard, S., George, W. D. & Maguire, G. P. (1992). Psychological morbidity in the first year after breast surgery. *Eur J Surg Oncol* 18, 327-31.

Golden-Kreutz, D. M. & Andersen, B. L. (2004). Depressive symptoms after breast cancer surgery: relationships with global, cancer-related, and life event stress. *Psycho-oncology* 13, 211-20.

Hartl, K., Janni, W., Kastner, R., Sommer, H., Strobl, B., Rack, B. & Stauber, M. (2003). Impact of medical and demographic factors on long-term quality of life and body image of breast cancer patients. *Ann Oncol* 14, 1064-71.

Hartl, K., Schennach, R., Muller, M., Engel, J., Reinecker, H., Sommer, H. & Friese, K. Quality of life, anxiety, and oncological factors: a follow-up study of breast cancer patients. *Psychosomatics* 51, 112-23.

Hoekstra, H., Ormel, J. & De Fruyt, F. (1996). *Handleiding NEO persoonlijkheidsvragenlijsten NEO-PI-R en NEO-FFI [Manual NEO personality questionnaires NEO-PI-R and NEO-FFI]*. Swets Test Services: Lisse, The Netherlands.

Hopwood, P., Fletcher, I., Lee, A. & Al Ghazal, S. (2001). A body image scale for use with cancer patients. *Eur J Cancer* 37, 189-97.

Hopwood, P., Haviland, J. S., Sumo, G., Mills, J., Bliss, J. M. & Yarnold, J. R. Comparison of patient-reported breast, arm, and shoulder symptoms and body image after radiotherapy for early breast cancer: 5-year follow-up in the randomised Standardisation of Breast Radiotherapy (START) trials. *Lancet Oncol.*

Hortobagyi, G. N., de la Garza Salazar, J., Pritchard, K., Amadori, D., Haidinger, R., Hudis, C. A., Khaled, H., Liu, M. C., Martin, M., Namer, M., O'Shaughnessy, J. A., Shen, Z. Z. & Albain, K. S. (2005). The global breast cancer burden: variations in epidemiology and survival. *Clin Breast Cancer* 6, 391-401.

Janni, W., Rjosk, D., Dimpfl, T. H., Haertl, K., Strobl, B., Hepp, F., Hanke, A., Bergauer, F. & Sommer, H. (2001). Quality of life influenced by primary surgical treatment for stage I-III breast cancer-long-term follow-up of a matched-pair analysis. *Ann Surg Oncol* 8, 542-8.

Janz, N. K., Mujahid, M., Lantz, P. M., Fagerlin, A., Salem, B., Morrow, M., Deapen, D. & Katz, S. J. (2005). Population-based study of the relationship of treatment and sociodemographics on quality of life for early stage breast cancer. *Qual Life Res* 14, 1467-79.

Jolly, M., Pickard, A. S., Mikolaitis, R. A., Cornejo, J., Sequeira, W., Cash, T. F. & Block, J. A. Body Image in Patients with Systemic Lupus Erythematosus. *Int J Behav Med.*

Joly, F., Espie, M., Marty, M., Heron, J. F. & Henry-Amar, M. (2000). Long-term quality of life in premenopausal women with node-negative localized breast cancer treated with or without adjuvant chemotherapy. *Br J Cancer* 83, 577-82.

Kenny, P., King, M. T., Shiell, A., Seymour, J., Hall, J., Langlands, A. & Boyages, J. (2000). Early stage breast cancer: costs and quality of life one year after treatment by mastectomy or conservative surgery and radiation therapy. *Breast* 9, 37-44.

King, M. T., Kenny, P., Shiell, A., Hall, J. & Boyages, J. (2000). Quality of life three months and one year after first treatment for early stage breast cancer: influence of treatment and patient characteristics. *Qual Life Res* 9, 789-800.

Kraus, P. L. (1999). Body image, decision making, and breast cancer treatment. *Cancer Nurs* 22, 421-7; quiz 428-9.

Lindop, E. & Cannon, S. (2001). Experiences of women with a diagnosis of breast cancer: a clinical pathway approach. *Eur J Oncol Nurs* 5, 91-9.

Manne, S. & Badr, H. (2008). Intimacy and relationship processes in couples' psychosocial adaptation to cancer. *Cancer* 112, 2541-55.

Manne, S. & Badr, H. (2009). Intimacy processes and psychological distress among couples coping with head and neck or lung cancers. *Psychooncology.*

Meyer, L. & Aspegren, K. (1989). Long-term psychological sequelae of mastectomy and breast conserving treatment for breast cancer. *Acta Oncol* 28, 13-8.

Millar, K., Purushotham, A. D., McLatchie, E., George, W. D. & Murray, G. D. (2005). A 1-year prospective study of individual variation in distress, and illness perceptions, after treatment for breast cancer. *J Psychosom Res* 58, 335-42.

Montazeri, A., Harirchi, I., Vahdani, M., Khaleghi, F., Jarvandi, S., Ebrahimi, M. & Haji-Mahmoodi, M. (2000). Anxiety and depression in Iranian breast cancer patients before and after diagnosis. *Eur J Cancer Care (Engl)* 9, 151-7.

Morris, T., Greer, H. S. & White, P. (1977). Psychological and social adjustment to mastectomy: a two-year follow-up study. *Cancer* 40, 2381-7.

Movsas, B. (2003). Quality of life in oncology trials: a clinical guide. *Semin Radiat Oncol* 13, 235-47.

O'Carroll, R. E., Cossar, J. A., Couston, M. C. & Hayes, P. C. (2000). Sensitivity to change following liver transplantation: a comparison of three instruments that measure quality of life. *J Health Psychol* 5, 69-74.

Pikler, V. & Winterowd, C. (2003). Racial and body image differences in coping for women diagnosed with breast cancer. *Health Psychol* 22, 632-7.

Sarwer, D. B. & Cash, T. F. (2008). Body image: interfacing behavioral and medical sciences. *Aesthet Surg J* 28, 357-8.

Schou, I., Ekeberg, O., Sandvik, L., Hjermstad, M. J. & Ruland, C. M. (2005). Multiple predictors of health-related quality of life in early stage breast cancer. Data from a year follow-up study compared with the general population. *Qual Life Res* 14, 1813-23.

Schover, L. R., Yetman, R. J., Tuason, L. J., Meisler, E., Esselstyn, C. B., Hermann, R. E., Grundfest-Broniatowski, S. & Dowden, R. V. (1995). Partial mastectomy and breast reconstruction. A comparison of their effects on psychosocial adjustment, body image, and sexuality. *Cancer* 75, 54-64.

Sprangers, M. A. (2002). Quality-of-life assessment in oncology. Achievements and challenges. *Acta Oncol* 41, 229-37.

Sprangers, M. A., Groenvold, M., Arraras, J. I., Franklin, J., Te Velde, A., Muller, M., Franzini, L., Williams, A., de Haes, H. C., Hopwood, P., Cull, A. & Aaronson, N. K. (1996). The European Organization for Research and Treatment of Cancer breast cancer-specific quality-of-life questionnaire module: first results from a three-country field study. *J Clin Oncol* 14, 2756-68.

White, C. A. (2000). Body image dimensions and cancer: a heuristic cognitive behavioural model. *Psychooncology* 9, 183-92.

WHOQOL Group (1998). The World Health Organization Quality of Life Assessment (WHOQOL): development and general psychometric properties. *Soc Sci Med* 46, 1569-85.

Wolberg, W. H., Romsaas, E. P., Tanner, M. A. & Malec, J. F. (1989). Psychosexual adaptation to breast cancer surgery. *Cancer* 63, 1645-55.

Yeo, W., Kwan, W. H., Teo, P. M., Nip, S., Wong, E., Hin, L. Y. & Johnson, P. J. (2004). Psychosocial impact of breast cancer surgeries in Chinese patients and their spouses. *Psychooncology* 13, 132-9.

Yun, Y. H., Bae, S. H., Kang, I. O., Shin, K. H., Lee, R., Kwon, S. I., Park, Y. S. & Lee, E. S. (2004). Cross-cultural application of the Korean version of the European Organization for Research and Treatment of Cancer (EORTC) Breast-Cancer-Specific Quality of Life Questionnaire (EORTC QLQ-BR23). *Support Care Cancer* 12, 441-5.

Zimmermann, T., Scott, J. L. & Heinrichs, N. (2010). Individual and dyadic predictors of body image in women with breast cancer. *Psychooncology* 19, 1061-8

4

Surgical Prevention of Arm Lymphedema in Breast Cancer Treatment

Corradino Campisi, Corrado C. Campisi and Francesco Boccardo
Department of Surgery – Unit of Lymphatic Surgery,
S. Martino Hospital, University of Genoa,
Italy

1. Introduction

Disruption of the axillary nodes and closure of arm lymphatics can explain the significantly high risk of early and late lymphatic complications after axillary dissection, especially the most serious complication that is arm lymphedema which occurs in about 25% (ranging from 13 to 52%) of patients. Sentinel lymph node (SLN) biopsy has reduced the severity of swelling to nearly 6% (from 2 to 7%) and, in case of positive SLN, complete axillary dissection (AD) is still required. That is why ARM method was developed aiming at identifying and preserve lymphatics draining the arm. It consists in injecting intradermally and subcutaneously a small quantity (1-2 ml) of blue dye at the medial surface of the arm which helps in locating the draining arm lymphatic pathways. ARM technique allowed to find variable clinical anatomical conditions from what was already generally known, that is the most common location of arm lymphatics below and around the axillary vein. In about one-third of the cases, blue lymphatics can be found till 3-4 cm below the vein, site where SLN can easily be located, justifying the occurrence of lymphedema after only SLN biopsy. ARM procedure showed that blue nodes were almost always placed at the lateral part of the axilla, under the vein and above the second intercostals brachial nerve. Leaving in place lymph nodes related to arm lymphatic drainage would decrease the risk of arm lymphedema, but not retrieving all nodes, the main risk is to leave metastatic disease in the axilla. Conversely, arm lymphatic pathways when they enter the axilla, cannot be site of breast tumoral disease and their preservation would certainly bring about a significant decrease of lymphedema occurrence rate (1-4).

2. Lymphangiogenesis and other local changes

Another important aspect to point out is that, in the axilla, new lymphatic vessel formation (lymphangiogenesis) occurs in response to the ligation of lymphatic vessels involved in lymph node retrievement. Lymphangiogenesis and lymphatic hypertension were demonstrated experimentally in case of lymphatic drainage obstruction. And, in response to lymphatic hypertension, lympho-venous shunts open and provide alternative lymphatic pathways when the main ones are obstructed. These mechanisms represent an adaptive response to lymphatic hypertension but are not enough to restore normal flow parameters. Furthermore, chronic obstruction to lymph flow progressively leads to a reduced lymphatic contractility, lymphatic thrombosis and fibrotic changes, at a different degree according to variable constitutional predisposition (5-9)

3. Surgical preventive procedures

Recent advances in the treatment of breast cancer, specifically as concerns the prevention of lymphatic complications following sentinel lymph node biopsy and axillary dissection brought to the proposal of a new technique to primarily prevent lymphedema by microsurgical lymphatic-venous anastomoses. ARM technique allows to identify arm lymphatics and lymph nodes which can therefore be preserved even though there is the risk to leave undetected metastatic disease in the axilla. But, it is almost impossible to preserve efferent lymphatics from the blue nodes because they join the common axillary nodal basin draining the breast. Thus, not preserving efferent lymphatics makes practically impossible to preserve arm lymphatic flow. So, on the basis of our wide experience in the treatment of lymphedema by microsurgical lymphatic-venous anastomoses (LVA), we thought to perform LVA immediately after finishing nodal axillary excision. The surgical technique proposed for patients with operable breast cancer requiring an axillary dissection consisted in carrying out LVA between arm lymphatics identified by injecting blue dye in the arm and an axillary vein branch simultaneously (Lymphatic Microsurgical Preventive Healing Approach - LY.M.P.H.A.) (10). It is almost always possible to find blue lymphatics and also to find a vein branch long enough to be connected to arm lymphatics which are usually locate very laterally.

Patients are followed up both clinically by volumetric assessment and by lymphangioscintigraphy performed before surgery and after 18 months. Blue nodes in relation to lymphatic arm drainage can be identified in almost all patients after blue dye injection at the arm. All blue nodes must be resected and 2 to 4 main afferent lymphatics from the arm can be prepared and used for anastomoses. Lymphatics are introduced inside the vein cut-end by a U-shaped stitch. Other few stitches are given to fix the lymphatic adventitia to the vein wall. The operation takes only 15-20 minutes averagely, since both lymphatics and the vein are prepared during nodal dissection. LVA proved not only to prevent lymphedema but also to reduce early lymphatic complications (i.e. lymphorrhea, lymphocele) thanks to the reduced regional intralymphatic pressure. Drain tubes can be removed after about 7-10 days at the utmost. Post-op lymphangioscintigraphy allowed to demonstrate the patency of microvascular anastomoses after over 1 year and half from operation.

4. Clinical experience

Study design

Among fortynine consecutive women from March 2008 to September 2009 addressed to complete AD, performed by surgeons of the same Beast Unit, who used the same technique, 46 were randomly divided in two groups, the other 3 were not analyzed because refused to perform lymphoscintigraphy (LS) pre-operatively. Twentythree underwent LYMPHA technique, performed by a surgeon skilled in lymphatic microsurgery, for the prevention of arm lymphedema (LYMPHA group - LG). The other 23 patients had no preventive surgical approach (control group - CG). No wrapping neither compression therapy was used in any of the patients of both groups.

The average age was 57 years (range 39-80 years). In order to be included in this prospective study, patients with unilateral breast cancer had to be addressed to complete AD due to clinically or ultrasonographic positive axillary limph nodes or positive SLN. Exclusion criteria were cases in whom only SLN biopsy technique was performed and SLNs were negative.

In the LYMPHA group (LG), 16 patients there were lymph nodal metastasis and therefore lymphatic venous anastomosis were performed during the primary surgery together with breast cancer treatment, sentinel lymph node biopsy, intraoperative frozen sections (showing the metastasis) and axillary dissection (AD). In other 7 patients there were no lymph nodal metastasis demonstrated by intraoperative frozen sections and therefore LYMPHA technique was planned after finding micrometastasis by following immunohistochemical investigations. Thus, in this last group of patients we could perform LYMPHA during the complete lymph nodal dissection in the second time surgery.

Operating technique

Patients signed a specific consent form indicating the kind of operation, possible risks, and complications to participate or not in the LYMPHA procedure. The blue dye (Lymphazurin) was injected in the volar surface of the upper third of the arm in a quantity of about 1-2 ml intradermally, subcutaneously and under muscular fascia. Usually after 5-10 minutes it is already possible to visualize arm blue lymphatics. Axillary nodal dissection was performed usually starting far from the upper lateral part of the axilla which was removed nearly at the end of the dissection in order not to damage the lymphatic pathways coming from the arm. This lymphatics were temporally clipped near their afference to the nodal capsule and thus prepared for anastomosis.

During lymph nodal dissection also one or two collateral branches of the axillary vein are prepared with a length suitable for reaching the lymphatic vessels. The microsurgical technique of lymphatic venous anastomosis has already been described (11). The vein was averagely 2 mm in diameter and lymphatics about half mm. the number of lymphatics anastomosed varied from 2 to 4. The technique is the "sleeve" procedure: lymphatics are put into the vein cut-end. A collateral of the axillary vein is used for anastomoses. In some cases a big gap inbetween the vein and the lymphatics can be found, but in these cases it is usually enough to better dissect the vein and above all the lymphatics from the surrounding tissues. In case it is necessary one of the subscapular or thoraco-dorsal veins which are usually long enough can also been used. A particular attention must be paid in placing the drain tube in order not to damage the anastomosis (Fig.1). Lymphatic-venous anastomoses take only 15-20 minutes to be performed and in our study were performed by a surgeon skilled in lymphatic microsurgery. There is no increased rate of blood loss, wound infection and seromas compared to standard ALND (Fig. 2).

Clinical and lymphoscintigraphic assessment

All patients of the two groups were preoperatively studied clinically by volume measurements (using the formula of a truncated cone according to Kuhnke method) (10) and by lymphoscintigraphy. Lymphedema, was defined as a difference in excess volume of at least 100 ml compared to preoperative VOL measurements. The follow up included volumetry at 1, 3, 6, 12 and 18 months postoperatively in both groups.

Lymphoscintigraphy was carried out in 21 cases in the LG and in 20 cases of the CG after 18 months postoperatively (Fig. 3).

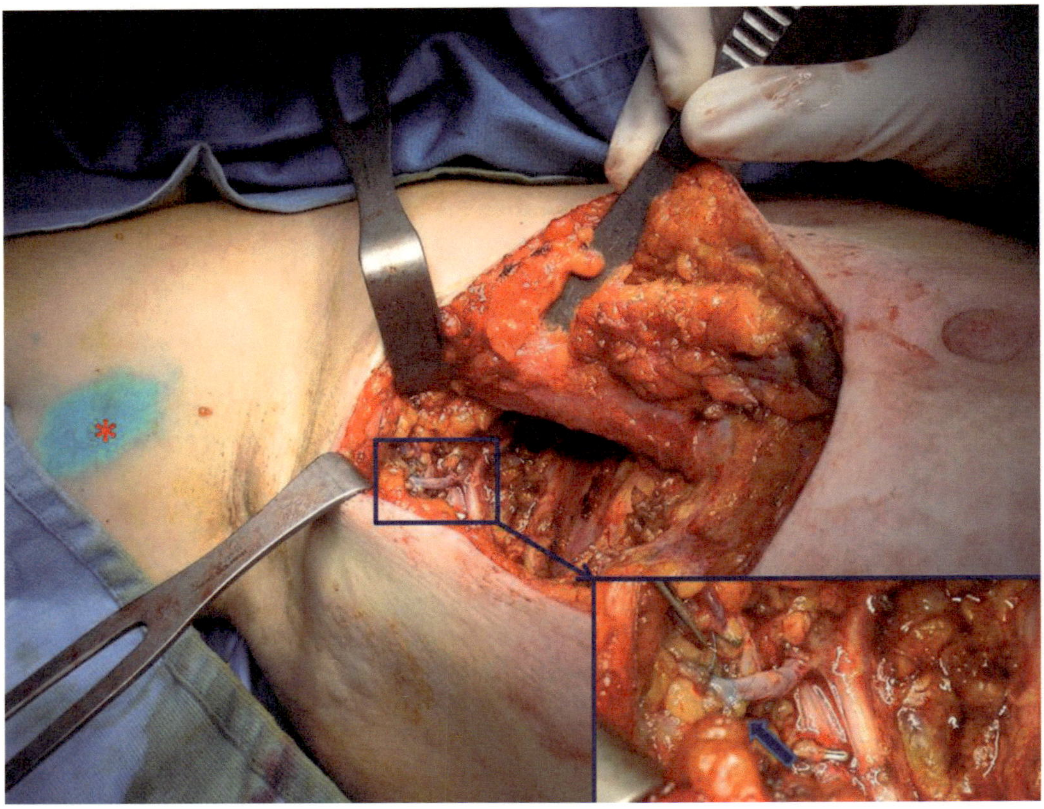

Fig. 1. Lymphatic-venous-anastomoses (rectangle) to prevent arm lymphedema (LYMPHA). Note the blue dye (*) injected at the upper third of the volar surface of the arm to visualise arm lymphatics. The patency of lymphatic-venous anastomosis is proved by the passage of the blue dye into the vein branch (arrow).

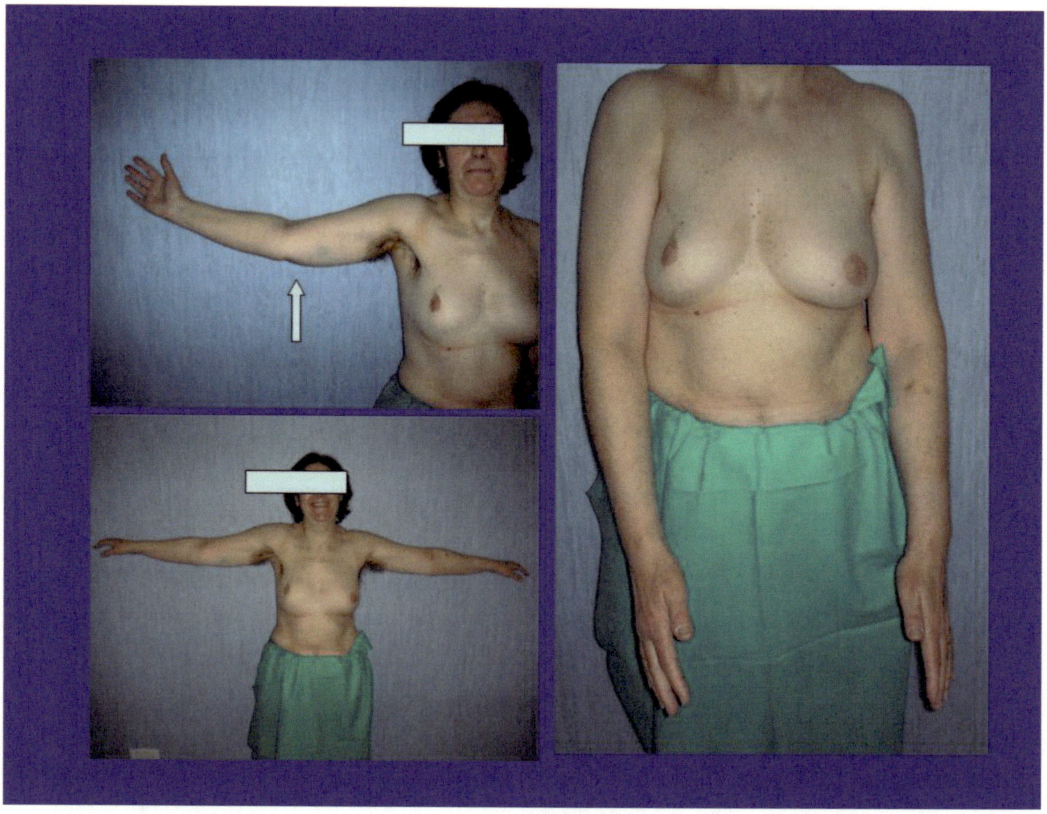

Fig. 2. Patient who underwent axillary lymphnodal dissection and primary surgical prevention of secondary lymphedema by LYMPHA procedure.

Statistical analysis

Non-parametric tests were used to explore the variable relationships between groups and between timing. The comparison between groups of quantitative variables age, BMI, Preop LS, lymphonodes retrived, metastatic lymphnodes (MLS LN) and volume at baseline was performed using Wilcoxon test. Nominal baseline variables surgical procedure, radiotherapy and presence of cellulitis were compared using Chi square or Fisher's Exact Test.

The comparison of difference between baseline and volume after 1, 3, 6, 12 and 18 months from operation in LG and CG was performed using Wilcoxon test (between groups) and matched pair test (between timing). The volume difference between baseline and different timing in LG and CG was represented by box plots showing 10°, 25°, 75° and 90° percentiles. Number of patients with lymphedema, defined as a difference in excess volume of at least 100 ml, at 18 months in PG and CG were compared using 2-sided Fischer's Exact Test.

Results

Lymphedema appeared in 1 patient in the LG after 6 months from the operation (4,34 %) and persisted till 18 months later. It occurred in a patient who underwent radiotherapy and became stable with time without any inflammatory complications. In the CG lymphedema occurred in 7 patients (30,43 %) and appeared mostly after 3 months from operation.

Beginning from month 3, the proportion of patients with lymphedema was statistically higher in CG (p-value=0.047). Table 1 summarizes baseline characteristics of all participants, according to treatment group. There were no significant differences between the two groups in the baseline values of measures of demographic and anthropometric data, in disease characteristics and in type of surgery, and in the proportion of women who undertook to radiotherapy and had a cellulitis. In Figure 4, volume difference between baseline and different timing in LG and CG is represented by box plots showing 10°, 25°, 75° and 90° percentiles.

When compared with previous volume measure, no significant difference in the arm volume were observed in LG during follow-up, while the arm volume in CG showed a significant increase after 1 (mean difference 11.61 ml, S.E. 3.87, p-value<0.01) , 3 (mean difference 22.82 ml, S.E. 5.9, p-value<0.01) and 6 months (mean difference 31.56 ml, S.E. 5.78, p-value<0.01) from operation. No significant changes in arm volume were observed at month 12 and 18, in comparison with data registered at month 6 and 12, respectively, in CG. Significant higher volume with respect to baseline after 1, 3, 6, 12 and 18 months from operation (every timing p-value<0.01) was detected in CG in comparison with LG.

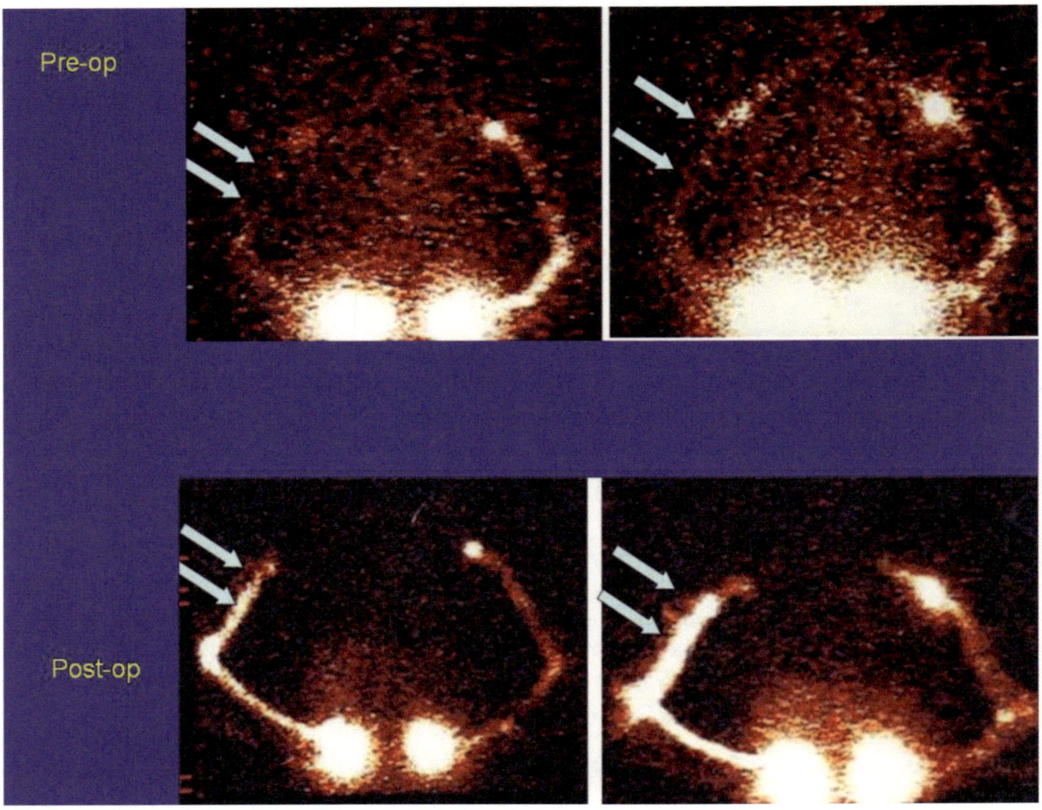

Fig. 3. Lymphoscintigraphic patterns before and after axillary lymphnodal dissection associated with LYMPHA technique.

Duplex scan allowed to exclude a venous pathology in all patients. LS allowed to confirm the lymphostatic nature of the edema. To quantify visual findings in LS, the Kleinhans transport index (TI) was used (4,13,14). The TI includes the following parameters: transport kinetics (K), distribution of the tracer (D), appearance time of lymph nodes in minutes (T), visualization of lymph nodes (N), visualisation of lymph vessels (V); TI = K + D + (0,04 x T) + N + V (Table 2). Normal lymphoscintigraphy pattern corresponded to TI less than 10. An impaired LS pattern in our study had a mean TI of 16 (range 12-19).
Moreover, pre-operatively LS had a significant predictive value (TI) in terms of risk of lymphedema appearance. To this regard LS proved to be an instrumental criteria to select patients at risk for secondary lymphedema.
Post-operatively LS demonstrated the patency of microlymphaticvenous anastomosis (patency rate: 95,6%) both through direct (visualization of preferential lymphatic pathway, disappearance of the tracer passing into the blood stream) and indirect (early liver uptake of the tracer) parameters in the LG group. In the CG on the other hand LS allowed to point out lymphatic drainage impairment in patients with secondary lymphedema.

5. Discussion

Notwithstanding the wide variability in lymphedema prevalence, the incidence of secondary arm lymphedema is significant. Sentinel lymph node biopsy (SLNB) was introduced and carried out to prevent lymphedema but, recent studies demonstrated that even with SLNB alone lymphedema rates are not negligible (13,17).
Therefore, prevention is of key importance to avoid lymphedema occurrence.
Axillary Reverse Mapping (ARM) procedure represents an attempt to identify and preserve arm lymphatic drainage. Success of this technique in preventing lymphedema will require ongoing follow-up and studies (6). Blue nodes were always located in the same position, at the lateral part of the dissection, under the axillary vein and just above the second intercostal brachial nerve (7). The main issue remains to make sure that the nodes identified are not metastatic and can be preserved during AD. Since the lymphatic pathways from the arm cannot be involved by metastatic process of the primary breast tumor, its preservation should not imply any risk of leaving undetected diseases in the axilla (1). With ARM technique the detection rate of blue lymphatics and nodes is 61-71%, and the preservation rate of 47% (1,6,7). The question is: can we spare what we find? The identification of afferent lymphatics and nodes belonging to the arm lymphatic pathways appears feasible. Nevertheless, the identification of the efferent lymphatics, which is mandatory to truly preserve the lymphatic flow of the arm, is almost impossible since the lymphatics departing from the blue nodes join the common lymphatic pathways draining the breast. Therefore, the preservation is practically impossible. That's why we conceived and carried out LYMPHA technique, which consist in performing LVA between arm lymphatics and collateral branches of the axillary vein at the same time as AD. Lymphatic-venous anastomoses are performed at the upper lateral part of the axilla, thus somehow protected from the negative effect of postop radiation. In fact, postop radiation did not cause any relevant problem in the patients with lymphatic-venous anastomoses in this study. Only in two patients, a transitory (for 3 and 5 days respectively) slight arm edema was observed which disappeared spontaneously. Patients were followed by volume measurements which allowed to demonstrate the absence of any negative effect of postop radiation. Furthermore, postop lymphoscintigraphy proved the patency of anastomoses long after surgery and

radiation. The preservation of arm lymphatics carries no risk of leaving disease in the axilla undetected, and it permits the prevention of lymphedema (10). Patients candidate for LYMPHA are those one addressed to AD with either clinical axillary N+ or SLN+. In pre-operative patients selection for LYMPHA clinical and instrumental criteria were evaluated (Fig.4).

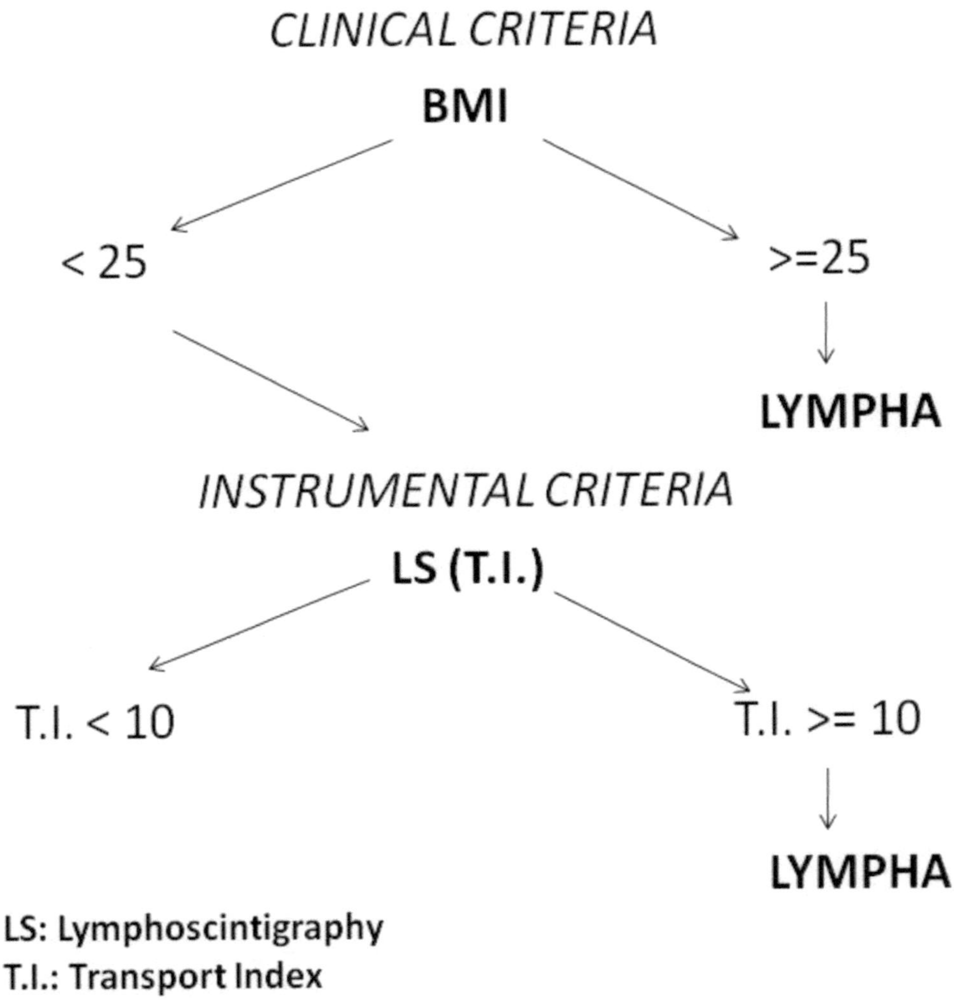

Fig. 4. Clinical and instrumental criteria to select patients for LYMPHA technique

History and physical esamination of the patients, together with BMI, could allow to select patients at risk for lymphedema and this suspect could be confirmed by LS, using semiquantitative evaluation which is represented by TI (15-19). Preop lymphoscintigraphy is useful to select patients at risk for arm lymphedema. LS shows lymphatic impairment (in terms of transport index) compared to the contralateral arm already present pre-operatively.

The quality of life is gaining more and more importance thanks to the prolongation of survival brought about by advanced and combined treatment of different tumors. Surgery has to be more and more conservative and try to maintain organ function and reduce morbility. LYMPHA technique proved to represent a new strategy of treatment to reduce morbility of axillary lymph nodal dissection when it is not possible to preserve arm lymphatic pathways due to the risk to leave tumoral diseases correlated to the breast cancer.

6. References

[1] M.Thompson, S.Korourian, R.Henry-Tillman, L.Adkins, S.Mumford, K.C. Westbrook, and V.S.Klimberg. Axillary Reverse Mapping (ARM): A New Concept to Identify and Enhance Lymphatic Preservation. Annals of Surgical Oncology 2007; 14(6):1890–1895.

[2] Britton TM, Buczacki SJ, Turner CL, et al. Venous changes and lymphedema 4 years after axillary surgery for breast cancer. Br J Surg 2007.

[3] Soran A, D_Angelo G, Begovic M, et al. Breast cancer-related lymphedema—what are the significant predictors and how they affect the severity of lymphedema. Breast J 2006; 12(6):536–43.

[4] Purushotham AD, Bennett Britton TM, Klevesath MB et al. Lymph node status and breast cancer-related lymphedema. Ann Surg. 2007 Jul;246(1):42-5.

[5] Sakorafasa GH, Perosa G, Cataliotti L, et al. Lymphedema following axillary lymph node dissection for breast cancer. Surg Oncol 2006; 15(3):153–165.

[6] C.Nos, B.Lesieur, K.B.Clough, F.Lecuru. Blue Dye Injection in the Arm in Order to Conserve the Lymphatic Drainage of the Arm in Breast. Cancer Patients Requiring an Axillary Dissection. Annals of Surgical Oncology 14(9):2490–2496

[7] R.Ponzone,, P.Mininanni, E.Cassina, P.Sismondi. Axillary Reverse Mapping in Breast Cancer: Can we Spare what we Find? Annals of Surgical Oncology 2007.

[8] Jila A, Kim H, Nguyen VP, Dumont DJ, Semple J, Armstrong D, Seto E, Johnston M. Lymphangiogenesis following obstruction of large postnodal lymphatics in sheep. Microvasc Res 2007; 73:214-223.

[9] Modi S, Stanton AWB, Svensson WE, Peters AM, Mortimer PS, Levick JR. Human lymphatic pumping measured in healthy and lymphoedematous arms by lymphaticcongestion lymphoscintigraphy. J Physiol 2007; 583.1:271-285.

[10] Boccardo F, Casabona F, De Cian F, Friedman D, Villa G, Bogliolo S, Ferrero S, Murelli F, Campisi C. Lymphedema microsurgical preventive healing approach: a new technique for primary prevention of arm lymphedema after mastectomy. Ann Surg Oncol 2009;16:703–708.

[11] Boccardo FM, Casabona F, Friedman D, Puglisi M, De Cian F, Ansaldi F, Campisi C. Surgical Prevention of Arm Lymphedema After Breast Cancer Treatment. Ann Surg Oncol. 2011 Mar 3.

[12] Campisi C, Boccardo F. Microsurgical techniques for lymphedema treatment: derivative lymphatic-venous microsurgery. World J Surg. 2004 Jun;28(6):609-13.

[13] Sitzia J. Volume measurement in lymphedema treatment: examination of formulae. Eur J Cancer Care 1995; 4:11-16.

[14] Casley-Smith JR. Measuring and representing peripheral oedema and its alterations. *Lymphology*. 1994;27:56 -70.

[15] Sener SF, Winchester DJ, Martz CH, et al. Lymphedema after sentinel lymphadenectomy for breast carcinoma. Cancer 2001; 92(4):748–52.

[16] Wilke LG, McCall LM, Posther KE, et al. Surgical complications associated with sentinel lymph node biopsy: results from a prospective international cooperative group trial. Ann Surg Oncol 2006; 13(4):491–500.
[17] Ververs JM, Roumen RM, Vingerhoets AJ, et al. Risk, severity and predictors of physical and psychological morbidity after axillary lymph node dissection for breast cancer. Eur J Cancer 2001; 37(8):991–9.
[18] Kleinhans E, Baumeister RG, Hanh D et al. Evaluation of transport Kinetics in lymphoscintigraphy: follow-up study in patients with transplanted lymphatic vessels. Eur J Nucl Med. 1985; 10:349-52.
[19] Cambria RA, Gloviczki P, Naessens JM et al. Noninvasive evaluation of the lymphatic system with lymphoscintigraphy: a prospective, semiquantitative analysis in 386 extremities. J Vasc Surg. 1993;18:773-82.

5

Chemotherapy-Induced Alopecia

Sudjit Luanpitpong and Yon Rojanasakul
West Virginia University,
Department of Pharmaceutical Sciences, Morgantown, West Virginia,
USA

1. Introduction

Chemotherapy-induced alopecia (CIA) is a frequent toxicity and arguably the most feared side effect of cancer chemotherapy (Carelle et al., 2002). The incidence of CIA is approximately 65% of all patients (Wang et al., 2006). CIA could be easily noticeable by self and others in a relative short time, thus it is linked with having cancer and chemotherapy. CIA compromises patient quality of life, especially for female and children, leading to poor therapeutic outcome. Despite significant progresses and substantial efforts in CIA research and development, no reliable and effective preventive treatment has become available. This limitation has been attributed to the lack of basic understanding of CIA pathogenesis and appropriate experimental models. This chapter will provide an overview of the basic and clinical aspects of CIA including hair follicle biology, characteristics of CIA along with the state-of-the-art experimental models and treatment strategies. Experimental approaches for pharmacologic inhibition of CIA including drug-specific antibodies, hair growth cycle modifiers, cytokines, growth factors, antioxidants, cell cycle modifiers, and apoptosis inhibitors will be discussed. Current understanding in the molecular mechanisms of CIA and the role of specific genes, e.g. p53 and Fas, in the process will also be discussed. The chapter will conclude with the perspective on the prevention and management of CIA.

2. Hair follicle biology

Chemotherapy causes structural damage of human scalp hairs. The effects may vary from altered hair appearance, decreased rate of hair growth, partial or complete hair loss (alopecia). To discuss the advances in the pathogenesis of CIA, an overview of hair follicle biology is first covered.

2.1 Hair follicle structure

Hair follicle structure changes during the various stages of hair growth cycle (see *Section 2.2* for review). In the anagen phase, hair structure is composed of two distinct components, hair follicle and hair shaft (Fig. 1a). The hair follicle is embedded in the connective tissue and subcutaneous fat. Contained within the hair follicle bulb is the pluripotent keratinocytes of hair matrix. Matrix cells in the lower part of hair bulb constantly divide at a high mitotic rate, whereas the matrix cells in the upper part of hair bulb have a low mitotic rate and could differentiate to form the inner root sheath (IRS) and hair shaft (HS), which are the middle and innermost layer of hair follicle, respectively. Outer root sheath (ORS), is the outermost layer of hair follicle that separates the whole organ from dermis and is believed to contain epithelial stem cells at its bulge region (Hardy, 1992; Krause and Foitzik, 2006; Alonso and Fuchs, 2006). Pigmentation of hair shaft depends on melanocytes, which reside in the hair matrix of hair follicle. Melanocytes transfer the melanin granule to keratinocytes of the growing hair shaft (Ohnemus et al., 2006). Besides the epithelial cells, hair follicle also contains the mass of mesenchymal dermal papilla (DP) cells at its base (Fig. 1b). The DP cells are connected to capillaries to derive nutrients from the blood and also function as a regulator of hair cycle (Sakita et al., 1995). Moreover, substantial evidence supports the correlation between DP cell number and the size of hair follicle and shaft (Elliot et al., 1993; Ishino et al., 1997).

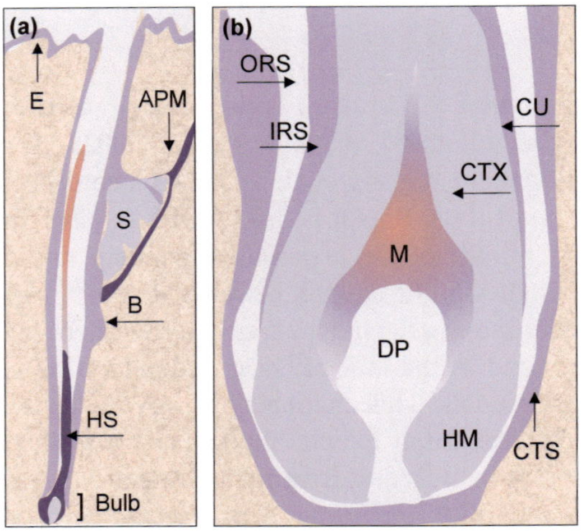

Fig. 1. Diagrammatic representation of hair follicle structure in its mature anagen phase. (a) A full-length longitudinal view of hair follicle. (b) Hair follicle bulb. Abbreviations: APM, arector pili muscle; B, bulge; CTS, connective tissue sheath; CTX, cortex of hair shaft; CU, cuticle of hair shaft; DP, dermal papilla; E, epidermis; HM, hair matrix; HS, hair shaft; IRS, inner root sheath; M, melanocytes; ORS, outer root sheath; S, sebaceous gland.

2.2 Hair growth cycle

Each hair follicle undergoes rhythmic changes through the three phases of hair cycle, which are anagen, catagen and telogen (Fig. 2). Anagen is an active growth phase of hair follicle. During anagen, daughter cells of pluripotent keratinocytes move upwards and adapt into one of the six epithelial lineages, namely Henley, Huxley and cuticle of the IRS and cuticle, cortex and medulla of the HS. As the HS cells become fully differentiated, they extrude their organelles and are tightly packed to form cysteine-rich hair keratins. The IRS and HS interlock via their cuticle structures, however, the IRS degenerates in the upper follicle, thereby releasing the HS that continues to move towards the skin surface. Subsequently, the hair follicle enters the catagen or regression phase. During catagen, there are extensive apoptosis of epithelial cells in the hair follicle bulb and ORS, leading to the formation of epithelial strands. The HS hence stops differentiation and forms the club hair, which moves up until it reaches the bulge region. Dermal papilla cells are condensed and move upwards to the bulge region. After that, the hair enters the telogen or resting phase. In this phase, the

HS exhibits no significant proliferation, apoptosis or differentiation. The transition from telogen to anagen occurs when the bulge stem cells are activated (Cotsaleris and Millar, 2001; Krause and Foitzik, 2006; Alonso and Fuchs, 2006; Ohnemus et al., 2006).

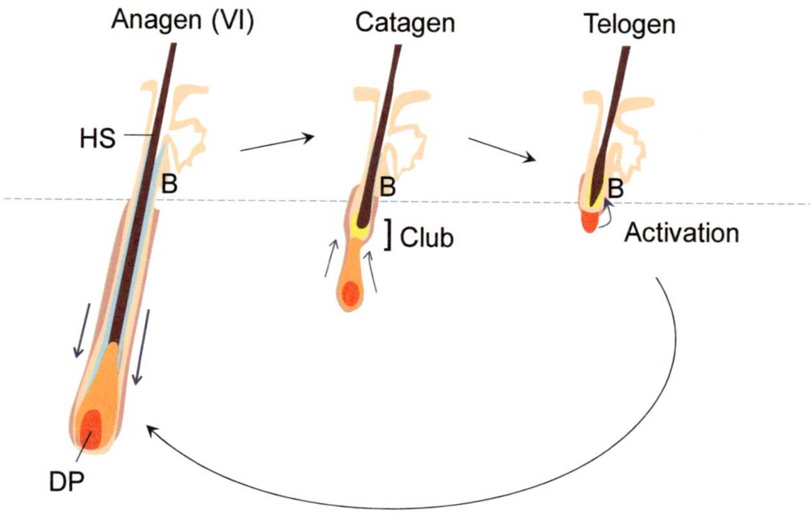

Fig. 2. Hair growth cycle. A new hair shaft is produced during anagen, and the old hair is released from the follicle as the new shaft develops. Anagen VI (mature anagen) is the stage where new HS reaches the skin surface and continues to grow through the rest of anagen. During catagen, the lower two thirds of the epithelial follicle are regressed. The hair develops a club structure, which retains the hair in the follicle. Then, the follicle enters a telogen phase until a new growth cycle is activated. Abbreviations: B, bulge; DP, dermal papilla; HS, hair shaft.

3. Chemotherapy-induced alopecia

CIA or hair loss caused by chemotherapy is the most common cutaneous side effect of chemotherapy. CIA ranks among patients as a severe side effect that affects their quality of life.

3.1 Impact on cancer therapy

CIA has an enormous psychological and social impact on patients, which can be summarized as: (i) symbol of cancer for self (constant reminder of their treatment) and others (outwardly visible); (ii) personal confrontation of being ill or mortality; (iii) vulnerability; (iv) powerlessness; (v) shame; (vi) loss of privacy; (vii) punishment, and (viii) change in self and other perception (Freedman, 1994; Pozo-Kaderman et al., 1999). Female and children have more difficulties coping with the CIA. Indeed, up to 8% of women are reported to reject chemotherapy for fear of CIA (Mundstedt et al., 1997; McGarvey et al., 2001). CIA also results in reduced social activities since hair partly plays a role in social and sexual communications (Batchelor, 2001). Additionally, these negative impacts of CIA may contribute to poor therapeutic outcome, as stress and depression lowers the body's immune function and is highly associated with cancer progression (Spiegel and Giese-Davis, 2003; O'Leary, 1990).

3.2 Pathophysiology

The basic principle of chemotherapy is to impair the mitotic and metabolic process of cancer cells. Unfortunately, certain normal cells and tissues with rapid metabolic and mitotic rates such as the hair follicles are also affected by the chemotherapy. Up to 90% of hair follicles undergo anagen, an active growth phase, at a given time. The rapid hair growth as well as the high blood flow rate around the hair bulb leading to the accumulation of drugs is a key predisposing factor for rapid and extensive alopecia (Batchelor, 2001). In humans, CIA usually begins approximately 2 to 4 weeks and is complete at 1 to 2 months after the initiation of chemotherapy (Batchelor, 2001). Hair might be easily depilated as early as 1 to 2 weeks after the treatment due to the weakening and breakage of hair shaft. The hair would fall out upon combing and in the bedding area. The degree of CIA depends on the type of chemotherapy, dosage regimen and route of administration. Almost all chemotherapies cause alopecia but with varying degrees of severity and frequency (Apisanthanarax and Duvic, 2003) as summarized in Table 1.

More common or severe		Less common or severe	
Bleomycin	Cyclophosphamide	Amscarine	Busulfan
Cytarabine	Cisplatin	Carmusine	Chlorambucil
Dacarbazine	Dactinomycin	Carboplatin	Epirubicin
Docetaxel	Doxorubicin	Gemcitabine	Hydroxyurea
Etoposide	Fluorouracil	Interleukin-2	Melphalan
Idarubicin	Ifosfamide	Mercaptopurine	Methotrexate
Interferon-α	Irinotecan	Mitomycin	Mitoxantrone
Mechlorethamine	Nitroureas	Procarbazine	Teniposide
Paclitaxel	Thiotepa	Vinorelbine	
Topotecan	Vinblastine		
Vincristine	Vindesine		

Table 1. Chemotherapeutic agents associated with alopecia.

A high-dose intravenous chemotherapy is commonly associated with more rapid and extensive alopecia. By contrast, oral therapy at lower doses on a weekly schedule tends to cause less alopecia even though the total dose may be large (Wilkes, 1996). Combination therapy consisting of two or more chemotherapeutic agents normally causes a higher incidence and more severe CIA compared to single agent therapy. Long-term chemotherapy may also result in the loss of pubic, axillary and facial hair.

CIA is usually reversible with the hair regrowth generally occurring 3 to 6 months after the end of treatment. However, in most cases the new hair is grey or differs in color, representing the distortion of pigmentation process. Moreover, the new hair typically exhibits some changes in hair structure and texture, e.g. coarser, slow growth, and reduced density (Wang et al., 2006; Trueb, 2009). Permanent alopecia has been reported but rarely occurs (Betcheler, 2001).

4. Experimental models

4.1 Animal models

Due to the ethical problems in obtaining scalp biopsies from chemotherapy patients, little is known about the mechanisms of CIA in humans. In the last decade, important information about the CIA comes mostly from animal models. The commonly used animal models are neonatal rats and adult mice. However, there are some differences in human and rat/mouse hair growth pattern. In humans, the hair growth cycle occurs in a mosaic or asynchronous pattern, where the growth cycle of individual hair follicles is independent of neighbouring hair follicles. In contrast, rodent hair growth occurs in a wave pattern, beginning from the head and moving towards the tail. A group of hair follicles at a specific area are usually in the same stage of hair cycle. In general, only 10% of hair follicles in adult mice or rats are in the anagen phase as compared to 90% in adult humans. Some animals including guinea pigs and Angora rabbits exhibit a mosaic hair growth pattern but are not commonly used due to their insensitivity to CIA.

4.1.1 Neonatal rat model

The early model for CIA was established in newborn rats (Hussein et al., 1990; Hussein, 1993). Seven to eight-day old Sprague Dawley rats exhibit spontaneous anagen hair growth for about a week. In this model, administration of chemotherapeutic agents such as cytosine arabinoside, doxorubicin, cyclophosphamide, and etoposide induces alopecia one week after the treatment with the severity of CIA depending on the agents (Hussein et al., 1990; Hessein, 1991; Jimenez and Yunis, 1992).

The major advantage of neonatal rat model is the rapid and easily noticeable CIA due to progressive hair loss from the head and throughout the body in about 2 days. Several drawbacks and limitations of this animal model have been reported. For examples, the level of growth factors and cytokines and the hair follicle structure in neonatal rats differ substantially from those in mature animals, thus altering the response of hair follicles to treatment agents. Also, the lack of hair pigmentation in Sprague Dawley rats, which have a white fur, limits the study of drug effects on melanocytes. Indeed, some observations in newborn rats appear irrelevant to humans. For instance, the protective effect of topical application of 1,25-dihydroxyvitamin D3 on alopecia induced by cyclophosphamide was observed in neonatal rats but not in humans (Jimenez and Yunis, 1992; Hidalgo et al., 1999).

4.1.2 Adult mouse model

The adult black C57BL/6 mouse model for CIA was first developed in 1994 (Paus et al., 1994). In this mouse strain, the skin melanocytes are confined to hair follicles and the stage of hair growth is indicated by the skin color, i.e., pink during the telogen phase and black during the anagen phase. To mimic human hair scalp, depilation is performed to induce the mouse hair follicles at telogen phase to enter anagen phase, which is normally achieved in about 9 days. At around 16 days after the depilation, morphological signs of catagen are detectable. At day 20 after the depilation, all hair follicles are in the telogen phase. The CIA model was used to study the effect of cyclophosphamide (120-150 mg/kg, ip) on day 9 after the depilation (anagen phase). Cyclophosphamide was found to induce premature catagen development, dystrophic follicles, and complete alopecia in 6 days. In the past decade, progress in the understanding of hair follicle damage and pathogenesis of CIA has been obtained largely by using this model. On a cellular level, cyclophosphamide induces massive apoptosis of keratinocytes and melanocytes, although the precise mechanism of induction is largely unknown (Hendrix et al., 2005).

4.2 Culture models

4.2.1 Organ culture model

Although animal models have provided valuable information regarding the pathogenesis of CIA, the animal physiological and pathological conditions do not necessarily mimic human conditions. The first human organ-culture hair follicle model for CIA was developed in 2007 (Bodo et al., 2007). In this model, mature anagen (anagen VI) human hair follicles are micro-dissected intact from the occipital scalp of healthy adults. The isolated hair follicles are maintained in William's E medium containing L-glutamine, hydrocortisone, and insulin. 4-Hydroperoxycyclophosphamide (4-HC), a key cyclophosphamide metabolite, was used to verify key *in vivo* characteristics of CIA since clinical and animal data of cyclophosphamide-induced CIA are well established. 4-HC was shown to induce melanin clumping and incontinence, reduce keratinocyte proliferation, induce keratinocyte and dermal papilla cell apoptosis, and induce premature catagen, resembling *in vivo* hair follicle dystrophy. Comparison of the test results in adult mouse model and organ culture model in response to cyclophosphamide is shown in Table 2. The human organ-culture hair follicle system could be used to study the pathogenesis and potential treatment of CIA, i.e., to identify key molecular targets and inhibitors of CIA.

Key clinical parameters	Adult mouse model	Organ culture model
Inhibition of hair shaft elongation	Not directly	Yes
Increased apoptosis of matrix keratinocytes	Yes	Yes
Decreased proliferation of matrix keratinocytes	Not assessed	Yes
Catagen induction	Yes	Yes
Disrupted melanogenesis and melanin transfer	Yes	Yes

Table 2. Comparison of adult mouse model and organ culture model.

4.2.2 Cell culture model

Keratinocytes, dermal papilla cells, and melanocytes constitute the major cell types in the hair follicle. In CIA, massive apoptosis of keratinocytes occurs; thereby cultured keratinocytes are commonly used as a predictive model for chemotherapy-induced hair follicle damage. Primary and immortalized normal human keratinocytes (HaCaT) have been used to test the effects of chemotherapeutic agents and protectants (Matsumoto et al., 1995; Braun et al., 2006; Janssen et al., 2008). However, since different hair follicle cells interact and affect each other cell growth and cycling (Rogers and Hynd, 2001), the effects of chemotherapeutic agents on other cell types, e.g., dermal papilla cells and melanocytes, should also be evaluated, i.e., through the use of a co-culture system. Furthermore, current cell culture models lack biological measures of hair growth and cycling; however, they offer the advantages of gene manipulation, ease of use, high throughput, and low cost.

5. Approaches to prevent CIA

Several approaches have been investigated to overcome CIA. These approaches can be broadly classified as physical and pharmacological, as described below.

5.1 Physical prevention

5.1.1 Scalp torniques

Scalp torniques are the application of bands around the head to occlude the superficial blood flow to scalp, thus reducing the amount of drugs delivered to the hair follicles. The torniques range from 10 mmHg above systolic pressure to 300 mmHg around the scalp. These torniques are applied 5-10 minutes prior to or at the time of chemotherapy until up to 30 minutes after the drug administration (Cline, 1984). Although reports described mild to moderate prevention of CIA induced by vincristine, cyclophosphamide, and doxorubicin, this technique is no longer recommended due to patient discomfort (Wang et al., 2006).

5.1.2 Scalp cooling

Scalp cooling or hypothermia is the application of cold to the scalp using a device (cap) that is pre-cooled in a freezer or exchanges coolant with reservoir. A period of cooling lasts from 5 minutes prior to chemotherapy until an hour or more after the drug administration. Many studies have shown that the efficacy of scalp cooling can range from 0-90% (for review, *see* Grevelman and Breed, 2005). A recent study reported that scalp cooling helps reduce major CIA in patients receiving doxorubicin (60 mg/m^2), docetaxel (80 mg/m^2), or combination of 5-fluorouracil (600 mg/m^2), epirubicin (60 mg/m^2), and cyclophosphamide (600 mg/m^2) for 6 to 9 cycles (Auvinen et al., 2010). The current hypotheses of the protective effect are: (i) cooling reduces blood flow to hair follicles by vasoconstriction, resulting in a decrease in the amount of drugs available for uptake; and (ii) cooling decreases cellular metabolism and drug uptake. Scalp cooling to 20°C was shown to reduce blood flow to 20% of normal flow; however, further decrease in the temperature (<18°C) did not result in further decrease in scalp blood flow (Janssen et al., 2007). Recent *in vitro* studies indicate the significant role of temperature on keratinocyte cell viability upon doxorubicin chemotherapy; however, there is no difference in cell survival between 10°C and 22°C (Janssen et al., 2008). Based on these findings, it appears that there is an optimal temperature for scalp cooling (~20°C), and that increasing the cooling will only result in patient discomfort. Other factors affecting the effectiveness of this method include drug regimen, application and duration of cooling, and the cool conductivity (Betcheler, 2001).

Scalp cooling is practically ineffective if the chemotherapeutic agent is administered as a continuous infusion over a prolonged period. Additionally, scalp cooling increases the risk of scalp metastasis, and is therefore contraindicated in patients with hematological malignancies and cutaneous T-cell lymphoma (Dean et al., 1979; Apisanthanarax and Duvic, 2003).

5.1.3 Heat treatment

Stress protein response is one of the cellular protective mechanisms against various adverse conditions. Enhanced expression of stress proteins such as Hsp90, Hsp70, and Hsp25 has been observed in response to certain physical and chemical stresses, which has been linked to increased stress tolerance. Previous *in vitro* studies have shown that heat treatment and overexpression of stress response proteins, e.g., Hsp70 and Hsp27, could protect against the cytotoxic effects of anticancer drugs such as doxorubicin, cyclophosphamide, etoposide, and taxol (Kampinga, 1995; Jaattela et al., 1998; Kwak et al., 1998; Ito et al., 1999; Xia et al., 1999), leading to the investigation of the protective effect of stress protein activation on CIA in neonatal rats (Jimenez et al., 2008). In this study, heat was locally applied to the skin with a copper cylinder through which heated water was circulated. Conducting gel (Vaseline) was applied to the skin to improve heat conductance. Heat treatment at 48-48.5°C for 20 minutes increases Hsp70 and subsequently protects against CIA in response to various treatments as summarized in Table 3. The protective effect of heat treatment was confirmed in an adult mouse model receiving cyclophosphamide. Additionally, localized heat treatment was shown not to interfere with the anti-tumor activity of drugs. These findings suggest that localized activation of stress proteins in the hair follicles might be an effective strategy against CIA without affecting the anti-tumor efficacy.

Chemotherapeutic agents	Dosing	Protective Frequency
Etoposide	I.P. 2.5 μg/g twice	0.94 (45/48)
Cyclophosphamide	I.P. 35.5 μg/g twice	0.97 (29/30)
Cyclophosphamide/doxorubicin	I.P. 20-30 μg/g once/2.5-4.5 μg/g twice	1.0 (56/56)
Taxol	S.C. 5 μg/animal, twice	1.0 (7/7)

Table 3. Localized, heat-induced protection against CIA in neonatal rats.

5.2 Pharmacological prevention

Currently, there are no FDA-approved drug treatments for CIA but several pharmacological strategies have been proposed. Many of these strategies have shown promising results in animals but their clinical use will require further investigations.

5.2.1 Tumor targeting delivery

Differences in the molecular machinery of normal cells and tumor cells as a result of cell transformation dominate the tumor targeting delivery arena. Tumor-specific ligands and antibodies have been used to provide targeting ability to drug carriers such as liposomes. Accordingly, these liposomes can protect patients from the side effects of chemotherapy, including hair loss. Examples of the targeting moieties are folate receptor (FR) for ovarian, colorectal, and breast cancer; transferrin for pancreatic cancer; anti-HER2 antibody for breast cancer; anti-CD19 for malignant B cells; anti-GD2 for neuroblastoma and melonoma; and prostate-specific membrane antigen (PMSA) aptamer for prostate cancer and tumor vascular endothelium (Huges et al., 2001; Yu et al., 2009).

5.2.2 Drug-specific antibodies

MAD11 monoclonal antibody (MAb) is an anti-anthracycline antibody that reacts with doxorubicin and other anthracycline chemotherapeutics. Topical administration of liposomes containing MAD11 MAb was shown to prevent CIA in doxorubicin-treated neonatal rats at the frequency of 31 in 45 rats (Balsari et al., 1994). MAD11 MAb was encapsulated into liposomes to facilitate absorption through the stratum corneum and to delay systemic distribution of the antibody. Topical MAD11 MAb was found to be nontoxic and does not induce systemic activation of cytokines. Thus, MAD11-loaded liposomes might be an effective strategy in preventing anthracycline-induced alopecia in cancer patients. However, the advantage of this strategy is limited in combination therapy since the antibody could not react with the other drugs in combination.

5.2.3 Hair growth cycle modifiers

5.2.3.1 Cyclosporine A

Cyclosporine A is an immunosuppressive immunophilin ligand used in the treatment of autoimmune diseases and in post-organ transplantation to reduce patients' graft rejection. In T-lymphocytes, cyclosporine A forms complex with cyclophilin and inhibits calcineurin, leading to the inhibition of Go to G1 cell cycle transition and proliferation. The use of cyclosporine A in alopecia originates from its common side effect of excessive hair growth called hypertrichosis. Cyclosporin A induces anagen and inhibits catagen of the hair cycle, leading to the promotion of hair growth under normal and pathologic conditions such as alopecia areata and androgenetic alopecia (Paus et al., 1989; Taylor et al., 1993; Lutz et al., 1994).

The effect of cyclosporine A on CIA has been investigated in neonatal rat and adult mouse models. In neonatal rats, topical administration of cyclosporine A prevents CIA induced by cyclophosphamide, cytosine arabinoside and etoposide (Hussein et al., 1995). In adult mice given cyclophosphamide, topical or systemic administration of cyclosporine A retards CIA, prevents the progression of damaged hair into telogen, and thus induces faster hair regrowth.

5.2.3.2 AS101

AS101, ammonium trichloro (dioxoethylene-o,o') tellurate, is a synthetic immunomodulator that has been shown to protect mice from hemopoietic damage caused by chemotherapeutic agents such as cyclophosphamide, 5-fluorouracil, doxorubicin and etoposide. In phase II clinical trials, AS101 was shown to protect against CIA in patients with non-small cell lung cancer (NSCLC) receiving a combination therapy of carboplatin and etoposide (Sredni et al., 1996). The results of this study are summarized in Table 4.

Treatments	No. of patients	% of patients in alopecia grade				
		No	Mild	Moderate	Severe	Total
Carboplatin and etoposide	30	20.4	5.1	28.2	38.5	7.7
+ AS101	28	37.2	16.2	27.9	13.9	4.6

Table 4. Prevention of alopecia in AS101-treated NSCLC patients.

The mechanism of action of AS101 was investigated in neonatal rats receiving cytosine arabinoside (Sredni et al., 1996). The study demonstrated that the protective effect of AS101 was through macrophage-derived factors such as interleukin-1 (IL-1). IL-1 induces the secretion of other cytokines such as keratinocyte growth factor (KGF) which stimulate the proliferation and differentiation of keratinocytes within the hair follicles.

5.2.3.3 Minoxidil

Minoxidil is one of the FDA approved drug for the treatment of androgenetic alopecia. Topical minoxidil shortens the telogen phase by inducing the entry of resting hair follicles into the anagen phase, thereby stimulating hair growth (Messenger and Rundegren, 2004). Minoxidil also prolongs the duration of anagen phase and enlarges hair follicles, probably by its proliferative and anti-apoptotic effects on dermal papilla cells (Han et al., 2004). Several studies have also investigated the effect of minoxidil on CIA. In neonatal rats, local injection of minoxidil protects against CIA induced by cytosine arabinoside but not by cyclophosphamide. However, topical minoxidil (2%) does not protect against CIA. In one randomized clinical trial, topical minoxidil (2%) was shown to shorten the duration of CIA in breast cancer patients receiving 5-fluorouracil, doxorubicin, and cyclophosphamide (Duvic et al., 1996). The results of this study is summarized in Table 5.

Interval	**Mean (days)**		***p*-value**
	Minoxidil	Placebo	
Baseline to maximal hair loss	61.8	50.3	0.15
Baseline to maximal regrowth	148.5	187.2	0.07
Maximal hair loss to first regrowth (period of baldness)	86.7	136.9	0.03
Baseline to first moderate or dense hair growth	131.2	155.3	0.40

Table 5. Minoxidil shortens duration of CIA.

5.2.4 Cytokines and growth factors

Hair follicle cells express receptors for multiple cytokines and growth factors that regulate hair growth cycle (Trueb, 2002). These regulators include fibroblast growth factors (FGF), transforming growth factors (TGF), insulin-like growth factors (IGF), epidermal growth factors (EGF), interferon and interleukins (Stenn and Paus, 2001). Moreover, hair cycle is regulated by androgens and parathyroid hormone (PTH) (Sawaya, 2001).

IL-1 and ImuVert, a biological response modifier derived from *S. Marcescens*, were reported to protect against CIA induced by cytosine arabinoside and doxorubicin in neonatal rats (Hussesin, 1993). Both agents can induce the release of multiple cytokines and growth factors. It was suggested that the protection of CIA by ImuVert is mediated through IL-1. Similarly, EGF and FGF-1 have been shown to protect against CIA induced by cytosine arabinoside but not by cyclophosphamide in neonatal rats (Jimenez and Yunis, 1992). In contrast, FGF-7 and KGF partially protect against CIA by cytosine arabinoside by retarding hair loss (Danilenko et al., 2000). In organ-culture human scalp hair follicles and HaCaT keratinocytes, KGF protects against the cytotoxicity of mafosfamide, the cell culture active derivative of cyclophosphamide (Braun et al., 2006). The mechanism of action of KGF has been proposed to involve specific signaling pathways including PI3K and ERK1/2.

PTH antagonists reduce cell apoptosis in the hair bulb matrix and delay the onset of CIA in adult mice, whereas PTH agonists enhance the apoptosis and accelerate hair regrowth after CIA. However, neither PTH agonists nor antagonists prevent CIA (Peters et al., 2001).

5.2.5 Antioxidants

Broad spectrum antioxidant *N*-acetyl cysteine (NAC), an analog and precursor of glutathione, when administered topically or parenterally, protects against CIA induced by cyclophosphamide in neonatal rats. In contrast, NAC could not protect adult mice from CIA induced by doxorubicin (Wang et al., 2006).

α-Tocopherol or vitamin E is an important lipid-soluble antioxidant. Several studies have reported the protective effect of high-dose vitamin E in patients receiving doxorubicin; however, conflicting results have also been reported. For example, A clinical study reported that 69% of the patients did not experience CIA when co-treated with vitamin E, while others reported no protective effect of vitamin E (Batchelor, 2001).

5.2.6 Cell cycle or proliferation modifiers

Rapid proliferation of keratinocytes during the anagen phase of hair follicle is one the main predisposing factors of CIA. Thus, one approach to protect against CIA is to arrest the cell cycle and inhibit cell proliferation.

5.2.6.1 Calcitriol

Multiple effects of calcitriol (1,25-dihydroxyvitamin D3) on keratinocytes, i.e., inhibition of DNA synthesis, Go/G1 cell cycle arrest, and induction of cell differentiation, have been reported (Kobayashi et al., 1998; Wang et al., 2006). Thus, it is likely that calcitriol induces changes in keratinocyte proliferation and/or terminal differentiation, subsequently altering cellular susceptibility to apoptosis. In neonatal rats, topical administration of calcitriol reduces CIA induced by cyclophosphamide, etoposide, and a combination treatment of cyclophosphamide and doxorubicin (Jimenez and Yunis., 1992). In adult mice receiving cyclophosphamide, topical calcitriol however fails to prevent or retard CIA, but somehow reduces massive apoptosis of hair matrix keratinocytes, a key feature of CIA, and enhances the regrowth of normal hair shaft. (Paus et al., 1996; Schilli et al., 1998). In humans, calcitriol has a protective effect against CIA induced by paclitaxel (Jimenez and Yunis, 1996), but not by a combination of 5-fluorouracil, doxorubicin and cyclophosphamide (Hidalgo et al., 1999)

5.2.6.2 CDK2 inhibitor

Cyclin-dependent kinase 2 (CDK2) is a member of the serine/threonine protein kinase family that plays a key role from late G1 to late G2 of the cell cycle. Potent small inhibitors of CDK2 have been synthesized and tested for their effect on CIA. One of these synthetic inhibitors was shown to inhibit the progression from late G1 into S phase in human diploid fibroblasts and also inhibit apoptosis induced by etoposide, 5-fluorouracil, taxol, cisplatin and doxorubicin. In neonatal rats, topical application of the inhibitor reduces hair loss at the site of application in 50% of the rats having etoposide-induced CIA and in 33% of the rats with CIA induced by cyclophosphamide and doxorubicin (Davis et al., 2001). Histological examinations of the skin from etoposide-treated rats show that the inhibitor increases the number of viable hair follicles and dermal papilla, reduces the level of inflammation and amount of damage to epithelium, reduces the thickening of epidermis and decreases the number of apoptotic cells in the hair follicle matrix. However, in subsequent studies the authors reported that they were unable to reproduce the results in the neonatal rat model (Davis et al., 2002), thus the use of this inhibitor in CIA becomes questionable, although the idea of using CDK2 inhibitors is still ongoing.

5.2.7 Inhibitor of apoptosis

5.2.7.1 Caspase3 inhibitor

Various chemotherapeutic agents induce apoptosis of hair follicle cells and cause CIA, although the underlying mechanisms are unclear. Caspase-3 is a key executor of apoptosis and its activation is normally used as an indicator of caspase-dependent apoptosis (Porter and Janicke, 1999). M50054, 2,2′-methylenebis, is an inhibitor of caspase-3 activation that was shown to inhibit etoposide-induced apoptosis in human monocytes. In neonatal rats, topical administration of M50054 reduces CIA induced by etoposide (Tsuda et al., 2001).

5.2.7.2 Anti-death FNK protein

FNK protein constructed from rat Bcl-xL by site-directed mutagenesis (Y22F/Q26N/R165K) localizes to mitochondria and functions to maintain mitochondrial membrane potential (Aosh et al., 2000). Mitochondrial membrane potential regulates the release of cytochrome C, which once binds to caspase-activating proteins such as Apaf-1 initiates the intrinsic caspase cascade and apoptosis (Li et al., 1997). Recently, FNK protein has been fused to protein transduction domain (PTD) to improve its cellular entry. Subcutaneous injection of PTD-FNK protects against CIA induced by etoposide in the neonatal rat model. The fusion protein helps retain hair follicle structures, prevent hair follicle regression and maintain the anagen duration upon etoposide treatment (Nakashima-Kamimura et al., 2008). Indeed, its protective effect on CIA suggests that it could penetrate the epidermis and reach the dermal hair follicles. Localized administration of FNK fusion protein has been suggested as a potential protein therapy for CIA without affecting the chemotherapy efficacy.

6. Molecular mechanisms of CIA

Molecular mechanisms of CIA are not well understood, in part due to the lack of appropriate experimental models that mimic human CIA. Much of our understanding on CIA is based on animal and cell culture models, some of which are described below.

6.1 DNA damage

Most chemotherapeutic agents including cyclophosphamide, doxorubicin and cisplatin induce DNA damage and kill both normal and cancer cells by apoptosis (Muller et al., 1998). p53 is a transcription factor and tumor suppressor protein that plays a critical role in cell cycle progression and apoptosis. Activation of p53 in response to DNA damage is associated with the degradation of Mdm2/p53 complex, leading to increased availability of p53 to bind DNA and consequently transcriptional activation of p53 target genes. Many p53 target genes, including Fas, Bax, Bcl-2, insulin-growth factor receptor type I (IGFR1), and insulin-like growth factor binding protein 3 (IGF-BP3), are expressed in the hair follicles (Lindner et al., 1997). In the adult mouse model for CIA, p53 was shown to be essential in the hair follicle response to DNA damage induced by cyclophosphamide. Specifically, hair loss was not observed and hair follicle cells remained active in p53-deficient mice, as shown by a large volume of hair bulb and dermal papilla, and active keratinocyte proliferation in the hair matrix (Botchkarev et al., 2000).

6.2 Apoptosis

Chemotherapy-induced apoptosis of hair follicle cells is one of the major findings from CIA animal studies. Although the mechanism of apoptosis is not well understood, p53 and Fas signaling pathways are believed to play a key role.

In adult mice, cyclophosphamide-treated hair follicles show a strong up-regulation of p53 in the hair matrix, particularly in TUNEL-positive apoptotic keratinocytes (Botchkarev et al., 2000). By contrast, in p53-deficient mice, apoptosis in the matrix keratinocytes was not detected after cyclophosphamide treatment, indicating the involvement of p53 in the apoptotic process. The precise mechanism of p53-dependent apoptosis in the hair follicles remains unclear, but likely involves several p53 target genes. Cyclophosphamide-treated p53-deficient mice show strongly down-regulated Fas in the hair follicle keratinocytes and highly up-regulated Bcl-2 in the dermal papilla as compared to wild-type mice. The role of Fas in the control of cyclophosphamide-induced apoptosis in keratinocytes was also investigated using Fas-deficient mice (Sharov et al., 2004). These mice show significantly reduced CIA and a parallel decrease in apoptotic keratinocytes and FADD and caspase-8 expression. Similarly, anti-Fas ligand neutralizing antibody inhibits cyclophosphamide-induced keratinocyte apoptosis. These studies indicate that Fas signaling is an important pathway in mediating the apoptosis induced by cyclophosphamide and suggest the cross-talk between p53 and Fas death signaling. However, the eventual hair loss observed in Fas-deficient mice points to the lower resistance of hair follicles to cyclophosphamide as compared to p53-deficient mice. Thus, it is likely that Fas signaling represents only a component of the p53-dependent apoptosis machinery in the hair follicles and that other p53 targets are also involved. Cyclophosphamide treatment also alters the expression of melanogenic proteins and causes apoptosis of hair follicle melanocytes (Sharov et al., 2003). In contrast to matrix keratinocytes, the melanocytes undergo apoptosis primarily through Fas signaling but not p53 signaling.

6.3 Reactive oxygen species

The observation that antioxidants such as NAC protect against CIA in animals suggest the involvement of reactive oxygen species (ROS) in CIA. Various chemotherapeutic agents induce oxidative stress through multiple mechanisms, i.e., activation of NADPH oxidase system and mitochondrial respiration chain. Agents that induce a high level of ROS include anthracyclines (e.g., doxorubicin, epirubicin, and daunorubicin), alkylating agents (e.g., cyclophosphamide), platinum coordination complexes (e.g., cisplatin, carboplatin, and oxaliplatin), and epipodophyllotoxins (e.g., etoposide) (Conklin, 2004). Interestingly, anthracyclines, alkylating agents, platinum complexes, and epipodophyllotoxins also induce CIA more frequently and more severely than most other agents, suggesting a relationship between ROS generation and CIA. The exact mechanism of how ROS induces or promotes CIA is unclear, but likely involves apoptosis regulation since apoptosis of hair follicles is a hallmark of CIA and since ROS generation is generally required for the induction of apoptosis by chemotherapeutic agents (Simon et al., 2000).

7. Perspectives

CIA is a major side effect that compromises patient quality of life, particularly for females and children. Overcoming CIA remains a major challenge in the management of cancer patients. Significant progresses in the pathobiology and molecular mechanisms of CIA have been made during the past decade, and several physical and pharmacological approaches to treat CIA have been attempted. However, effective treatment strategies have yet to be developed. A key to this success is a better understanding of the human CIA mechanisms which requires the development of more predictive experimental models. Animal models have been useful but have limitations and may not be predictive of human CIA. The newly developed organ culture system using human hair follicles is promising and could lead to the development of more effective treatment strategies for CIA. The recent success in combination chemotherapy also provides mechanistic insights to combating CIA through the use of different combination strategies.

Even if CIA cannot be completely prevented, it can be managed. Healthcare providers and patient family could help patients prepare for the sudden loss of hair, thus minimizing the negative impact on patients. Patients should receive the information regarding self-care strategies to take control and cope with CIA. Patients with long hair should be encouraged to try short hair style to make a better transition to total CIA. Patients are also advised to avoid physical and chemical trauma to the hair (e.g. bleaching, coloring and perming) and to shave their hair once the hair loss becomes prominent. Appropriate head covering may be used, depending on individual preference (Bachelor, 2001; Trueb, 2010).

8. Acknowledgment

This work was supported by the NIH grants HL076340, HL076340-04S1, and HL095579.

9. References

Alonso, L. & Fuchs, E. (2006) The hair cycle. *Journal of Cell Science* Vol.119, No.3 (January 2006), pp. 391-393.

Aosh, S.; Ohtsu, T. & Ohta, S. (2000) The super anti-apoptotic factor Bcl-xFNK constructed by disturbing intramolecular polar interactions in rat Bcl-x_L. *The Journal of Biological Chemistry* Vol.275, No.47, (November 2000), pp. 37240-37245.

Apisanthanarax, N. & Duvic, M. (2003) Dermatologic complications of cancer chemotherapy, In: *Frei Cancer Medicine*, R. C. Bast; D. W. Kufe; R. E. Pollock; R. R. Weichsellbaum; J. F. Holland & E. Frei, (5), 2271-2278, BC Decker, Hamilton, London.

Batchelor, D. (2001). Hair and cancer chemotherapy: consequences and nursing care—a literature study. *European Journal of Cancer Care* Vol.10, No.3, (September 2001), pp. 147-163.

Bodo, E.; Tobin, D. J.; Kamensich, Y.; Biro, T.; Berneburg, M.; Funk, W. & Paus, R. (2007) Dissecting the impact of chemotherapy on the human hair follicle. A pragmatic in vitro assay for studying the pathogenesis and potential management of hair follicle dystrophy. *The American Journal of Pathology* Vol.171, No.4, (October 2007), pp. 1153-1167.

Botchkarev, V. A.; Komarova, E. V.; Siebenhaar, F.; Botchkareva, N. V.; Komarov, P. G.; Maurer, M.; Gilchrest, B. A. & Gudkov, A. V. (2000) p53 is essential for chemotherapy-induced hair loss. *Cancer Research* Vol.60, No.18, (September 2000), pp. 5002-5006.

Braun, S.; Krampert, M.; Bodo, E.; Kumin, A.; Born-Berclaz, C.; Paus, R. & Werner, S. (2006) Keratinocyte growth factor protects epidermis and hair follicles from cell death induced by UV irradiation, chemotherapeutic or cytotoxic agents. *Journal of Cell Science* Vol.110, No.Pt 23, (November 2006), pp. 4841-4849.

Balsari, A. L.; Morelli, D.; Menard, S.; Veronesi, U. & Colnagho, M. I. (1994) Protection against doxorubicin-induced alopecia in rats by liposome-entrapped monoclonal antibodies. *The FASEB Journal* Vol.8, No.2, (February 1994), pp. 226-230.

Carelle, N.; Piotto, E.; Bellanger, A.; Germanaud, J.; Thuillier, A.; & Khayat, D. (2002) Changing patient perceptions of the side effects of cancer chemotherapy. *Cancer* Vol.95, No.1, (July 2002), pp. 155-163.

Cline, B. W. (1984) Prevention of chemotherapy-induced alopecia: A review of the literature. *Cancer Nursing* Vol.7, No.3, (June 1984), pp. 221-228.

Conklin, K. A. (2004) Chemotherapy-associated oxidative stress: impact on chemotherapeutic effectiveness. *Integrative Cancer Therapies* Vol.3, No.4, (December 2004), pp. 294-300.

Corsarelis, G. and Millar, S. E. (2001) Towards a molecular understanding of hair loss and its treatment. TRENDS *in Molecular Medicine* Vol.7, No.7, (July 2001), pp. 293-301.

Danilenko, D. M.; Ring, B. D.; Yanagihara, D.; Benson, W.; Wiemann, B.; Starnes, C. O. & Pierce, G. F. (1995) Keratinocyte growth factor is an important endogenous mediator of hair follicle growth, development, and differentiation. Normalization of the nu/nu follicular differentiation defect and amelioration of chemotherapy-induced alopecia. *American Journal of Pathology* Vol.147, No.1, (July 1995), pp. 145-154.

Davis, S. T.; Benson, B. G.; Bramson, H. N.; Chapman, D. E.; Dickerson, S. H.; Dold, K. M.; Eberwein, D. J.; Edelstein, M.; Frye, S. V.; Gampe Jr., R. T.; Griffin, R. J.; Harris, P. A.; Hassel, A. M.; Holmes, W. D.; Hunter, R. N.; Knick, V. B.; Lackey, K.; Lovejoy, B.; Luzzio, M. J.; Murray, D.; Parker, P.; Rocque, W. J.; Shewchuk, L.; Veal, J. M.; Walker, D. H. & Kuyper, L. F. (2001) Prevention of chemotherapy-induced alopecia in rats by CDK inhibitors. *Sciences* Vol.291, No.5501, (January 2001), pp. 134-137.

Davis, S. T.; Benson, B. G.; Bramson, H. N.; Chapman, D. E.; Dickerson, S. H.; Dold, K. M.; Eberwein, D. J.; Edelstein, M.; Frye, S. V.; Gampe Jr., R. T.; Griffin, R. J.; Harris, P. A.; Hassel, A. M.; Holmes, W. D.; Hunter, R. N.; Knick, V. B.; Lackey, K.; Lovejoy, B.; Luzzio, M. J.; Murray, D.; Parker, P.; Rocque, W. J.; Shewchuk, L.; Veal, J. M.; Walker, D. H. & Kuyper, L. F. (2002) Retraction. *Sciences* Vol.298, No.5602, (December 2002), pp. 2327.

Dean, J. C.; Salmon, S. E. & Griffiith, K. S. (1979) Prevention of doxorubicin-induced hair loss with scalp hypothermia. *New England Journal of Medicine* Vol.301, No.26, (December 27), pp. 1427-1429.

Duvic, M.; Lemak, N. A.; Valero, V.; Hymes, S. R.; Farmer, K. L.; Hortobagyi, G. N.; Trancik, R. J.; Bandstra, B. A. & Compton, L. D. (1996) A randomized trial of minoxidil in chemotherapy-induced alopecia. *Journal of the American Academy of Dermatology* Vol.35, No.1, (July 1996), pp. 74-78.

Elliott, K.; Stephenson, T. J. & Messenger, A. G. (1999) Differences in hair follicle dermal papilla volume are due to extracellular matrix volume and cell number: implications for the control of hair follicle size and androgen responses. *The Journal of Investigative Dermatology* Vol.113, No.6, (December 1999), pp. 873-877.

Freedman, T. G. (1994) Social and cultural dimensions of hair loss in women treated for breast cancer. Cancer Nursing Vol.17, No.4, (August 1994), pp. 334-341.

Grevelman, E. G. & Breed, W. P. M. (2005) Prevention of chemotherapy-induced hair loss by scalp cooling. *Annals of Oncology* Vol.16, No.3, (January 2006), pp. 352-358.

Han, J. H.; Kwon, O. S.; Chung, J. H.; Cho, K. H.; Eun, H. C. & Kim, K. H. (2004) Effect of minoxidil on proliferation and apoptosis in dermal papilla cells of human hair follicle. *Journal of Dermatological Science* Vol.34, No.2, (April 2004), pp. 91-98.

Hardy, M. H. (1992) The secret life of the hair follicle. *Trends in Genetics* Vol.8, No.2, (February 1992), pp. 55-61.

Hendrix, S.; Handjiski, B.; Peters, E. M. J. & Paus, R. (2005) A guide to assessing damage response pathways of the hair follicle: Lessons from cyclophosphamide-induced alopecia in mice. *The Journal of Investigative Dermatology* Vol.125, No.1, (July 2005), pp. 42-51.

Hidalgo, M.; Rinaldi, M.; Medina, G.; Griffin, T.; Turner, J. & Van Hoff, D. D. (1999) A phase I trial of topical topitriol (calcitriol, 1,25-dihydroxyvitamin D3) to prevent chemotherapy-induced alopecia. *Anticancer Drugs* Vol.10, No.4, (April 1999), pp. 393-395.

Huges, M. D.; Hussain, M.; Nawaz, Q.; Sayyed, P. & Akhtar, S. (2001) The cellular delivery of antisense oligonucleotides and ribozymes. *Drug Discovery Today* Vol.6, No.6, (March 2001), pp. 305-315.

Hussein, A. M.; Jimenez, J. J.; McCall, C. A. & Yunis, A. A. (1990) Protection from chemotherapy-induced alopecia in a rat model. *Science* Vol.249, No.4976, (September 1990), pp.1564-1566.

Hussein, A. M. (1991) Interleukin-1 protects against 1-beta-D-Arabinofuranosylcytosine-induced alopecia in the newborn rat model. *Cancer Research* Vol.51, No.12 , (June 1995), pp. 3329-3330.

Hussein, A. M. (1993) Chemotherapy-induced alopecia: New developments. *Southern Meidcal Journal* Vol.86, No.5, (May 1993), pp. 489-496.

Hussein, A. M.; Stuart, A. & Peters, W. P. (1995) Protection against chemotherapy-induced alopecia by cyclosporine A in the newborn rat animal model. *Dermatology* Vol.190, No.3, (1995), pp. 192-196.

Ishino, A.; Uzuka, M.; Tsuji, Y.; Nakanishi, J.; Hanzawa, N. & Imamura S. (1997) Progressive decrease in hair diameter in Japanese with male pattern baldness. *Journal of Dermatology* Vol.24, No.12, (Dec 1997), pp. 758-764.

Ito, H.; Shimojo, T.; Fujisaki, H; Tamamori, M.l Ishiyama, S.; Adachi, S.; Abe, S.; Marumo, F. & Hiroe, M. (1999) Thermal preconditioning protects rat cardiac muscle cells from doxorubicin-induced apoptosis. *Life Sciences* Vol.64, No.9, (January 1999), pp. 755-761.

Jaattela, M.; Wissing, D.; Kokholm, K.; Kallunki, T. & Egeblad, M. (1998) Hsp70 exerts its anti-apoptotic function downstream of caspase-3-like proteases. *The EMBO Journal* Vol.17, No.21, (November 1998), pp. 6124-6134.

Janssen, F. E. M.; Rajan, V.; Steenbergen, W.; van Leeuwen, G. M. J. & van Steenhoven, A. A. (2007) The relationship between local scalp skin temperature and cutaneous perfusion during scalp cooling. *Physiological Measurement* Vol.28, No.8, (August 2007), pp. 829-839.

Janssen, F-P. E. M.; Bouten, C. V. C.; van Leeuwen, G. M. J. & van Steenhoven, A. A. (2008) Effects of temperature and doxorubicin exposure on keratinocyte damage in vitro. *In Vitro Cellular and Developemental Biology. Animal* Vol.44, No.304, (March-April 2008), pp. 81-86.

Jimenez, J. J. & Yuniz A. A. (1992) Protection from chemotherapy-induced alopecia by 1,25-dihydroxyvitamind D3. *Cancer Research* Vol.52, No.18, (September 1992), pp. 5123-5125.

Jimenez, J. J. & Yunis, A. A. (1996) Vitamin D3 and chemotherapy-induced alopecia. Nutrition Vol.12, No.6, (June 1996), pp. 448-449.

Jimenez, J. J.; Roberts, S. M.; Mejia, J.; Mauro, L. M.; Munson, J. W.; Elgart, G. W.; Connelly, E. A.; Chen, Q.; Zou, J.; Goldenberg, C. & Voellmy, R. (2008) Prevention of chemotherapy-induced alopecia in rodent models. Cell Stress and Chaperones Vol.13, No.1, (February 2008), pp. 31-38.

Kampinga, H. H. (1995) Hyperthemia, thermotolerance and topoisomerase II inhibitors. *British Journal of Cancer* Vol.72, No.2, (August 1995), pp. 333-338.

Kobayashi, T.; Okumura, H.; Hashimoto, K.; Asada, H.; Inui, S. & Yoshikawa, K. (1998) Synchronization of normal human keratinocytes in culture: its application to the analysis of 1,25-dihydroxyvitamin D3 effects on cell cycle. *Journal of Dermatological Science* Vol.17, No.2, (June 1998), pp. 108-114.

Krause, K. & Foitzik, K. (2006) Biology of the hair follicle. *Seminars in Cutaneous Medicine and Surgery* Vol.25, No.1, (March 2006), pp. 2-10.

Kwak, H. J.; Jun, C. D., Pae, H. P., Yoo, J. C.; Park, Y. C.; Choi, B. M.; Na, Y. G.; Park, R. K.; Chung, H. T.; Chung, H. Y.; Park, W. Y. & Seo, J. S. (1998) The role of inducible 70-kDa heat shock protein in cell cycle control, differentiation, and apoptotic cell death of the human myeloid leukemic HL-60 cells. *Cellular Immunology* Vol.187, No.1, (July 1998), pp. 1-12.

Li, P.; Nijhawan, D.; Budihardjo, I.; Srinivasula, S. M.; Ahmad, M.; Alnemn, E. S. & Wang, X. (1997) Cytochrome c and dATP-dependent formation of Apaf-1/caspase-9 complex initiates an apoptotic protease cascade. *Cell* Vol.91, No.4, (November 1997), pp. 479-489.

Lindner, G.; Botchkarev, V. A.; Botchkareva, N. V.; Ling, G.; van der Veen, C. & Paus, R. (1997) Analysis of apoptosis during hair follicle regression (catagen). *American Journal of Pathology* Vol.151, No.6, (December 1997), pp. 1601-1617.

Lutz, G. (1994) Effects of cyclosporin A on hair. *Skin Pharmacology* Vol.7, No.1-2, (1994), pp. 101-104.

Matsumoto, Y.; Hayakawa, A.; Tamada, Y.; Mori, H. & Ohashi, M. (1996) Upregulated expression of Fas antigen on cultured human keratinocytes with induction of apoptosis by cisplatin. *Archieves for Dermatological Research* Vol.288, No.5-6, (May 1996), pp. 267-269.

McGravey, E. L.; Baum, L. D.; Pinkerton, R. C. & Rogers L. M. Psychological sequelae and alopecia among women with cancer. *Cancer Practise* Vol.9, No.6, (November/December 2001), pp. 283-289.

Messenger, A. G. & Rundegren, J. (2004) Minoxidil: mechanisms of action on hair growth. *British Journal of Dermatology* Vol.150, No.2, (February 2004), pp. 186-194.

Muller, M.; Wilder, S.; Bannasch, D.; Israeli, D.; Lehlbach, K.; Li-Weber, M.; Friedman, S. L.; Galle, P. R.; Stremmel, W.; Oren, M. & Krammer, P. H. (1998) p53 activates the CD95 (Apo-1/Fas) gene in response to DNA damage by anticancer drugs. *The Journal of Experimental Medicine* Vol.188, No.11, (December 1998), pp. 2033-2045.

Munstedt, K.; Manthey, N.; Sachsse, S. & Vahrson, H. (1997) Changes in self-concept and body image during alopecia induced cancer chemotherapy. *Support Care Cancer* Vol.5, No.2, (March 1997), pp. 139-143.

Nakashima-Kamimura, N.; Nishimaki, K.; Mori, T.; Asoh, S. & Ohta, S. (2008) Prevention of hemotherapy-induced alopecia by anti-death FNK protein. *Life Sciences* Vol.82, No.3-4, (January 2008), pp. 218-225.

O'Leary, A. (1990) Stress, emotion, and human immune function. Psychological Bulletin Vol.108, No.3, (November 1990), pp. 363-382.

Ohnemus, U.; Uenalan, M.; Inzunza, J.; Gustafsson, J. A. & Paus, R. (2006) The hair follicle as an estrogen target and source. *Endocrine Reviews* Vol.27, No.6, (July 2006), pp. 677-706.

Paus, R.; Stenn, K. S. & Link, R. E. (1989) The induction of anagen hair growth in telogen mouse skin by cyclosporine A administration. *Laboratory Investigation* Vol.60, No.3, (March 1989), pp. 365-369.

Paus, R.; Handjiski, B.; Eichmuller, S. & Czarnetzki, B. M. (1994) Chemotherapy-induced alopecia in mice induction by cyclophosphamide, inhibition by cyclosporine A, and modulation by dexamethasone. *American Journal of Pathology* Vol.144, No.4, (April 1994), pp. 719-734.

Paus, R.; Schilli, M. B.; Handjiski, B.; Menrad, A.; Henz, B.M. & Plonka, P. (1996) Topical calcitriol enhances normal hair regrowth but does not prevent chemotherapy-induced alopecia in mice. *Cancer Research* Vol.56, No.19, (October 1996), pp. 4438-4443.

Peters, E. M.; Foitzik, K.; Paus, R.; Ray, S. & Holick, M. F. (2001) A new strategy for modulating chemotherapy-induced alopecia, using PTH/PTHrP receptor agonist and antagonist. *Journal of Investigative Dermatology* Vol.117, No.2, (August 2001), pp. 171-178.

Porter, A. G. & Janicke, R. U. (1999) Emerging roles of caspase-3 in apoptosis. *Cell Death and Differentiation* Vol.6, No.2, (February 1999), pp. 99-104.

Pozo-Kaderman, C.; Kaderman, R. A. & Toonkel R. (1999) The psychological aspects of breast cancer. *Nursing Practitioner Forum* Vol.10, No.3, (September 1999), pp. 165-174.

Sakita, S.; Ohtani, O. & Morohashi, M. (1995) Dynamic changes in the microvascular architecture of rat hair follicles during the hair cycle. *Medical Electron Microscopy* Vol.28, No.3-4, (November 1995), pp. 187-192.

Sawaya, M. E. (2001) Regulation of the human hair cycle. *Current Problem in Dermatology* Vol.13, No.3, (May 2001), 206-210.

Schilli, M. B.; Paus, R. & Menrad, A. (1998) Reduction of intrafollicular apoptosis in chemotherapy-induced alopecia by topical calcitriol-analogs. *Journal of Investigative Dermatology* Vol.111, No.4, (October 1998), pp. 598-604.

Sharov, A. A.; Li, G. Z.; Palkina, T. N.; Sharova, T. Y.; Gilchrest, B. A. & Botchkarev, V. A. (2003) Fas and c-kit are involved in the control of hair follicle melanocyte apoptosis and migration in chemotherapy-induced hair loss. *Journal of Investigative Dermatology* Vol.120, No.1, (January 2003), pp. 27-35.

Sharov, A. A.; Siebanhaar, F.; Sharova, T. Y.; Botchkareva, N. V.; Gilchrest, B. A. & Botchkarev, V. A. (2004) Fas signalling is involved in the control of hair follicle response to chemotherapy. *Cancer Research* Vol.64, No.17, (September 2004), pp. 6266-6270.

Simon, H. U.; Haj-Yehia, A. & Levi-Schaffer, F. (2000) Role of reactive oxygen species (ROS) in apoptosis induction. *Apoptosis* Vol.5, No.5, (November 2000), pp. 415-418.

Spiegel, D. & Giese-Davis, J. (2003) Depression and cancer: mechanisms and disease progression. *Biological Psychiatry* Vol.54, No.3, (August 2003), pp. 269-282.

Sredeni, B.; Xu, R. H.; Albeck, M.; Gafter, U.; Gal, R.; Shani, A.; Tichler, T.; Shapira, J.; Bruderman, I.; Catanae, R.; Kaufman, B.; Whisnant, J. K.; Mettinger, K. L. & Kalechman, Y. (1996) The protective role of immunomodulator AS101 against chemotherapy-induced alopecia studies on human and animal models. International Journal f Cancer Vol.65, No.1, (January 1996), pp. 97-103.

Stenn, K.S. & Paus, R. (2001) Control of hair follicle cycling. *Physiological Reviews* Vol.81, No.1, (January 2001), pp. 449-494.

Taylor, M.; Ashcroft, A. T. & Messenger, A G. (1993) Cyclosporin A prolongs human hair growth *in vitro*. *Journal of Investigative Dermatology* Vol.100, No.3, (March 1993), pp. 365-369.

Trueb, R.M. (2002) Molecular mechanisms of androgenetic alopecia. *Experimental Gerontology* Vol.37, No.8-9, (August-September 2002), pp. 981-990.

Tsuda, T.; Ohmori, Y.; Muramatsu, H.; Hosaka, Y.; Takigushi, K.; Saitoh, F.; Kato, K.; Nakayama, K.; Nakamura, N.; Nagata, S. & Mochizuki, H. (2001) Inhibitory effect of M50054, a novel inhibitor of apoptosis, on anti-Fas-antibody-induced hepatitis and chemotherapy-induced alopecia. European Journal of Pharmacology Vol.433, No.1, (December 2001), pp. 43337-43345.

Trueb, R. M. (2009) Chemotherapy-induced alopecia. *Seminars in Cutaneous Medicine and Surgery* Vol.28, No.1, (March 2009), pp. 11-14.

Trueb, R. M. (2010) Chemotherapy-induced alopecia. *Current Opinion in Supportive and Palliative Care* Vol.4, No.4, (December 2010), pp. 281-284.

Wang, J.; Lu, Z. & Au, J. L. S. (2006) Protection against chemotherapy-induced alopecia. *Pharmaceutical Research* Vol.23, No.11, (November 2006), pp. 2505-2514.

Wilkes, G. M. (1996) Potential toxicities and nursing management, In: *Cancer Chemotherapy: a Nursing Process Approach*, M. Barton Burke; G. M. Wilkes & K. Inguersen, (2), 130-135, Jones & Bartlet, Boston.

Xia, W.; Vilaboa, N.; Martin, J. L.; Mestril, R.; Guo, Y. & Voellmy, R. (1999) Modulation of tolerance by mutant heat shcok transcription factors. *Cell Stress and Chaperones* Vol.4, No.1, (February 1999), pp. 8-18.

Yu, B.; Zhao, X.; Lee, L. J. & Lee, R. J. (2009) Targeted delivery systems for oligonucleotide therapeutics. *The AAPS Journal* Vol.11, No.11, (March 2009), pp. 195-203.

6

Sexuality and Intimacy in the Context of Cancer

J. M. Ussher, J. Perz, E. Gilbert,
Y. Hawkins and W. K. T. Wong
*University of Western Sydney,
Australia*

1. Introduction

1.1 The impact of cancer on sexuality and intimacy: A key aspect of quality of life

In 2006, more than 106,000 new cases of cancer were diagnosed in Australia, with the number of new cases in New South Wales alone expected to grow to 40,116 by 2011 (AIHW et al., 2007, Tracey et al., 2005). It is now widely recognised that cancer and its treatment can have a significant effect on the quality of life of both people with cancer (Stommel et al., 2004) and their family members, in particular their intimate partner (Hodges et al., 2005). Sexuality and intimacy are important aspects of an individual's quality of life (World Health Organisation, 1995), and there is a growing body of evidence to show that cancer can result in dramatic changes to sexuality, sexual functioning, relationships, and sense of self, regardless of cancer type. Indeed, these changes can be experienced as the most significant in the person with cancer's life (Anderson et al., 2000).

For women, treatments for gynaecological, colorectal, or breast cancer can alter patterns of fertility, have a negative impact on arousal and orgasm, reduce vaginal lubrication and elasticity (Jvaskova et al., 2003), precipitate negative changes to body image and sense of self, or precipitate 'sexual dysfunction' (Maughan et al., 2002, Sundquist, 2002, Baider et al., 2000). For men, prostate and testicular cancer can impact on fertility, ejaculatory capacity, and erectile potential (Gurevich et al., 2004), as well as provoking diminished confidence, fear, and embarrassment associated with sexual ability (Bokhour et al., 2001). The fatigue caused by cancer and certain treatments, such as chemotherapy and radiotherapy, is also typically associated with diminished desire (Rolland, 1994).

Changes to sexuality post-cancer have ramifications beyond sex as an activity. It has been argued that when sexual intercourse ceases after illness, touching and other forms of affectionate physical contact also diminish (Kuyper et al., 1998), because of a perception amongst some couples that these forms of affection necessarily lead to sexual intercourse, which is either not possible, or deemed inappropriate (Hughes, 2000). Equally, if all forms of sexual intimacy within the couple relationship disappear, couples facing cancer can feel isolated, anxious, depressed (Germino et al., 1995), inadequate (Anllo, 2000), or emotionally distant from their partner (Rolland, 1994). Conversely, sexual intimacy has also been found to make the experience of cancer more manageable and assist in the recovery process (Schultz et al., 2003), or be central to couple closeness and quality of life in palliative care (Lemieux et al., 2004).

1.2 The experience of cancer on partners' sexuality

Whilst the experiences of partners are often neglected in research on sexuality and intimacy post-cancer (Reichers, 2004), there is growing acknowledgement of their unmet needs in this area (De Groot et al., 2005, Perez et al., 2002, Soothill et al., 2003). Reported disruptions, include decreases in their own sex drive; fear of initiating sex with their partner; difficulty regaining a level of 'normality' within the sexual relationship; and feeling unwanted and unattractive because of cessation of sex (Maughan et al., 2002, Harden et al., 2002, Sanders et al., 2006).

Whilst the inclusion of partners in research on sexuality and cancer goes someway to addressing the issue of 'carer blindness' (Parker, 1990), one of the limitations of existing research in this area is the focus on cancers that affect sexual organs, primarily prostate, breast and gynaecological cancer. There is a need for research examining the experiences of partners across a range of cancer types, as cancers that do not involve parts of the body designated as 'sexual' may also impact on sexuality (Reichers, 2004). Equally, the focus of research to date has been on the physiological effects of cancer and its treatment upon the sexuality of partners. However, sexuality is a material-discursive phenomenon (Ussher, 1997a), and thus the dynamics of the care-giving relationship, and social constructions surrounding what constitutes 'appropriate' or 'taboo' sexual conduct post-cancer, may also interfere with a couples' sexual relationship. Partners who provide a great deal of intimate physical care to the person with cancer (such as helping with toileting or feeding) can experience difficulties in continuing to see them as a sexual person (Pope, 1999), repositioning them as a 'patient' (Kelly, 1992) or as asexual (D'Ardenne, 2004).

Broader cultural constructions of normative sexuality may also be influential in determining the ability of couples to renegotiate sexuality and intimacy post-cancer, particularly when sexual intercourse is no longer possible. As Judith Butler (1993) has argued, our understanding of sexual subjectivity is confined within a 'heterosexual matrix', within which masculinity and femininity are performed through engagement in normative sexual practices, described as the "coital imperative" (Gavey et al., 1999), with failure to perform coitus positioned as 'dysfunction', and other practices as not "real sex" (Few, 1997). This provides a theoretical framework for understanding why many heterosexual couples who cannot physiologically engage in sexual intercourse following diagnosis and treatment of cancer cease all expression of sexual intimacy. It also suggests that the dynamics and pressures of the caring role, as well as constructions and beliefs about what is acceptable or appropriate sexually post-cancer, are worthy of investigation across cancer types. This is one of the aims of the present chapter.

1.3 Pathways to difficulty or re-negotiation of sexuality post-cancer

Much of the existing research in this area simply documents changes in sexuality and intimacy post-cancer, however, there have been some attempts to examine pathways to difficulty or re-negotiation, primarily within a uni-linear model, with each study focusing on one specific construct. Qualitative research has reported associations between cessation of sexuality and intimacy post-cancer and difficulties in couple communication about sexual matters (Arrington, 2003, Foy et al., 2001, Holmberg et al., 2001), often for fear of creating feelings of guilt in the person with cancer (Kuyper et al., 1998), and one quantitative study reported an association between communication, relationship satisfaction, and sexuality (Hannah et al., 1992). Equally, interviews with partners of a person with cancer, recently conducted by the authors, revealed that successful re-negotiation of intimacy post-cancer was associated with good communication and positive relationship context (Gilbert et al., 2010a).

Until recently, research examining the impact of cancer on sexual wellbeing and intimacy has focused on the physical changes (Wilmoth, 2001), using quantitative methods of data collection - primarily surveys. Whilst quantitative methods can provide information on changes in large samples of individuals, they negate the lived experience and negotiation of sexual wellbeing after cancer (Gilbert et al., 2010b). At the same time, research has focused narrowly on ability to engage in satisfying sexual activity, satisfaction with the frequency of that activity (Wilmoth, 2001, Hensen, 2002), and the level of their sexual 'dysfunction' post-cancer, where functional sexuality is narrowly conceptualised as penile/vaginal intercourse (Fobair et al., 2006). Recent research has shown, however, that engaging in sexual intercourse may not be the primary focus of sexual concern after a cancer diagnosis, and that engagement in sexual intercourse does not necessary equate to sexual satisfaction (Wilmoth, 2001). Moreover, the primary focus on the physical effects of cancer or cancer treatment on sexual behaviour assumes that the experience of sexuality is limited to its corporeal dimensions, negating the influence of the social and relational construction of sexuality and illness (Meyerowitz et al., 1999), and the ways in which the meaning of sex is negotiated by individuals (Gilbert et al., 2010a).

1.4 Prevention and intervention for issues of sexuality and intimacy post-cancer

Recognition of sexual changes and their consequences, and of pathways to difficulty, is only the first step: We then need to use this knowledge to develop, and evaluate, programs of prevention and intervention to ameliorate difficulty and facilitate re-negotiation of sexuality post-cancer. Equally, whilst a range of psycho-social interventions have been developed for both people with cancer and their carers, few interventions include consideration of sexuality and intimacy, and even if they do, sexuality is positioned as merely one aspect of the cancer experience that couples need assistance with (e.g. Helgeson et al., 2006, Wardle et al., 2003). It has thus been argued that there is a need for psycho-education, which focuses specifically on the effects of cancer and its treatments on sexuality and intimacy (Rees et al., 1998). Since 2003, psychosocial guidelines for the care of people with cancer include recognition of the need for support in relation to changes in sexual functioning post-cancer (Initiative, 2003). However, these guidelines do not provide practical strategies for the application of such support in clinical practice, and sexuality is still rarely addressed by health professionals (Hordern et al., 2007b).

Equally, those psycho-educational interventions that do exist tend to focus on restoring sexual functioning, rather than on examining the quality of intimate physical contact, or renegotiation of sexual relationships through the development of alternative practices (Hordern et al., 2007b). Interventions also focus on 'sexual' cancers, such as prostate (Manne et al., 2004), or breast cancer (Manne et al., 2007, Marcus et al., 1998, Lethborg et al., 2003), with little offered to address the needs and concerns of couples living with other types of cancer, and no analysis of the relative efficacy of interventions across cancer types. This chapter will address this significant gap in the research literature, by outlining the issues that need to be considered in psycho-educational interventions which address issues of intimacy and sexuality with people with cancer and their partners.

2. Methods

2.1 Design

The study described in this chapter is part of a larger cross sectional project evaluating the needs and experiences of informal cancer carers in New South Wales, Australia. This chapter focuses on the experiences of a sub-set of carers who were caring for their partners. All participants completed standardised questionnaires measuring depression and anxiety, burden of care, as well as questions regarding changes in sexuality post-cancer. Participants who reported changes in sexuality after the diagnosis of cancer, completed open-ended questions describing the changes. From these participants, a sample was selected to take part in in-depth interviews to examine these issues in more detail.

2.1.1 Recruitment and participants

The larger study from which the participants were drawn was advertised via cancer and carer-specific newsletters, websites, and organisations, as well as through media releases, cancer support groups and cancer clinics across New South Wales. Family members, partners or friends of people with cancer, who self identified as providing care, and who volunteered to take part in the research, were asked to complete an online or postal questionnaire. A subset of the participants, who indicated willingness, were invited to take part in an in-depth interview. Ethical approval was granted from all relevant Committees including 10 Area Health Services across New South Wales, Australia, The Cancer Council New South Wales, and the University of Western Sydney. Three hundred and twenty nine carers participated in this larger study. This paper draws upon a sub-sample of 156 (55 men, 101 women) participants who were caring for their partners and responded to the question 'does their cancer impact on your sexual relationship?'. One hundred and twenty-two participants (43 men, 79 women), or 78% of this sub-sample reported that the onset of cancer had negatively impacted upon their sexuality and their sexual relationship and completed open-ended questions describing the changes. When we examined the type of cancers associated with changes to sexuality post-cancer, the rate was 90% for partners of men with prostate cancer, 71% for partners of women with gynaecological cancer, and 78% for partners of women with breast cancer. Overall, the percentage of partner carers of partners with 'non-sexual' cancers who reported an impact on the sexual relationship was 76%, and the percentage of those caring for partners with cancers involving 'sexual' sites was 84%. Forty-six percent of partner carers indicated a willingness to be interviewed about sexuality and 20 were selected on the basis of whether they had been involved in, or were currently involved in, a sexual or intimate relationship with the person for whom they care/d, and self-reported changes to sexuality since the diagnosis of their partner's cancer, stratified by gender, cancer stage and type.

Sample characteristics are presented in Table 1. Ninety-six percent of the participants reported being in a heterosexual relationship, with the remaining in a lesbian relationship, and 1 participant in a gay male relationship. Participant ages ranged from 28 to 79, with a mean age of 57 (SD = 10.73; skewness = -.47), with their partner ages (person with cancer) displaying a comparable profile ranging from 29 to 93, with a mean age of 59 (SD = 11.83; skewness = -.15). Colorectal/digestive, breast and haematological cancer types account for 44.2% of the reported cancer types, 35% indicating an advanced stage of cancer, and the average time since diagnosis was 3.49 years. Carer partners reported spending an average of 10 hours per day providing direct care. There were 26 bereaved participants (11 men, 15 women), with the time of partner's death ranging from 1 month to 4 years, who reported retrospectively on their experience of caring for their partner.

2.2 Quantitative methods and analyses

2.2.1 Measures

The Hospital Anxiety and Depression Scale (HADS) (Zigmond et al., 1983), was used to provide a brief measure of the presence of anxiety and depression. The HADS has very well established psychometric properties and is a reliable and valid instrument, with Cronbach alphas at .80 to .93 for the anxiety and .81 to .90 for the depression subscales (Herrmann, 1997, Janda et al., 2008). Higher scores indicate higher psychological disturbances.
The Caregiver Reaction Assessment Scale (CRA) (Nijboer, 1999) was used to examine caregiver burden. Subscales include: Disrupted Schedule, Financial Problems, Lack of Family Support, Health Problems, and Self-Esteem. As an assessment of both positive and negative reactions to care-giving by partners of patients with cancer, the CRA has been described as a reliable and valid instrument, with Cronbach alpha coefficients ranging from .62 to .83 for the separate subscales (Nijoboer, 1999). A higher score indicates a stronger impact of the attribute.
Questions on sexuality were also developed for the study, in consultation with the study's steering advisory committee, which comprised of two carer representatives from an independent advocacy organisation (Cancer Voices New South Wales), professionals providing support services to cancer patients and their carers, an oncologist, and researchers working in the field of psycho-oncology, sexuality, health, and gender. Three dichotomous questions (no, yes), asked participants: if they were in a sexual relationship with the patient; have there been changes to the sexual relationship post-cancer; and if so, have issues about sexuality been discussed with a health care provider?

2.2.2 Statistical analyses

Cronbach alpha coefficients were calculated to assess the internal consistency of HADS and CRA subscales. Cronbach alpha values above .80 were considered estimates of good reliability, while scores above .60 were considered adequate. A multivariate logistic regression with backward selection was conducted to determine the relationship between CRA subscales and impact on the sexual relationship to test the research question of the impact of burden of care on changes to the sexual relationship post-cancer. Univariate linear regressions with impact on the sexual relationship as a predictor and HADS Anxiety and Depression subscales as outcome variables, were conducted to assess the association between changes to the sexual relationship and psychological well-being. This analysis excluded data from the 26 bereaved participants, given that the HADS measures psychological well-being over last 7 days. To examine the potential moderating influence of participant gender, age, hours of provided direct care, and cancer type (dichotomised as non-sexual or sexual type), a series of multiple regressions were conducted where interactions with these variables were examined in addition to the main effect of impact on the sexual relationship. Cancer stage was not examined, due to the small cell size in early stage cancer. Equations with continuous predictor variables were centred as suggested by Howell (2002). An alpha level of .05 was used for all analyses.

2.3 Qualitative methods and analysis

2.3.1 Measures

Two open-ended questionnaire items concerning changes in sexuality post-cancer were: please describe the changes to your sexual relationship; and, if your role as carer has made any difference to your sexual relationship, please describe this difference. Participants who were interviewed were asked the same set of questions, with scope to elaborate on topics or issues as they arose.

A semi-structured interview, audio-recorded and conducted on a face-to-face or telephone basis, lasting approximately 1 hour, was used to examine in depth partners' experiences of sexuality post-cancer. The interview discussion focused on: changes to partners' intimate/sexual relationship; feelings about their intimate/sexual relationship; communication with the person with cancer about intimacy; and experiences with health care professionals. In accordance with established protocols in qualitative research, sampling was discontinued when information redundancy was reached, and no additional information was forthcoming (Miles et al., 1994).

2.3.2 Analysis of open-ended questions and interviews

All of the interviews were transcribed verbatim, and thematic analysis was used to analyse the data (Braun et al., 2006). After transcription, the interviews and open-ended questionnaire responses were independently read by two researchers, in order to ascertain the major themes, and to develop a coding frame. Following discussion between the researchers, and other members of the research team, the coding system was used to organise the data into conceptual categories which were based on participants' stories and responses. The research was, therefore, largely inductive, where the concepts and categories came from the data, rather than being deductive or informed by existing preconceptions about cancer caring and sexuality (Janesick, 1994). The interviews and responses were then coded thematically by two of the researchers, using consensus discussion, with a third researcher available to discuss any disagreements. NVivo software, a program which allows for qualitative data to be organised thematically, as well as across demographic, or other key variables, was used to organise the coded data. The coding frame focused on the following major themes: Nature of changes to sexuality (cessation; reduction; renegotiation); Reasons given for changes to sexuality (Impact of cancer or cancer treatment: caring role; re-positioning of person with cancer as patient); and Feelings about such changes (positive and negative). Discussion and competing explanations between the two researchers during the coding process, as well as discussions with the broader team, allowed the coding frame to be refined (Barbour, 2001). Responses from the questionnaire were also tabulated and counted to identify frequency and patterning within and across groups, specifically gender and cancer type.

3. Results

3.1 Quantitative results

3.1.1 Reliability estimates

HADS Anxiety and Depression subscales displayed good reliability with Chronbach alpha scores >.80 (.87 and .81 respectively), while the CRA subscales 'Disrupted Schedule' (.77) and 'Lack of Family Support' (.67) had adequate internal consistency with scores >.60). Cronbach alpha scores for the remaining CRA subscales were <.60 ('Self Esteem' at .56; 'Financial Problems' at .44; and 'Health Problem' at -.17). Descriptive statistics for the HADS and CRA subscale scores are presented in Table 1.

Variable	*N*	Mean	S.D.	Range
Partner carer age	153	57	10.63	28 - 79
Person with cancer age	154	59	11.83	29 - 93
Hours of direct care per day	116	10.25	9.06	0 – 24
Years since diagnosis	153	3.48	4.36	2mths – 23yrs
CRA subscale scores:				
• Disrupted schedule	152	17.17	5.18	0 – 25
• Health problems	153	13.23	2.56	3 - 19
• Lack of family support	155	9.28	4.75	0 - 25
• Financial problems	152	8.30	3.26	0 - 15
• Self esteem	152	26.19	4.49	5 - 35
• HADS subscale scores:				
• Anxiety	126	10.79	4.40	1 - 20
• Depression	125	7.38	4.11	0 - 19
	N	%		
Sexual orientation:				
• Heterosexual	149	95.5		
• Lesbian / Gay	7	4.5		
Ethnicity:				
• White European /Aust	141	90.4		
• Asian	3	1.3		
• Not stated	12	7.7		
Cancer type:				
• Colorectal/Digestive	24	15.4		
• Breast	23	14.7		
• Haematological	22	14.1		
• Multiple Non-Sexual	15	9.6		
• Multiple Sexual	10	6.4		
• Prostrate	10	6.4		
• Other*	52	33.4		
Stage of disease:				
• No longer detectable	29	18.6		
• Early	10	6.4		
• Advanced	56	35		
• Not sure/applicable	61	39		

* "Other" includes: Respiratory, Gynaecological, Brain, Mesothelioma, Pancreatic and missing.

Table 1. Sample characteristics for partner carer and person with cancer

3.1.2 Predictors of changes to the sexual relationship

Table 2 summarises the odds ratios (*Exp(B)*) for CRA subscales as predictor variables in a model predicting changes to the sexual relationship post-cancer. The CRA subscale "Disrupted Schedule' was the single significant predictor of changes to the sexual relationship (*Exp(B)* = 1.20, p = .002, CI = 1.05 - 1.22), indicating that a person with a one-point increase in CRA "Disrupted Schedule' would be 1.2 times more likely to report that the sexual relationship had changed post-cancer. No other CRA subscales emerged as predictors of change to the sexual relationship post-cancer.

CRA Subscale	*Exp(B)*	Significance	95% CI
Variables in the model			
Disrupted Schedule	1.20	.002	1.05 - 1.22
Variables not in the model			
Health Problems	.02	.86	.85 - 1.22
Lack of Family Support	.07	.16	.97 - 1.19
Financial Problems	.03	.73	.88 - 1.20
Self Esteem	-.02	.64	.89 - 1.07
Constant	-.73	.26	

Note: Model significant at the level of 0.01; -2 log likelihood = 145.84; X^2 = 10.21.

Table 2. Multivariate logistic regression results for factors associated with a change in the sexual relationship post cancer (N = 146)

3.1.3 Impact of changes in the sexual relationship upon psychological well-being

Table 3 presents the results of univariate regression analyses conducted to examine the contribution of the predictor variable 'changes to the sexual relationship post-cancer' on participant's HADS Anxiety and Depression scores. Changes to the sexual relationship was a significant predictor of HADS Anxiety scores ($t_{(124)}$ = 2.04, p = .04) and HADS Depression scores ($t_{(124)}$ = 2.02, p = .04) respectively. Multiple regressions testing the main effect of changes to the sexual relationship and interaction terms representing potential moderating variables were conducted separately for gender, age, hours of provided direct care, and cancer type. No significant interaction effects were found predicting either HADS Anxiety or HADS Depression scores.

	B	*SE B*	*ß*
HADS Anxiety Subscale			
Change in the sexual relationship	1.82	.89	.18*
HADS Depression Subscale			
Change in the sexual relationship	1.68	.83	.18*

Note: For HADS Anxiety, R^2 = .03; For HADS Depression, R^2 = .03. * $p < .05$.

Table 3. Univariate regression results for change in the sexual relationship upon psychological wellbeing (N = 124)

3.2 Qualitative results

One hundred and twenty two partners, including 26 who were bereaved, elaborated on the changes to their sexual relationship they had experienced post-cancer, in open-ended responses. These responses concerned the status of the sexual relationship, perceived reasons for the changes, and partners' feelings about the changed relationship. Each theme is reported below, illustrated by extracts from the questionnaires and the interviews. Demographic information is provided for longer quotes stemming from the interviews. For readability, these specific details are not provided for every questionnaire and interview quote. Percentages cited refer to the open ended questionnaire responses, completed by 122 participants.

3.2.1 Status of current sexual relationship

Two major themes characterised accounts of the current status of the sexual relationship: cessation or decreased frequency of sex or intimacy; and re-negotiation of sex or intimacy.

Cessation or decreased frequency of sex and intimacy. Complete cessation of sex, decrease in the frequency of sex, or a reduction in the frequency or quality of intimacy and closeness, was reported by 59% of women and 79% of men. The complete 'end' of the sexual relationship was reported by some participants as a sudden event: "Our sex life disappeared overnight"; "Gone from fantastic sex life to none". For other participants, it was a gradual change: "Initially we found other ways to be intimate, however over time our sex life has ceased". The impact of both the cessation of sex, and the loss of intimacy, was evident in the following interview extract:

> A big… big chunk of your life is lost, And I don't just mean the physical aspects of it… I mean that's… you can live with that or you can… or go without, but… the whole package is gone and I think that's hard that, you're a widow with somebody that's still around.
>
> *57 year old woman caring for 53 year old husband with brain cancer*

Of the participants who reported decreased sexual frequency, rather than complete cessation, many positioned their sexual relationship in ways that indicated that they had previously enjoyed an active sex life: "We had a very strong physical relationship up until the cancer was discovered and after it, it just faded away"; "Very poor, we use to have sex 5 times a week, now maybe once in 3 or 4 months". Others simply described a change in frequency: "Virtually non-existent"; "This aspect of our marriage has nearly stopped". Many participants also reported decreased closeness and intimacy. Responses included: "…I couldn't cuddle like we used to" and, "Often feel frustrated that it doesn't happen like it used to - he is not as romantic either". Participants also shared these sentiments in the interviews, for example:

> I don't know whether you just take this huge step back and you're not feeling that intimacy, because I think it comes from fear that you start to think well, maybe they won't be around, and if this is the way it's going to be then I should start preparing myself rather than being clingy and wanting to be in their space.
>
> *52 year old woman caring for 55 year old husband with prostate cancer*

Renegotiation of sexual and non-sexual intimacy post-cancer. Renegotiation of their sexual relationship, in terms of non-coital sexual practices, or the development of non-sexual intimacy, was reported by 19% of women and 14% of men. Men (12%) were more likely than women (1%) to report having developed alternative sexual behaviours to those practiced prior to the cancer. This consisted of changed sexual positions when attempting intercourse: "I am obviously more careful, having adjusted positions"; as well as the development of "workable alternatives to achieve partner satisfaction... within restrictions caused by the treatments", including oral sex, massage, masturbation, or the use of a vibrator.

Women (18%) were more likely than men (5%) to report that re-negotiation involved non-sexual intimacy, such as hugging and cuddling: "I'd put my legs up on his lap, and he'd put his arms around me, and I'd cuddle into him, and we'd watch TV".

> The last week of my husband's life, he wanted to make love, but physically could not due to his illness. We talked this over as we always did and he knew that hugs, cuddles and closeness were far more important than the actual act of making love.
>
> *64 year old woman who cared for 64 year old husband with pancreatic cancer, bereaved*

The importance of this closeness to the well-being of both the partner and the person with cancer was emphasized by many of the interviewees. In the excerpt below, one partner describes how important it was to maintain physical closeness with her husband, despite the significant physical barriers that could have served to restrict the expression of intimacy.

> We deliberately had kept the double bed. And then, when he got sick, and they needed a more supportive bed, I brought my single bed in, and we got this special height, set at the same height, so that we was always next to me. ... I remember the morning he died, I remember cuddling him all night. (...) Just to have your... to have your arm around him was just so, so good.
>
> *59 year old woman who cared for 69 year old husband with mesothelioma, bereaved*

3.2.2 Reasons for changes in sexual relationships

Many of the participants provided reasons for changes in their sexual relationship post-cancer. These were: the impact of cancer treatment; exhaustion resulting from the caring role; and the re-positioning of the person with cancer as a patient, rather than as a sexual partner.

Impact of cancer treatment. Participants referred to "cancer" and then specified the impact of cancer treatment as the major reason for changes to the sexual relationship. Within this theme, reports of physical barriers to sex were reported by 30% of men and 33% of women. For some, the physical barriers were directly related to the physical outcomes of cancer treatment on sexual functioning, for example: "Hormonal treatment has the effect of chemical castration, i.e. my husband has no sexual function"; "her poor body has been so cut and chemo has affected her so much that sex is not even possible"; "...non-existent due mainly to the chronic pain syndrome and a less than full confidence in colostomy bags!" For others, abstinence was due to overall bodily restrictions: "... He is physically unable to position himself for sex now".

> In June an epidural catheter was inserted into my husband's chest and commenced on morphine 30 mgs three times a day. Not only was there no energy or inclination, because of the pain and reduced energy, there was now a 'physical barrier' to our relationship as well as all the side effects of morphine.
>
> *59 year old woman who cared for 56 year old husband with mesothelioma, bereaved*

Many of the participants also described side effects of the treatment such as pain, fatigue, and exhaustion. Pain was described thus: "When he is unwell because of treatment I tend to be very careful in touching him in case it causes further pain/discomfort". Descriptions of fatigue being given as a reason for changes to the sexual relationship included: "As a result of treatment (chemotherapy) my wife is tired more of the time and her libido is reduced";

"He was just too exhausted". The impact of cancer treatment on the self-esteem and self-image of their partner was also identified as a reason for changes to the sexual relationship in a number of cases. For example, one partner commented that:

> As her health declined she had very low self esteem caused by loss of hair and muscle tone. When I did have sex at the beginning she would accuse me of not treating her the same as I did in the past and get depressed.
>
> *61 year old man caring for 43 year old female partner with lung cancer, bereaved*

Exhaustion resulting from the caring role. In citing reasons for changes to the sexual relationship, exhaustion resulting from the caring role was positioned as the cause by 16% of the women and 9% of the men. The responses included: "We don't really have any intimacy anymore for reasons including his health and my exhaustion"; "Exhaustion, brain still ticking about things to be organised"; "Even if he was still interested in the sexual side of our marriage I think I would have been too exhausted to have taken part". Participants also commented on revised prioritisation, centred on coping and survival, leaving no time for sex or intimacy.

> ...sexual relations of any sort were not an option as I had to be on the go all the time, looking after her. My sexual desires, needs or wants were not in my mind.
>
> *62 year old man who cared for 64 year old wife with liposarcoma, bereaved*

Re-positioning of person with cancer as patient. For 28% of women and 47% of men caring for a partner with cancer, the caring role was reported to have resulted in a re-positioning of the person with cancer as a patient, which subsequently influenced their sexual relationship. Many partners described emotional effects of the caring role, or concern for their partner's feelings and health status. Comments included: "With all the worry and stress that my husband is most likely to die, I now have very little desire for sex"; "Curbed by concerns about inflicting pain or discomfort";

> I just wanted to treat her the same as I always did but I couldn't get the thought out of my head that she was terminally ill.
>
> *61 year old man caring for 43 year old female partner with lung cancer, bereaved*

Participants also reported a redefined role or status as carer rather than lover. Examples included: "My role as a carer has overridden my role as a wife..."; "Having to spend more time on house/garden chores and be carer/nurse, one feels more like a housekeeper than a lover".

> When you are a carer it's hard to be a lover, for either party, when dealing with incontinence of both bowel and bladder infections, along with the daily grind of showering, dressing, shaving, etc, then transferring from bed to wheelchair and return.
>
> *59 year old woman who cared for 63 year old male partner with haematological cancer, bereaved*

A number of male participants gave accounts which suggested sex was 'inappropriate' with a person with cancer: "I was very aware of my role as carer and never did anything to embarrass my wife. There was never any inappropriate behaviour". This could result in ambivalent feelings in the face of the partners' own desires.

> I feel disgusted with myself that I would inflict sex upon a dying woman, having said that my wife does not object and occasionally welcomes it, saying it is a life giving and loving act and a part of our sacrament.... I was never a fast lover, but now I try and get it over and done with for her.
>
> *45 year old man caring for 44 year old wife with breast cancer*

In the interviews, a number of the women participants also described now positioning their partner as a child, which was antithetical to sexuality:

> it's like looking after ...one of your children now. That's the feelings that you have, you know, you don't have any ..sexual feelings for your children ... (so) I just don't have them anymore.
> *57 year old woman, caring for 53 year old husband with advanced brain cancer.*

3.2.3 Partners' feelings about their changed sexual relationship

In the open-ended questions, a number of the participants made comments about the emotions they experienced in response to these changes in their sexual relationship post-cancer. These were evenly divided between positive and negative responses.

Positive responses. Positive accounts were provided by 17% of women and 16% of men. Within this theme, participants described feelings of understanding or acceptance of the effects of cancer or caring on their sexual relationship.

> Treatment makes my partner feel sick and makes me worry about him so this means we don't feel up to sex... This is not an issue - just a fact/reality of current situation.
> *39 year old woman caring for 53 year old male partner with lung cancer*

A number of participants also reported affection and companionate devotion:

> Sexual urge had gone but my husband made me feel the most loved and cared for woman on this earth by his loving actions, his consideration, his caring attitude and the advice I sought even up till 12 hours before he died. I loved this man totally and he me.
> *68 year old woman who cared for 69 year old husband with brain cancer, bereaved*

In the interviews, a number of participants reported that the cancer experience had actually brought them closer together, with one man saying he "probably has a more affectionate relationship at this point in our lives, and marriage" than prior to the onset of cancer, and another commenting "with the exclusion of sex, our intimacy is closer probably than it's been for a long time". A third male participant said that whilst he and his wife "haven't had sex (intercourse) as frequently", he feels that his relationship is "better", he feels "happier", and feels as if he is a "more attentive partner" and a "better father". Increased emotional closeness, despite absence of sex, was also evident in a number of the women participants' interviews:

> We are so much closer now than we were....we wouldn't be as close now and we wouldn't be able to talk about absolutely anything now...Just seeing him at night, just makes my heart just go hshshsh.... Whereas before I don't think we appreciated that about each other.
> *29 year old woman caring for 33 year old husband with brain cancer*

Negative responses. Negative feelings were reported by 13% of the women and 21% of the men who said that there had been a change in their sexual relationship. These responses included self-blame, "No sex for 12 months - more my fault", and rejection by their partners "I felt excluded and unwanted. Sex became a chore and mechanical"; "She has absolutely no sexual interest in me whatsoever". A number of woman participants also expressed rejection toward their partners:

> I don't feel the desire to have a physical relationship with my husband. It almost makes me feel ill to even contemplate it. His whole physical appearance repels me.
> *52 year old woman caring for 55 year old husband with prostate cancer*

Participants also reported lack of fulfilment in relation to sex: "Not able to relax and enjoy"; "Often feel frustrated that it doesn't happen like it used to"; "At times, I have considered having an affair purely for sexual gratification".

> …leaves me less satisfied - there was a time shortly a few weeks after she was diagnosed with breast-bone cancer where I found it hard to orgasm/ejaculate - I would fail twice after some minutes, then succeed the next day.
> *45 year old man caring for 44 year old wife with breast cancer*

Some participants mentioned feelings of perceived obligation. For men, it was usually in relation to feeling that their partner felt obliged to provide sex. Examples included: "On the infrequent occasions we now have sex she wants it over and done with as quickly as possible"; "She became less interested in sex and only accommodated me as if it was a wifey duty". For women participants, obligation was positioned in terms of themselves feeling obliged to engage in sex.

> At the early stages of the diagnosis I felt that I couldn't say no to him which put a lot of pressure on me. I had to make sure that I could respond to him and not give him any chance of feeling that I didn't want to make love to him.
> *59 year old woman caring for 63 year old husband with gastric adenocarcinoma*

A small number of women participants shared negative feelings regarding family planning and fertility:

> Prostate cancer has required removal of the sac that produces sperm. I am 36 and had always taken for granted I would fall pregnant in the most natural and intimate way. Once my partner is stronger, we will seek advice from an IVF Clinic regarding artificial insemination (hence my partner has secured enough in the sperm bank!). Still this whole traumatic experience has left me feeling very upset.
> *36 year old woman caring for 59 year old husband with prostate cancer*

Some participants reported feeling angry that their sexual relationship was 'lost', as one woman commented, "(I'm) so much crosser…because a big part of our relationship had just gone out the window". Sadness at the loss of their sexual relationship was also evident in many of the accounts: "There is just an enormous sadness that we can no longer have this intimacy…"; "Still this whole traumatic experience has left me feeling very upset"; "it's profound sadness, I mean very, very sad", resulting in feeling "terribly fragile and vulnerable and sad, and so sorry that it was all going".

3.2.4 Discussions of sexuality with health professionals

In response to a question regarding whether there had been discussion of sexuality with a health professional, 20% of partners indicated that there had. The rate of discussion differed across cancer types, ranging from 50% of prostate cancer partner carers, to 0% of respiratory cancer. The rates across the other main cancer types were: 33% brain; 33% pancreatic; 30% breast; 29% gynaecological; 20% multiple - sexual; 17% colorectal/digestive; 17% mesothelioma; 15% multiple - non sexual; 15% other; and 9% haematological. Of those who had discussed sexuality with health care providers, 30% stated that they were not at all or not very satisfied, 33% said that they were neither satisfied nor dissatisfied, and 37% indicated that they were satisfied or very satisfied.

In the interviews, a number of the partners commented on their discussions with health professionals, in each case giving a critical account. When they asked about sexual matters, partners reported being told "Oh you don't need to know that and things like that", or told that they were "irresponsible to be thinking about having children" in raising fertility as a concern. The majority, however, gave accounts of sexuality not being discussed at all: "I haven't got a lot of medical advice about how we should continue to conduct our intimate relationship"; "they did not educate us on anything… at all".

it's not properly addressed by the medical profession, it is just completely glossed over. And I can remember, you know, we were sitting when the diagnosis came through and the guy said well, you know, you'll get these hormone pills and we'll give you an injection into your stomach and of course that will be the end of your sex life; and we're just sitting there (...) That was the end of the discussion.
67 year old woman who cared for 85 year old husband with prostate, bowel, and lung cancer, bereaved.

4. Conclusion

This study examined changes to sexuality following the diagnosis and treatment of cancer, as well as the impact of such changes on psychological well-being, for informal carers who were the partner of a person with cancer. The mixed method design allowed for the extent and impact of changes to sexuality post-cancer to be measured using quantitative measures, and subjective experience of changes to sexuality to be evaluated using open-ended questionnaire items and interviews. Within a Critical Realist epistemological standpoint, each methodology is treated as equally valid in providing insight into the phenomenon under investigation.

The majority of participants reported that the cancer experience had impacted on their sexual relationship, resulting in a cessation or reduction of sexual activity, with only a minority renegotiating sexual intimacy post-cancer. This supports previous research which demonstrated that the impact of cancer and cancer treatment extends beyond the person with cancer (Baider et al., 2000, Gurevich et al., 2004, Juraskova et al., 2003, Maughan et al., 2002, Rolland, 1994, Walsh et al., 2005), reinforcing the need for acknowledgement of the sexual and intimate needs of partners, as well as of people with cancer. Rather than restricting our sample to partners caring for person with cancer affecting the reproductive areas of the body, we examined changes to sexuality post-cancer across a range of cancer types. The majority of participants who were providing support to a person with prostate, breast or gynaecological cancer cited an impact, confirming previous research (Maughan et al., 2002, Harden et al., 2002, Sanders et al., 2006). However the finding that a high proportion of partners of a person with 'non-sexual' cancer also reported changes highlights the pressing need to attend to and further investigate the sexual concerns and needs of all partners who care for a person with cancer.

The finding that partners who reported changes in sexuality post-cancer reported significantly higher levels of depression and anxiety than those who reported no sexual changes, adds support to the notion that sexuality is associated with cancer carers' quality of life and psychological well-being (Foy et al., 2001). Depression and anxiety may be a cause, or a consequence, of changes in sexuality post-cancer; further research is needed to examine this issue in more depth, looking at the factors which may moderate and mediate changes to the sexual relationship in cancer carers and their partners, as well as the consequences of such changes for the couple. Future research would also benefit from examining changes in sexuality and their impact across cancer stage, which was not possible in the present study due to the low numbers participants caring for someone with early stage cancer.

Whilst gender was not a significant moderator of impact of changes to sexuality on psychological well-being, there were some gender differences in the accounts of the nature of changes to the sexual relationship post-cancer. Reports of complete cessation of sex were more common for women than men, and very few women gave accounts of developing alternative sexual practices if intercourse was no longer possible. This could be attributed to women being more likely to assume that they should subordinate their own needs to the needs of their partner (O'Grady, 2005), and to cultural constructions of normative heterosexuality which expect men to initiate sex (Ussher, 1997b). Previous research has found that partners are reluctant to initiate sexual intimacy if the person with cancer does not initiate (Maughan et al., 2002), and that heterosexual women partners do not wish to initiate sex, or discuss alternatives to coital sex, for fear of emasculating their partner if he can not 'perform' through sexual intercourse (Boehmer et al., 2001). This is consistent with research that has demonstrated that sexual performance is positioned as central to heterosexual constructions of 'manhood', with failure having negative consequences in terms of a man's sense of self (Tiefer, 1994).

Equally, the 'male sex drive discourse' which positions men as 'needing' sex (Hollway, 1989, Potts, 2002), may result in the sexual needs of male partners being classified by either or both members of the couple as being 'important enough' for sex to continue post-cancer, or for alternative sexual practices to be developed, in contrast to women partners who were more likely to report that re-negotiated intimacy was non-sexual. The phallocentric bias evident in the research and clinical literature on cancer and sexuality (Hyde, 2006), which serves to reinforce the notion that 'normal' sex = coitus, and emphasises sexual 'functioning' with little attention to alternative practices, needs to be challenged, as this potentially plays a significant role in the construction of truths about sexuality which people with cancer and their partners take up, limiting their exploration of alternatives to coitus post-cancer. However, in the present study, four of the six lesbian partners all reported complete cessation of sex, suggesting that even couples positioned outside of a heterosexual matrix (Butler, 1990) can experience changes to sexuality post-cancer.

Whilst previous research has attributed changes in sexuality and intimacy post-cancer to the physiological effects of cancer or cancer treatment, a finding confirmed by many of the accounts in the present study, our findings also showed that the caring role also had an impact on the sexual relationship (Hawkins et al., 2009). Participants who reported changes in sexuality post-cancer reported significantly higher scores on the disrupted schedule sub-scale of the Caregiver Reaction Assessment Scale, suggesting aspects of burden of care were associated with such changes. In the interviews and open ended questions, these participants also associated sexual changes with stress, fatigue and exhaustion, revised prioritisation centred on coping and survival, and a redefined status as carer rather than lover. Past research that has explored carers' experiences of stress and exhaustion primarily focuses on the impact upon carers' general health and well-being. For example, Brown and Stetz (1999, p. 186) found that the initial period of 'becoming a caregiver' is particularly stressful, as carers are focused not only on their new role, but also have to 'face the present', negotiate their choice/or lack thereof to care, develop competency around their caring tasks, and evaluate their future. It is important to further investigate how the stresses involved in being a caregiver impact upon a carer's sexuality, and how this may in turn impact on quality of life (Foy et al., 2001). The finding in the present study that women were more likely to report that exhaustion had an impact on sexuality is in line with previous research which found that women cancer carers experience greater personal costs from caring (Lutsky et al., 1994, Ussher et al., 2008). As these personal costs have been found to be associated with higher rates of depression and anxiety, as well as lower life satisfaction and quality of life ratings, (Hagedoorn et al., 2000, Bookwala et al., 2000), it is a serious health issue.

The impact of the re-positioning of the person with cancer as 'patient' or 'child', rather than as 'lover', is an important issue which requires further investigation. The finding that the physical symptoms of cancer, or the physical tasks associated with cancer caring, makes it difficult for many carers to continue to see their partner as a sexual person, confirms patterns found in other spheres of health care (Parker, 1990, Pope, 1999). This assignment of individuals with cancer with a 'sick' or 'childlike' identity, which is antithetical to an identity as a person with sexual desires and needs, can significantly impact on the sexual and intimate relationship of a couple facing cancer (Kelly et al., 1996). Sex can be positioned as 'inappropriate', or as a 'frivolous activity' (Holmberg et al., 2001), resulting in carers experiencing guilt in the face of their own sexual needs or desires, and the avoidance of any discussion or re-negotiation of sexual practices, as was reported in the present study. This could be seen as one aspect of a broader practice of self-silencing in cancer carers, where the needs of the carer are repressed, because the person with cancer has to be put first (Ussher et al., 2010). However, it is also associated with cultural discourses which position people with cancer as having limited sexual needs, or as asexual (D'Ardenne, 2004, Schildrick, 2005), resulting in a different set of norms being applied to what is acceptable behaviour (Wellard, 1998). The finding that male partners were more likely to report an impact of re-positioning the person with cancer as a patient may result from the role of carer being a more unfamiliar position for men to take up, given the congruence between femininity and the caring role (O'Grady, 2005). It may thus be more difficult for men to eroticize a partner with cancer who is in need of care. This matter is worthy of further investigation in future research.

As the majority of partners positioned these changes to their sexual relationship as problematic, confirming previous research (Kuyper et al., 1998, Perez et al., 2002, Reichers, 2004, Soothill et al., 2003, Thomas et al., 2002), this suggests that education and information about sexuality post-cancer which challenges myths and provides a framework for re-negotiation of sexual relationships, needs to be included in supportive interventions for partner carers. At present, there is a dearth of research in this area, with no published research examining cancer carer interventions with a sexual component (see Harding et al., 2003). The finding in the present study that some partners reported increased closeness and intimacy emphasises the importance of helping couples to re-negotiate intimacy and sexuality post-cancer, as well as the importance of recognising, and reinforcing, the rewards of cancer caring (Hudson et al., 2005, Sinding, 2003).

Whilst it has been recognised that health professionals need to discuss issues of sexuality and intimacy with patients in cancer and palliative care (Initiative, 2003), the findings of the present study confirm previous research which found that these discussions are not taking place for the majority of people with cancer or their partners (Stead et al., 2002), particularly for those outside the sphere of prostate cancer. Even when sexuality was discussed, this was not at a level which was satisfactory to the majority of participants in the present study. This confirms recent Australian research which reported mis-matched expectations and unmet needs in relation to communication about sexuality between health professionals and individuals with cancer (Hordern et al., 2007a, Hordern et al., 2007b), suggesting that further education and training of health professionals is required, in order that they will be able to advise couples affected by cancer on issues of sexuality and intimacy, and address their unmet needs in this arena (Rees et al., 1998). Without the legitimacy of being able to discuss potential or actual disruptions to the sexual relationship with a health care professional, partners may feel that they cannot discuss such issues with the person with cancer, and as a result, may experience sadness, anger, and isolation (Gilbert et al., 2008), as was reported by many of the participants in the present study.

A number of methodological issues need to be considered when evaluating the findings of this research. Firstly, the issue of selection bias needs to be examined. The present study used self-selection in response to advertisement or information sheets distributed by cancer organisations or clinics, and thus may not have tapped a representative sample of informal cancer carers. Indeed, as noted above, future research in this field needs to systematically examine sexuality post-cancer across cancer stage. However, there was a good distribution across cancer type, gender and age-group, in contrast to many previous studies of cancer and sexuality which focussed solely on cancers affecting the sexual organs. Equally, as the participants were recruited for a general study on cancer caring, answering questions on sexuality as part of a broader questionnaire or interview, it could be argued that we have recruited individuals who would not usually respond to requests to take part in a research study on sexuality, and thus have obtained a broader sample for our research. Secondly, this study did not use standardised measures of sexual functioning, sexual or relationship satisfaction, but rather focussed on subjective reports through open ended questionnaire items or interview. Future research in this field could usefully adopt these standardised measures along side qualitative measures, to allow for greater triangulation of data, in evaluating of the extent and impact of changes to sexuality post-cancer. Thirdly, the cross sectional design meant that all assessment of change were retrospective. A longitudinal design would more effectively allow for the evaluation of changes to sexuality across cancer stage, and allow pre-post cancer treatment changes to be evaluated more thoroughly.

In conclusion, sexuality and intimacy are central aspects of quality of life that have often been neglected in examinations of the well-being of partners of a person with cancer. The findings of the present study add further support to the suggestion that sex should not be positioned as 'inappropriate' or 'trivial' in the context of cancer care, but rather be recognised as an aspect of couple relationships which is associated with well-being (Cort et al., 2004). Having health care professionals legitimate sexuality by 'giving permission' for couples to be sexually active or physically intimate when undergoing and recovering from treatment for cancer is one of the key strategies that could assist in this repositioning (Schwartz et al., 2002). The positive consequences of this may include increased feelings of well-being on the part of the partner carer, and closeness between the couple, which will have positive consequences for the physical and psychological well-being of the person with cancer (Hodges et al., 2005), the central aim of professional cancer care. There is thus no justification for sexuality and intimacy being ignored or dismissed: partner cancer carers are telling us that it is important, it is time for health professionals to recognise this need and to act accordingly.

5. Acknowledgements

The larger cross sectional project evaluating the needs and experiences of informal cancer carers, from which this study was drawn, was funded by an Australian Research Council Linkage Grant, LP0560448, in conjunction with the Cancer Council New South Wales, Westmead Hospital, and Carers New South Wales. The chief investigators on the project were Jane Ussher and Phyllis Butow, the partner investigators were Gerard Wain, Gill Batt and Kendra Sundquist, Janette Perz and Emilee Gilbert were associate investigators. Thanks are offered to Angela Pearce, Caroline Joyce and Lisa Hallab for research support and assistance.

6. References

AIHW and AACR (2007), Vol. Cancer series no. 37 Canberra: AIHW.

Anderson, B., L and Golden-Kreutz, D., M (2000)*Sexual self-concept for the women with cancer,* In *Cancer and the Family* (Eds, Baider, L., Cooper, C., L and De-Nour, A., K) John Wiley and Sons, England.

Anllo, L., M (2000) Sexual life after breast cancer. *Journal of Sex and Marital Therapy,* 26, 241-248.

Arrington, M., I (2003) "I Don't Want To Be An Artifical Man": Narrative Reconstruction of Sexuality among Prostate Cancer Survivors. *Sexuality and Culture,* 7, 30-58.

Baider, L. and De-Nour, J. (2000) Cancer and the spouse: Gender-relared differences in dealing with health care and illness. *Critical Reviews in Oncology/Hematology,* 40, 115-123.

Barbour, R., S (2001) Checklists for improving rigour in qualitative research: A case of the tail wagging the dog? . *British Medical Journal,* 322, 1115-1117.

Boehmer, U. and Clarke, J., A (2001) Communication about prostate cancer between men and their wives. *The Journal of Family Practice,* 50, 226-231.

Bokhour, B., G, Clarke, J., A, Inui, T., S, Silliman, R., A and Talcott, J., A (2001) Sexuality after treatment for early prostate cancer. *Journal of General Internal Medicine,* 16, 649-655.

Bookwala, J. and Schulz, R. (2000) A Comparison of Primary Stressors, Secondary Stressors and Depressive Symptoms between Elderly Caregivers' Husbands and Wives: The Caregivers' Health Effects Study. *Psychology and Aging,* 15, 607-616.

Braun, V. and Clark, J., A (2006) Using thematic analysis in psychology. *Qualitative Research in Psychology,* 3, 77-101.

Brown, M., A and Stetz, K. (1999) The labour of caregiving: A theoretical model of caregiving during potentially fatal illness. *Qualitative Health Research,* 9, 182-197.

Butler, J. (1990) *Gender Trouble: Feminism and the Subversion of Identity,* Routledge, New York.

Butler, J. (1993) *Bodies that Matter: On the discursive limits of sex,* Routledge, New York London.

Cort, E., Monroe, B. and Oliviere, D. (2004) Couples in palliative care. *Sexual and Relationship Therapy,* 19, 337-354.

D'Ardenne, P. (2004) The couple sharing long-term illness. *Sexual and Relationship Therapy,* 19, 291-308.

De Groot, J., M, Mah, K., Fyles, A., Winton, S., Greenwood, S., De Petrillo, A., D and Devins, S. (2005) The psychosocial impact of cervical cancer among affected women and their partners. *International Journal of Gynecological Cancer,* 15, 918-925.

Few, C. (1997) The politics of sex research and constructions of female sexuality: what relevance to sexual health work with young women? *Journal of Advanced Nursing,* 25, 615-625.

Fobair, P., Stewart, S., L, Chang, S., D'Onofrio, C., Banks, P., J and Bloom, J., R (2006) Body image and sexual problems in young women with breast cancer. *Psycho-oncology,* 15, 579-594.

Foy, S. and Rose, K. (2001) Men's experiences of their partner's primary and recurrent breast cancer. *European Journal of Oncology Nursing,* 5, 42-48.

Gavey, N., McPhillips, K. and Braun, V. (1999) Interruptus Coitus: Heterosexuals account for intercourse. *Sexualities,* 2, 35-68.

Germino, B., B, Fife, B., L and Funk, S., G (1995) Cancer and the partner relationship: What is its meaning? *Seminars in Nursing Oncology,* 11, 43-50.

Gilbert, E. and Ussher, J. (2007) (Re)negotiating the sexual relationship in the context of cancer care: An examination of informal carers' experiences of caring and gender practices in couple relationships. *Archives of Sexual Behaviour,* forthcoming.

Gilbert, E., Ussher, J., M and Perz, J. (2010a) Re-negotiating sexuality and intimacy post-cancer: The experiences of carers in a couple relationship with a person with cancer. *Archives of Sexual Behavior* in press.

Gilbert, E., Ussher, J. M. and Perz, J. (2010b) Sexuality after breast cancer: A review. . *Mauritius,* 66.

Gurevich, M., Bishop, S., Bower, J., Malka, M. and Nyhof-Young, J. (2004) (Dis)embodying gender and sexuality in testicular cancer. *Social Science and Medicine,* 58, 1597-1607.

Hagedoorn, M., Buunk, B., Kuijer, R., Wobbes, T. and Sanderman, R. (2000) Couples Dealing With Cancer: Role and Gender Differences Regarding Psychological Distress and Quality of Life. *Psycho-Oncology,* 9, 232-242.

Hannah, M. T., Gritz, E., R, Wellisch, D., K, Fobair, P., Hoppe, R., T, Bloom, J., Sun, G., W, Varghese, A., Cosgrove, M., D and Spiegel, D. (1992) Changes in marital and sexual functioning in long-term survivors and their spouses: Testicular cancer versus hodgkin's disease. *Psycho-oncology,* 1, 89-103.

Harden, J., Schafenacker, A., Northouse, L., Mood, D., Smith, D., Pienta, K., Hussain, M. and Baranowski, K. (2002) Couples' Experiences with Prostate Cancer: Focus Group Research. *Oncology Nursing Forum,* 29, 701-709.

Harding, R. and Higginson, I. J. (2003) What is the Best Way to Help Caregivers in Cancer and Palliative Care? A Systematic Literature Review of Interventions and Their Consequences. *Palliative Medicine,* 17, 63-74.

Hawkins, Y., Ussher, J. M., Gilbert, E., Perz, J., Sandoval, M. and Sundquist, K. (2009) Changes in sexuality and intimacy after the diagnosis of cancer. The experience of partners in a sexual relationship with a person with cancer. *Cancer Nursing,* 34, 271-280.

Helgeson, V. S., Lepore, S. J. and Eton, D. T. (2006) Moderators of the Benefits of Psychoeducational Interventions for Men With Prostate Cancer. *Health Psychology,* 25, 348-354.

Hensen, H., K (2002) Breast cancer and sexuality. *Sexuality and disability,* 20, 261-275.

Herrmann, C. (1997) International experiences with the hospital anxiety and depression scale—a review of validation data and clinical results. *Journal of Psychosomatic Research,* 42, 17-41.

Hodges, L., J, Humphris, G., M and Macfarlane, G. (2005) A meta-analytic investigation of the relationship between the psychological distress of cancer patients and their carers. *Social Science and Medicine,* 60, 1-12.

Hollway, W. (1989) *Subjectivity and method in psychology: gender, meaning and science.,* Sage, London.

Holmberg, S., K, Scott, L., L, Alexy, W. and Fife, B., L (2001) Relationship issues of women with breast cancer. *Cancer Nursing,* 24, 53-60.

Hordern, A., J and Street, A., J (2007a) Communicating about patient sexuality and intimacy after cancer: mismatched expectations and unmet needs. *Medical Journal of Australia,* 186, 224-227.

Hordern, A., J and Street, A., J (2007b) Constructions of sexuality and intimacy after cancer: Patient and health professional perspectives. *Social Science and Medicine,* 64, 1704-1718.

Hudson, P. L., Aranda, S. and Hayman-White, K. (2005) A psycho-educational intervention for family caregivers of patients receiving palliative care: A randomized controlled trial. *Journal of Pain and Symptom Management,* 30, 329-341.

Hughes, M., K (2000) Sexuality and the cancer survivor: A silent coexistence. *Cancer Nursing,* 23, 477-482.

Hyde, A. (2006) The politics of heterosexuality - a missing discourse in cancer nursing literature on sexuality: A discussion paper. *International Journal of Nursing Studies,* 44, 315-325.

Initiative, N. B. C. C. a. N. C. C. (2003) *Clinical practice guidelines for the psychosocial care of adults with cancer.,* National Breast Cancer Centre, Camperdown, NSW.

Janda, M., Steginga, S., Dunn, J., Langbecker, D., Walker, D. and Eakin, E. (2008) Unmet supportive care needs and interest in services among patients with a brain tumour and their carers. *Patient Education and Counseling,* 71, 251-258.

Janesick, V., J (1994)*The dance of qualitative research design. Metaphor, Methodolatry and Meaning,* In *Strategies of Qualitative Inquiry* (Eds, Denzin, N., K and Lincoln, Y., S) Sage Publications, London.

Juraskova, I., Butow, P., Robertson, R., Sharpe, L., McLeod, C. and Hacker, N. (2003) Post-treatment sexual adjustment following cervical and endometrial cancer: A qualitative insight. *Psycho-oncology,* 12, 267-279.

Jvaskova, I., Butow, P., Robertson, R., Sharpe, L., McLeod, C. and Hacker, N. (2003) Post-treatment sexual adjustment following cervical and endometrial cancer: A qualitative insight. *Psycho-oncology,* 12, 267-279.

Kelly, M. (1992) Self, identity and radical surgery. *Sociology of Health and Illness,* 14, 390-415.

Kelly, M. and Field, D. (1996) Medical sociology, chronic illness and the body. *Sociology of Health & Illness,* 18, 241-257.

Kuyper, M., B and Wester, F. (1998) In the shadow: The impact of chronic illness on the patient's partner. *Qualitative Health Research,* 8, 237-253.

Lemieux, L., Kaiser, S., Pereira, J. and Meadows, L., M (2004) Sexuality in palliative care: Patient perspectives. *Palliative Medicine,* 18, 630-637.

Lethborg, C. E. and Kissane, D. W. (2003) 'It Doesn't End on the Last Day of Treatment': A Psychoeducational Intervention for Women After Adjuvant Treatment for Early Stage Breast Cancer. *Journal of Psychosocial Oncology,* 21, 25-41.

Lutsky, S. M. and Knight, B. G. (1994) Explaining Gender Differences in Caregiving Distress: The Roles of Emotional Attentiveness and Coping Styles. *Psychology and Aging,* 9, 513-519.

Manne, S., Babb, J., Pinover, W., Horwitz, E. and Ebbert, J. (2004) Psychoeducational group intervention for wives of men with prostate cancer. *Psycho-Oncology,* 13, 37-46.

Manne, S., Kendall, J., Patrick-Miller, L. and Winkel, G. (2007) Intimacy-enhancing intervention for women with early stage breast cancer and their partners. *Psycho-Oncology*, 16, S5-6.

Marcus, A. C., Garrett, K. M., Cella, D., Wenzel, L. B., Brady, M. J., Crane, L. A., McClatchey, M. W., Kluhsman, B. C. and Pate-Willig, M. (1998) Telephone counseling of breast cancer patients after treatment: A description of a randomized clinical trial. *Psycho-Oncology*, 7, 470-482.

Maughan, K., Heyman, B. and Matthews, M. (2002) In the shadow of risk. How men cope with a partner's gynaecological cancer. *International Journal of Cancer Studies*, 39, 27-34.

Meyerowitz, B., E, Desmond, K., Rowland, J., H, Wyatt, G., E and Ganz, P., A (1999) Sexuality following breast cancer. *Journal of Sex & Marital Therapy*, 25, 237-250.

Miles, M. B. and Huberman, A. M. (1994) *Qualitative data analysis: An expanded sourcebook*, Sage Publications Inc, Thousand Oaks, CA, US.

Nijboer, C., Triemstra, M., Temperlaar, R., Sanderman, R., & Van den Bos, G. A. M. (1999) Measuring both negative and positive reactions to giving care to cancer patients: Psychometric properties of the Caregiver Reaction Assessment (CRA). *Social Science & Medicine*, 48, 1259-1269.

O'Grady, H. (2005) *Women's relationship with herself: Gender, Foucault, therapy*, Routledge, London.

Parker, G. (1990)*Spouse carers: Whose quality of life?*, In *Quality of Life: Perspectives and Policies* (Eds, Baldwin, S., Godfrey, C. and Propper, C.) Routledge, London.

Perez, M., A, Skinner, E., C and Meyerowtiz, B., E (2002) Sexuality and Intimacy Following Radical Prostatectomy: Patient and Partner Perspectives. *Health Psychology*, 21, 288-293.

Pope, E. (1999) When illness takes sex out of a relationship. *Siecus report*, 27, 8-12.

Potts, A. (2002) *The Science/Fiction of Sex: Feminist Deconstruction and the Vocabularies of Heterosex*, Routledge, London.

Rees, C., E, Bath, P., A and Lloyd-Williams, M. (1998) The information needs of spouses of women with breast cancer: patients' and spouses' persepctives. *Journal of Advanced Nursing*, 28, 1249-1258.

Reichers, E., A (2004) Including Partners into the Diagnosis of Prostate Cancer: A review of the literature to provide a model of care. *Urologic Nursing*, 24, 22-38.

Rolland, J., S (1994) In sickness and in health: The impact of illness on couples' relationships. *Journal of Marital and Family Therapy*, 20, 327-335.

Sanders, S., Pedro, L., W, Bantum, E., O and Galbraith, M., E (2006) Couples Surviving Prostate Cancer: long-term intimacy needs and concerns following treatment. *Clinical Journal of Oncology Nursing*, 10, 503-508.

Schildrick, M. (2005) Unreformed Bodies: Normative Anxiety and the Denial of Pleasure. *Women's Studies*, 34, 327-344.

Schultz, W., C, M and Van de Wiel, H., B, M (2003) Sexuality, intimacy and gynaecological cancer. *Journal of Sex and Marital Therapy*, 29(s), 121-128.

Schwartz, S. and Plawecki, R., N (2002) Consequences of Chemotherapy on the Sexuality of Patients with Lung Cancer. *Clinical Journal of Oncology Nursing*, 6, 1-5.

Sinding, C. (2003) "Because you know there's an end to it": Caring for a relative or friend with advanced breast cancer. *Palliative and Supportive Care*, 1, 153-163.

Soothill, K., Morris, S., M, Thomas, C., Harman, J., C, Francis, B. and McIllmurray, M., B (2003) The universal, situational and personal needs of cancer patients and their main carers. *European Journal of Oncology Nursing,* 7, 5-13.

Stead, M., L, Brown, J., M, Fallowfield, L. and Selby, P. (2002) Communication about sexual problems and sexual concerns in ovarian cancer: A qualitative study. *Western Journal of Medicine,* 176, 18-19.

Stommel, M., Kurtz, M., E, Given, C., W and Given, B., A (2004) A longitundinal analysis of the course of depressive symptomatiology in geriatric patients with cancer of the breast, colon, lung or prostate. *Health Psychology,* 23, 564-73.

Sundquist, K. (2002) The Cancer Council New South Wales.

Thomas, C., Morris, S., M and Harman, J., C (2002) Companions through cancer: The care given by informal carers in cancer contexts. *Social Science and Medicine,* 54, 529-544.

Tiefer, L. (1994) The medicalization of impotence: Normalizing phallocentrism. *Gender and Society,* 8, 363-377.

Tracey, E., A, Roder, D., Bishop, J. and Chen, W. (2005) Cancer Institute NSW, Sydney.

Ussher, J. M. (1997a) *Body talk: The material and discursive regulation of sexuality, madness and reproduction,* Routledge, London.

Ussher, J. M. (1997b) *Fantasies of Femininity: Reframing the Boundaries of Sex,* Penguin/Rutgers, London/New York.

Ussher, J. M. and Sandoval, M. (2008) Gender Differences in the Construction and Experience of Cancer Care: The Consequences of the Gendered Positioning of Carers. *Psychology and Health* 23(8) 945-963.

Ussher, J. M. and Perz, J. (2010) Gender Differences in Self-Silencing and Psychological Distress in Informal Cancer Carers. *Psychology of Women Quarterly,* 228-242.

Walsh, S., R, Manuel, J., C and Avis, N., E (2005) The impact of breast cancer on younger women's relationships with their partner and children. *Families, Systems and Health,* 23, 80-93.

Wardle, J., Williamson, S., McCaffery, K., Sutton, S., Taylor, T., Edwards, R. and Atkin, W. (2003) Increasing attendance at colorectal cancer screening: Testing the efficacy of a mailed, psychoeducational intervention in a community sample of older adults. *Health Psychology,* 22, 99-105.

Wellard, S. (1998) Constructions of chronic illness. *International Journal of Nursing Studies,* 35, 49-55.

Wilmoth, M., C (2001) The aftermath of breast cancer: An altered sexual self. *Cancer Nursing,* 24, 278-286.

World Health Organisation (1995) The world health organisation quality of life assessment (whoqol) position paper. *Social Science and Medicine,* 41, 1403-1409.

Zigmond, A. S. and Snaith, R. P. (1983) The hospital anxiety and depression scale. *Acta Psychiatrica Scandinavica,* 67, 361-370.

7

Cancer-Associated Immune Deficiency: A Form of Accelerated Immunosenescence?

Chia-Ming Chang[1], Chien-Liang Wu[2] and Yen-Ta Lu[1,2]
[1]*Department of Medical Research, Mackay Memorial Hospital,*
[2]*Chest Division, Medical Department, Mackay Memorial Hospital,*
Taiwan

1. Introduction

Cancer (medical term: malignant tumor) is a major global health problem and a life-threatening disease that accounts for ~13% of all deaths annually. The number of cancer deaths gradually increases year by year, and it is estimated that more than 11 million people will die from malignances in 2030. Various definitions of cancer have been proposed over the last few decades. In general, cancer displays several malignant features including the uncontrolled proliferation of abnormal cells, local invasion of normal tissue, and metastasis to a distant organ via the circulatory or lymphatic system. Environmental and genetic factors are considered to be the major causes of cancer. Cancer is believed to originate from a single normal cell through a multistage transformation that is assumed to take decades of development. Continuous exposure to some environmental factors (e.g., tobacco, unhealthy diet, radiation, chemical toxins, viruses, etc.) can potentially interact with gene changes in our bodies to enhance the formation of cancer (see http:// www.who.int/mediacentre/fac tsheets/ fs297/en/index.html).

Conventional treatments include surgical resection, chemotherapy, and radiotherapy. Although these series of interventions can effectively control localized or disseminated tumors, there is still a high rate of metastatic recurrence, thus limiting a patient's survival. Other strategies, such as immunotherapy, cytokine therapy, and adoptive cell therapy, have shown some promising results for malignances in animal models. Unfortunately, several phase I/II clinical trials have shown that most patients still fail to completely eliminate cancer (Aldrich et al., 2010). It is becoming increasingly clear that cancer cells express immunogenic antigens that can induce an effective immune response against tumor formation (Lowe et al., 2007); therefore, during the initial stages of disease, cancer cells could essentially be recognized and rejected by the immune system, which exerts host-protective and tumor-modeling actions on developing tumors. Nonetheless, cancer cells also have numerous mechanisms to evade immunosurveillance (Burnet, 1970; Dunn et al., 2002), such as the downregulation of major histocompatibility complex (MHC) molecules or the antigen processing and presentation machineries, increasing the secretion of inhibitory cytokines, and the expression of inhibitory molecules to induce apoptosis in tumor-specific T cells (Dunn et al., 2004; Ferrara et al., 2003; Gabrilovich et al., 1996). On the basis of these phenomena, countless studies have confirmed the hypothesis that breaking self-tolerance and priming T lymphocytes are essential to treat cancer. Here, we discuss another possible immunosurveillance evasion mechanism in which the immune system fails to eliminate tumors not because tumor antigens are absent, but rather that an inappropriate proportion of T lymphocytes with an "accelerated immunosenescence" status are present in cancer patients (Chen et al., 2010). Although cancer patients are often considered to have poor immunity, very few attempts have been made to examine the dysfunctional immune profile of these patients in detail. Thus, it is not surprising that there is a vast discrepancy in the responses of cancer patients to immunotherapy. This chapter will cover selected aspects of cancer-associated immune deficiency, emphasizing the cause and effect of accelerated immunosenescence in cancer patients. A better understanding of the immune profiles of cancer patients may inform more successful therapeutic strategies for the treatment of malignancies.

2. Cancer-related immune deficiency

When patients are diagnosed with cancer, a phenotypic classification might be very useful to evaluate their immune status and track the progression of the disease. The immune system exhibits characteristic changes during cancer growth and progression, and these changes are significant in some specific T-cell populations. Compared with normal individuals, the immune profiles of cancer patients include the following characteristics (Fig. 1):

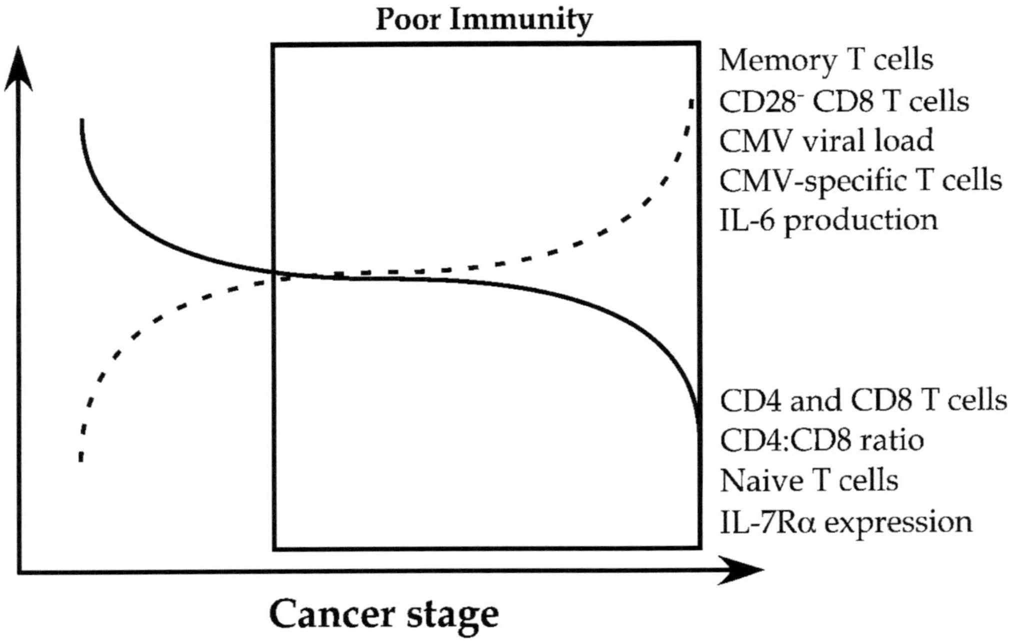

Fig. 1. Immune profiles of cancer patients over the disease progression. A significant trend of decreasing functional T-cell populations including CD4, CD8, CD4:CD8 ratio, naïve T cells with the progression of cancer, and the accumulation of memory T cells and dysfunctional populations such as $CD28^-$ and CMV-specific T cells are observed in cancer patients. The decreased expression of IL-7Rα in cancer patients could be associated with underlying inflammatory cytokines, e.g., IL-6, and CMV reactivation.

2.1 Inverted CD4/CD8 ratio

The antitumor immune responses are predominantly governed by the cell-mediated immunity. CD4 and CD8 T cells are the main types of lymphocytes in cell-mediated immunity and play a central role in the induction of efficient immune responses against tumors (Ho et al., 2002; Pardoll & Topalian, 1998; Toes et al., 1999). There are 2 different subsets of CD4 T cells, helper T cells (T_H cells) and regulatory T cells (T_{reg} cells), each with a different function. Once activated, T_H cells mediate the activation of CD8 T cells. Conversely, T_{reg} cells attenuate the immune reaction to maintain immunotolerance and suppress autoreactive T cells (Buckner, 2010). CD8 T cells, which are also called cytotoxic T cells (T_c cells), directly kill cancer and infected cells. Since CD4 T_H cells play an important role in optimizing CD8 T cells activation, an adequate number of CD4 T_H cells is therefore required to sustain the effector function against tumor cells by CD8 T cells.

In normal adults, CD4 and CD8 T cells each constitute well over 20% of the total lymphocyte population, whereas the proportion of these cells in cancer patients is lower and appears to decline according to the cancer stage (Chen et al., 2010; Mozaffari et al., 2007). An inadequate amount of T cells indicates that cancer patients cannot generate a sufficient immune response, resulting in an increase in the frequency and severity of infectious diseases. The ratio of CD4/CD8 T cells has indeed been used as an indicator for evaluating an individuals' immune function. In general, the CD4/CD8 ratio in healthy people is often >1; nonetheless, in patients with terminal cancer, this ratio drops significantly. Thus, an inverted CD4/CD8 ratio in cancer patients is one of the T-cell immune risk phenotypes (IRP) that is associated with increased morbidity and mortality (Wikby et al., 1998).

2.2 Subpopulation shifts in the T cells

The pattern of T cells differentiation may also serve as an important indicator for evaluating immune status in cancer patients. Naïve T cells are thought to be quiescent and capable of recognizing novel antigens (from tumor cells or pathogens) presented by antigen-presenting cells (APCs) to initiate the so-called adaptive immune response. Upon additional antigenic stimulation, primed T cells may start further differentiation leading to the clonal expansion of antigen-specific cells capable of executing immune response. Most of the activated T cells die rapidly through apoptosis; however, some may differentiate into memory T cells and survive for a long period of time. Once memory T cells encounter the same antigen, they will restart a faster and stronger immune response than the naïve T cells. Thus, it is of crucial importance for the immune system to have sufficient amounts of naïve T cells to respond to a variety of novel antigens.

In humans, the expression patterns of C-C chemokine receptor 7 (CCR7) and leukocyte common antigen isoform (CD45RA) are associated with the naïve, memory, and effector function of human T cells (Fig. 2, upper panel) (Sallusto et al., 1999). In general, naïve T cells express $CCR7^+$ and $CD45RA^+$. Effector T cells, in contrast, have a $CCR7^-$ and $CD45RA^+$ phenotype. Memory T cells can be further divided into 2 sub-populations according to the differential expression of CCR7. $CCR7^+$ T cells can be considered as precursors of the $CCR7^-$ subgroup. $CCR7^+$ T cells are identified as central memory (CM) cells that secrete the cytokine interleukin 2 (IL-2), while the $CCR7^-$ population has been referred to as effector memory (EM) cells that predominately express interferon−γ (IFN-γ) and interleukin-4 (IL-4). Both subgroups provide immunologic memory. T_{CM} cells generally localize in lymphoid tissues and generate a rapid and vigorous immune response when an identical antigen is encountered, whereas T_{EM} cells patrol peripheral organs where they may also reach local lymph nodes through afferent lymph vessels (Mackay et al., 1990). It has been shown that T_{CM} cells have a superior anti-cancer killing function than T_{EM} cells. (Klebanoff et al., 2005) The distribution of T-cell subpopulations varies substantially in patients with cancer, from being normal in some early-stage to being increasingly disturbed at more advanced disease and in those whom have undergone chemotherapy. Typically, patients have a relative shrinkage of early T cells populations including the naïve and T_{CM} cell, but an increased proliferation and differentiation toward T_{EM} and effector T cells, one of the characteristic features of T-cell exhaustion (Klebanoff et al., 2006) (Fig. 2, lower panel). The distribution of

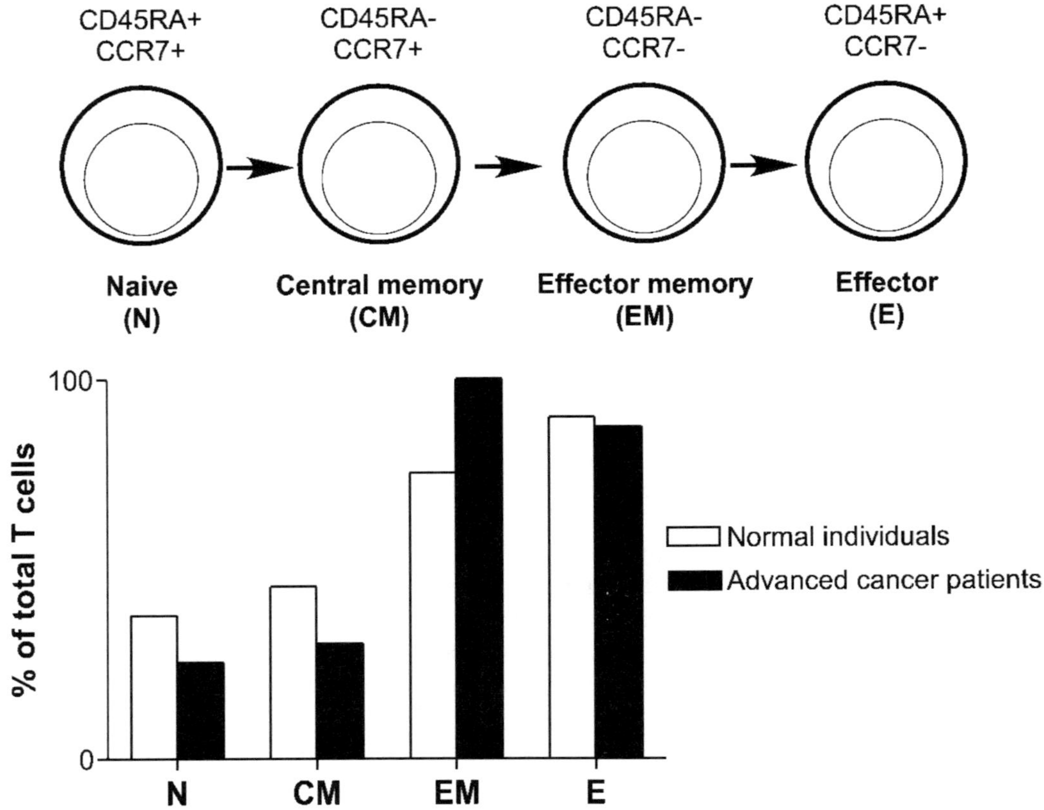

Fig. 2. Alteration of T-cell subpopulations in advanced cancer patients. The expression of the phenotypic markers CD45RA and CCR7 was used to define naïve, central memory, effector memory, and effector subpopulations (upper panel). The relative proportions of T-cell subpopulations in normal individuals and advanced cancer patients (lower panel). *N*, naïve T cells; *CM*, central memory T cells; *EM*, effector memory T cells; *E*, effector T cells.

T-cell subsets in cancer patients may explain the abnormal immune status that they suffer from: inadequate naïve and T_{CM} cells cause a shortage in the source of T cells with higher plasticity, while the accumulation of T_{EM} cells without appropriate T_H cells to prime an efficient immune response causes immune exhaustion. Another possible explanation has been advanced in which the T-cell pool shrinks as dysfunctional T cells accumulate and compete for survival with naïve and T_{CM} cells. While the total size of the T-cell pool remains unchanged, some memory T-cell subsets that are present at a low frequency may be lost (Akbar et al., 2004). These phenomena indicate that a patient's immune status is unfavorable against cancer. This is especially evident in advanced disease, particularly in patients extensively treated with chemotherapy. The immune system of such patients would suffer from chronic stimulation by relentless release of tumor or viral antigens resulted from disease progression and treatment. In time, this may lead to the impairment of naïve T-cell differentiation and a failure of adequate effector and proliferative capacity. Similar phenomena are observed in some chronic virus infection systems in humans (e.g., human immunodeficiency virus, and hepatitis C virus, etc.). Despite a vigorous immune response and subsequent generation of memory T cells in the early stages of viral infections, continue virus stimulation may serve as a driving force for the generation of virus specific T-cells. However, the activity of such T-cells is gradually lost during the persistent virus infection, eventually leading to the accumulation of exhausted T cells (Letvin & Walker, 2003; Pantaleo & Koup, 2004; Rehermann & Nascimbeni, 2005).

2.3 Down-regulation of CD28 on T cells

In general, the initiation of T-cell activation requires at least 2 signals. Antigen presenting cells (APCs) uptake foreign antigens (from tumor cells or infectious materials) and then present antigenic peptides that are bound to class I or class II MHC molecules to form the peptide-MHC complex. This complex and specific T-cell receptor (TCR) engagement provide a recognition signal (signal 1) for the activation of naïve T cells. However, signal 1 is not sufficient to fully activate an immune response on its own. Having received signal 1, the interaction of a co-stimulatory molecule with its ligand provides the verification signal (signal 2) (Allison, 1994; Liu & Linsley, 1992). Without signal 2, T cells will enter the anergy state (Harding et al., 1992; Mueller et al., 1989). CD28 is one of the co-stimulatory molecules on the surface of T cells and a critical component of the adaptive immune response against infections and tumors. Furthermore, naïve and T_{CM} cells express CD28 on their cell surface, whereas T_{EM} and effector T cells are predominantly $CD28^-$ (Pawelec et al., 2009). CD28 provides a co-stimulatory signal to interact with B7 molecules expressed on APCs and amplifies the signals delivered via the TCR, including increased cytokine expression, promotion of T-cell proliferation, and survival (Okkenhaug et al., 2001; Viola et al., 1999).
With cancer progression, the surface expression of CD28 on T cells is gradually downregulated, resulting in the accumulation of $CD28^-$ cells in the CD4 and CD8 T-cell populations. These cells, which are so-called senescent cells, have shortened telomeres, thus limiting the proliferative potential (Effros, 1997; Valenzuela & Effros, 2002) and may become apoptosis resistant (Brzezinska et al., 2004; Posnett et al., 1999). These indicate that cancer patients have a higher than normal proportion of mature T cells that are incapable of undergoing further differentiation. In addition, there is an irreversible loss of $CD28^+$ cells, the proliferation of which is either limited or has ceased completely during APC priming. This, in turn, may result in hyporesponsive immunity in cancer patients. Thus, it would appear that further T-cell clonal expansion is inhibited in patients with advanced stage cancer. An important concept in immunotherapy is that CD28 cells are necessary for T cells to interact with APCs and proliferate effectively; therefore, the down-regulation of CD28 in patients with advanced disease suggests that attempts at immunotherapy, such as dendritic cell vaccines, may not be very effective as they simply may not have enough $CD28^+$ T cells left to mount an adequate response to the antigen introduced by the vaccine.

2.4 Lower interleukin-7 receptor α chain (IL-7Rα) expression

Interleukin-7 (IL-7) is a pleiotropic cytokine that preferentially maintains B, natural killer, and T-cell survival and homeostasis (Kim et al., 2008; Kittipatarin & Khaled, 2007; Surh & Sprent, 2008). It shares the use of the interleukin-2 receptor γ chain (IL-2Rγ) with interleukin 2 (IL-2), but has its own IL-7Rα. IL-7Rα is mainly expressed by all naïve T cells (Fry & Mackall, 2005). IL-7Rα$^+$ T cells enhance their proliferation in response to homeostatic signals compared with IL-7Rα$^-$ cells. In cancer patients, the decrease in the naïve T-cell population has been found to be associated with the down-regulation of IL-7Rα, but not the plasma IL-7 level. Furthermore, the expression of IL-7Rα in naïve CD4 T cells is significantly lower than in naïve CD8 T cells. This may partly explain why CD4 is also at a lower level than CD8 in cancer patients. The mechanism underlying the down-regulation of IL-7Rα remains poorly understood. Some investigators suggested that the accumulation of T_{EM} cells and prosurvival cytokines, such as interleukin-6 (IL-6), may suppress the expression of IL-7Rα (Park et al., 2004; van Leeuwen et al., 2005). Indeed, plasma IL-6 levels are higher in cancer patients than in healthy individuals, suggesting a possible association with the down-regulation of IL-7Rα. Another possible explanation is that the down-regulation of IL-7Rα might be caused by a persistent viral infection as many persistent virus-specific T cells lack IL-7Rα (Wherry et al., 2004). In an in vitro study, van Leeuwen and colleagues showed that IL-7Rα$^-$ T cells fail to respond to IL-7, but survived and expanded after TCR stimulation. Therefore, it is suggested that IL-7Rα$^-$ T cells specific for persisting viruses are maintained via their intermittent contact with antigens derived from the latent virus (van Leeuwen et al., 2005). IL-7Rα$^-$ T cells may thus survive and accumulate in cancer patients because they are regularly triggered by antigens released during chemotherapy or due to the reduced immune status and, therefore, do not depend on IL-7 for their survival. Consequently, antigen-experienced effector and memory T subsets are replaced by expanded clones of cells that display a late differentiation phenotype, especially the CD8 subset. Likewise, the repertoire of cells available to respond to novel antigenic challenges shrinks.

2.5 Higher IL-6 production

IL-6 is one of the pro-inflammatory cytokines, e.g., interleukin-1 β (IL-1β), tumor necrosis factor-α (TNF-α), and IFN-γ, which regulate immune reactions to tissue damage and lead to inflammation (Kishimoto, 2010). IL-6 has been found to be a "two-edged sword" in a variety of human tumors, in that it can switch from behaving as a paracrine growth inhibitor to behaving as an autocrine growth stimulator with the same cells during malignant tumor cell proliferation (Knupfer & Preiss, 2007). Cancer patients often have prominent circulating levels of IL-6, but not TNF-α and IFN-γ, compared with the levels in healthy individuals. However, the source of the circulating IL-6 in patients is not clear, but it may be produced by macrophages and T cells reacting to the tumor or by the tumor itself (Ebrahimi et al., 2004). Recent reports showed a correlation between increased serum levels of IL-6 and advanced stage metastatic disease and poor outcomes in other types of cancer (Bellone et al., 2006). On the other hand, IL-6 is considered a crucial pro-inflammatory cytokine in immunosenescence and involved in induction acute-phase of C-reactive protein (CRP) in the liver that is associated with the increased morbidity of elderly (Krabbe et al., 2004; Wikby et al., 2006).

2.6 Human cytomegalovirus (CMV) reactivation and CMV-specific CTLs

CMV is a highly prevalent herpes virus that is chronically carried by more than 70% of the world's population (Rawlinson, 1999). It appears to be the most immunodominant antigen confronted by a carrier's immune system throughout life. The primary CMV infection usually occurs early in childhood, but seldom causes severe disease, and was long thought not to be a major human pathogen. However, the virus has mechanisms to evade immune surveillance and survive in an immunocompetent host. Once infected, the virus hides in the human body and the immune system is unable to eliminate it completely. A hallmark of latent CMV infection is its capacity to induce recurrent disease, mainly in immunocompromised individuals. Patients at high risk for reactivation of latent CMV include those with a human immunodeficiency virus infection, malignancies, organ transplant, or on immunosuppressive therapy (Alberola et al., 2001; Chemaly et al., 2004; Limaye et al., 2001). It has been suggested that CMV-specific effector T cells accumulate with aging in such large numbers that they may be the dominant T-cell population in the peripheral blood of healthy elderly individuals. In fact, CMV-specific CD8 T cells in such individuals may constitute as much as 50% of the entire CD8 T-cell repertoire (Khan et al., 2002).

In cancer patients, over 50% of patients on cancer chemotherapy experience CMV reactivation during the course of chemotherapy (Han, 2007; Kuo et al., 2008; Ogata et al., 2011), with the average viral load peaking after the third course of treatment (Kuo et al., 2008). Furthermore, CMV-specific IgG titers are simultaneously elevated with the increase in virus load. In addition, the clonal expansion of CMV-specific CD8 T cells is also observed in cancer patients; however, these cells are predominantly $CD28^-$, indicating that the expanded CMV-specific T-cell clones are terminally differentiated cells, i.e., essentially hyporesponsive to CMV (Chen et al., 2010). These T cells not only suppress other memory T-cell populations through competition for space or growth factors but also reduce the overall T-cell diversity and function (Effros et al., 2005; Messaoudi et al., 2004). The adverse impact of CMV on the immune status of cancer patients, thus, may be due to the presence of clonally expanded, highly differentiated, dysfunctional CMV-specific T cells that inhibit the diversity and ability of the immune system to respond to other antigens (Wherry et al., 2007). In extensively treated patients with terminal cancer, a decrease in the population of early-differentiated T cells, such as naïve and T_{CM} cells, is associated with the expansion of a CMV-specific T-cell clone. In addition, IL-7Rα expression of the immune cells was inversely correlated to the intracellular viral load of CMV. Following chemotherapy, CMV reactivation left a fingerprint on the T-cell population, i.e., a significantly enhanced number of circulating cytolytic T cells in CMV carriers. The clonal expansion of CMV-specific T cells may thus shrink the repertoire of immune cells available for other antigens. In fact, this may be a contributory factor to the disease progression frequently seen in cancer patients. Therefore, CMV drives the expansion of T-cell subsets that are linked with immunosenescence, which may add to the chemotherapy-associated deterioration of immune function (Messaoudi et al., 2004; Wherry et al., 2007).

3. Accelerated immunosenescence

"Immunosenescence" has often been described as age-associated deterioration of the immune system in the elderly. The Swedish OCTO/NONA longitudinal studies of the very elderly (>85 years) identified some immune parameters, the so-called "immune risk profile," which predict the 2, 4, and 6 year mortality rates. Immune risk profiles (IRP) mainly include (Ferguson et al., 1995; Pawelec et al., 2004; Pawelec et al., 2006; Wikby et al., 1998):

i. inverted CD4/CD8 ratio,
ii. poor T-cell proliferative activity,
iii. increased CD28⁻CD8 T cells,
iv. persistent CMV infection,
v. clonal expansion of dysfunctional CMV-specific CD8 T cells.

	Age-associated immunosenescence (>85 years)	Aggressively treated cancer patients[a] (45–75 years)
CD4/CD8 ratio	-	-
Naïve T cells	-	-
Memory T cells	+	+
$CD28^-$ T cells	+	+
CMV-specific T cells	+	+
IL-7Rα	Possible-	-
IL-6	+	+
CMV viral load	+	+

Table 1. Comparison of the immune profiles in age-associated immunosenescence and aggressively treated cancer patients. +, increase; -, decrease. [a]Patients with various types of cancer were enrolled in the Mackay Memorial Hospital. None of the patients had received immunotherapy when the blood samples were collected, but all had received chemotherapy according to the standard treatment regimen for their specific cancer (Chen et al., 2010).

It has been suggested that age-related dysfunction may not be the sole cause of immunosenescence, but the presence of an infectious component appears to be the force driving T cells towards senescence. Pawelec et al. has proposed that CMV infection is responsible for the development of immunosenescence in the elderly, not aging per se (Pawelec et al., 2006). The inflame-aging hypothesis in human ageing proposed by Franceschi et al. also suggests that immunosenescence is mainly driven by the chronic viral antigen stimulation (Franceschi et al., 2000). Repeated CMV infection induces significant expansion of late differentiated-stage of $CD28^-CD8$ effector cells, leading to alteration of homeostatic T-cell (i.e., inverted CD4/CD8 ratio and T-cell subpopulations, etc.). An analysis of immunosenescence data revealed that elderly individuals had a decreased number of naïve T cells and an increased number of effector/memory and effector CD8 T cells compared to young individuals; however, both had a similar amount of T_{CM} cells. Such large expansion would not only limit the number of clonal expansions of CMV-specific T cells but also result in shrinkage of clonal diversity (Hadrup et al., 2006; Pawelec et al., 2004). Thus, it is not surprising that old people have increased susceptibility to pathogens. The CMV-specific $CD28^-CD8$ effector cells can secret IL-6 cytokine that prolong inflammatory activity during pathogen infections (O'Mahony et al., 1998). The increased levels of circulating IL-6 would potentially induce CRP that is significantly correlated with mortality of elderly (Krabbe et al., 2004; Wikby et al., 2006). Patients with cancer are more vulnerable than healthy individuals to have CMV reactivation. In fact, the immune status of cancer patients is very similar to IRP seen in the elderly. Our previous data have shown that patients with cancer may suffer from a very high rate of CMV reactivation during chemotherapy (Kuo et al., 2008) that the pattern of IRP in age-associated immunosenescence can develop in a short period of time. Therefore, down-regulation of early differentiated subpopulations (naïve and T_{CM} cells), accumulation of the $CD28^-$ population and CMV-specific T cells, and high levels of CMV viral load and IL-6 secretion were observed in cancer patients who were extensively treated (Table 1). We propose that CMV reactivation (viral antigens) combined with cancer progression (tumor antigens) and treatment schedule may drive T cells toward senescence in cancer patients (Chen et al., 2010). These data refer a similar phenomenon of "accelerated immunosenescence". Thus, it is not surprising that several clinical trials of immunotherapy still fail to completely eliminate cancer. The immune exhaustion of advanced cancer patients could be one of the reasons for the poor clinical outcome of immunotherapy.

4. Conclusions

In summary, we propose that patients with advanced cancer who received extensive treatment have an accelerated immunosenescence that may be clinically relevant for cancer treatment. Typically, there is a decrease in naïve and T_{CM} cells, but an increase in the proliferation and differentiation of the T_{EM} population. The immune impairment in these patients is associated with multiple factors such as the stage of cancer, impact of treatment schedules, and consequence of CMV reactivation. It has been suggested that, with aging, CMV-specific effector T cells accumulate in such large numbers that they may be the dominant T-cell population in the peripheral blood of healthy elderly individuals. These T-cells are found to be specific for fewer epitope of CMV (Pawelec et al., 2005).

In addition, CMV infection may induce a decrease in T-cell telomere length and lead to a shift in the composition of the T-cell pool (van de Berg et al., 2010). The deleterious effect of CMV persistence on the human immune system is usually insidious and requires decades to be recognized. By contrast, the immune systems of cancer patients are somehow rapidly driven to an analogous state of immunosenescence. Therefore, it is conceivable that patients who receive extensive chemotherapy would have a greater risk of repeated CMV exposure, leading to the accumulation of CMV-specific immune cells. The clonal expansion of CMV-specific T cells may thus shrink the repertoire of immune cells available for other antigens and result in the chemotherapy-associated deterioration of immune function.

With a more complete understanding of the immune profile of cancer patients, clinical investigators will be able to provide strategies to restore a robust immune response in the tumor-bearing host (active tumor immunity) or, alternatively, promote immunity by the adoptive transfer of activated effector cells or tumor-specific antibodies into the tumor-bearing host (passive tumor immunity). In addition, certain biomarkers, such as the T-cell subpopulations, IL-7Rα, CD28, IL-6, CMV-specific T cells, CMV-specific IgG, and CMV viral load, may be useful for monitoring the immune status of patients during, or more importantly, before cancer treatment. Since CMV reactivation may in turn serve as the driving force for generating virus-specific T cells rather than tumor-specific T cells, we propose that even latent CMV infection may contribute to the immune tolerance of tumors. This raises the intriguing possibility that preemptive anti-CMV treatment could be an important adjunct in cancer treatment, especially during chemotherapy. Without consistent antigenic stimulation, T_{EM} cells undergo apoptosis, resulting in a decrease in this cell population and an increase in committed effector cells. Prevention of CMV reactivation before the initiation of conventional therapy or immunotherapy could promote immune reconstitution and therefore contribute to a better response once specific anti-cancer treatment is given. We believe that this strategy is worthy of further investigation.

5. References

Akbar, A. N., Beverley, P. C. & Salmon, M. (2004). Will telomere erosion lead to a loss of T-cell memory? Nat Rev Immunol, 4(9): 737-743.

Alberola, J., Tamarit, A., Cardenoso, L., Estelles, F., Igual, R. & Navarro, D. (2001). Longitudinal analysis of human cytomegalovirus glycoprotein B (gB)-specific and neutralizing antibodies in AIDS patients either with or without cytomegalovirus end-organ disease. *J Med Virol*, 64(1): 35-41.

Aldrich, J. F., Lowe, D. B., Shearer, M. H., Winn, R. E., Jumper, C. A. & Kennedy, R. C. (2010). Vaccines and immunotherapeutics for the treatment of malignant disease. *Clin Dev Immunol*, 2010: 697158.

Allison, J. P. (1994). CD28-B7 interactions in T-cell activation. *Curr Opin Immunol*, 6(3): 414-419.

Bellone, G., Smirne, C., Mauri, F. A., Tonel, E., Carbone, A., Buffolino, A., Dughera, L., Robecchi, A., Pirisi, M. & Emanuelli, G. (2006). Cytokine expression profile in human pancreatic carcinoma cells and in surgical specimens: implications for survival. *Cancer Immunol Immunother*, 55(6): 684-698.

Brzezinska, A., Magalska, A., Szybinska, A. & Sikora, E. (2004). Proliferation and apoptosis of human CD8(+)CD28(+) and CD8(+)CD28(-) lymphocytes during aging. *Exp Gerontol*, 39(4): 539-544.

Buckner, J. H. (2010). Mechanisms of impaired regulation by CD4(+)CD25(+)FOXP3(+) regulatory T cells in human autoimmune diseases. *Nat Rev Immunol*, 10(12): 849-859.

Burnet, F. M. (1970). The concept of immunological surveillance. Prog Exp Tumor Res, 13: 1-27.

Chemaly, R. F., Yen-Lieberman, B., Castilla, E. A., Reilly, A., Arrigain, S., Farver, C., Avery, R. K., Gordon, S. M. & Procop, G. W. (2004). Correlation between viral loads of cytomegalovirus in blood and bronchoalveolar lavage specimens from lung transplant recipients determined by histology and immunohistochemistry. *J Clin Microbiol*, 42(5): 2168-2172.

Chen, I. H., Lai, Y. L., Wu, C. L., Chang, Y. F., Chu, C. C., Tsai, I. F., Sun, F. J. & Lu, Y. T. (2010). Immune impairment in patients with terminal cancers: influence of cancer treatments and cytomegalovirus infection. *Cancer Immunol Immunother*, 59(2): 323-334.

Dunn, G. P., Bruce, A. T., Ikeda, H., Old, L. J. & Schreiber, R. D. (2002). Cancer immunoediting: from immunosurveillance to tumor escape. *Nat Immunol*, 3(11): 991-998.

Dunn, G. P., Old, L. J. & Schreiber, R. D. (2004). The immunobiology of cancer immunosurveillance and immunoediting. *Immunity*, 21(2): 137-148.

Ebrahimi, B., Tucker, S. L., Li, D., Abbruzzese, J. L. & Kurzrock, R. (2004). Cytokines in pancreatic carcinoma: correlation with phenotypic characteristics and prognosis. *Cancer*, 101(12): 2727-2736.

Effros, R. B. (1997). Loss of CD28 expression on T lymphocytes: a marker of replicative senescence. *Dev Comp Immunol*, 21(6): 471-478.

Effros, R. B., Dagarag, M., Spaulding, C. & Man, J. (2005). The role of CD8+ T-cell replicative senescence in human aging. *Immunol Rev*, 205: 147-157.

Ferguson, F. G., Wikby, A., Maxson, P., Olsson, J. & Johansson, B. (1995). Immune parameters in a longitudinal study of a very old population of Swedish people: a comparison between survivors and nonsurvivors. *J Gerontol A Biol Sci Med Sci*, 50(6): B378-382.

Ferrara, N., Gerber, H. P. & LeCouter, J. (2003). The biology of VEGF and its receptors. *Nat Med*, 9(6): 669-676.

Franceschi, C., Bonafe, M., Valensin, S., Olivieri, F., De Luca, M., Ottaviani, E. & De Benedictis, G. (2000). Inflamm-aging. An evolutionary perspective on immunosenescence. *Ann N Y Acad Sci*, 908: 244-254.

Fry, T. J. & Mackall, C. L. (2005). The many faces of IL-7: from lymphopoiesis to peripheral T cell maintenance. *J Immunol*, 174(11): 6571-6576.

Gabrilovich, D. I., Chen, H. L., Girgis, K. R., Cunningham, H. T., Meny, G. M., Nadaf, S., Kavanaugh, D. & Carbone, D. P. (1996). Production of vascular endothelial growth factor by human tumors inhibits the functional maturation of dendritic cells. *Nat Med*, 2(10): 1096-1103.

Hadrup, S. R., Strindhall, J., Kollgaard, T., Seremet, T., Johansson, B., Pawelec, G., thor Straten, P. & Wikby, A. (2006). Longitudinal studies of clonally expanded CD8 T cells reveal a repertoire shrinkage predicting mortality and an increased number of dysfunctional cytomegalovirus-specific T cells in the very elderly. *J Immunol*, 176(4): 2645-2653.

Han, X. Y. (2007). Epidemiologic analysis of reactivated cytomegalovirus antigenemia in patients with cancer. *J Clin Microbiol*, 45(4): 1126-1132.

Harding, F. A., McArthur, J. G., Gross, J. A., Raulet, D. H. & Allison, J. P. (1992). CD28-mediated signalling co-stimulates murine T cells and prevents induction of anergy in T-cell clones. *Nature*, 356(6370): 607-609.

Ho, W. Y., Yee, C. & Greenberg, P. D. (2002). Adoptive therapy with CD8(+) T cells: it may get by with a little help from its friends. *J Clin Invest*, 110(10): 1415-1417.

Khan, N., Shariff, N., Cobbold, M., Bruton, R., Ainsworth, J. A., Sinclair, A. J., Nayak, L. & Moss, P. A. (2002). Cytomegalovirus seropositivity drives the CD8 T cell repertoire toward greater clonality in healthy elderly individuals. *J Immunol*, 169(4): 1984-1992.

Kim, H. R., Hwang, K. A., Park, S. H. & Kang, I. (2008). IL-7 and IL-15: biology and roles in T-Cell immunity in health and disease. *Crit Rev Immunol*, 28(4): 325-339.

Kishimoto, T. (2010). IL-6: from its discovery to clinical applications. *Int Immunol*, 22(5): 347-352.

Kittipatarin, C. & Khaled, A. R. (2007). Interlinking interleukin-7. *Cytokine*, 39(1): 75-83.

Klebanoff, C. A., Gattinoni, L. & Restifo, N. P. (2006). CD8+ T-cell memory in tumor immunology and immunotherapy. *Immunol Rev*, 211: 214-224.

Klebanoff, C. A., Gattinoni, L., Torabi-Parizi, P., Kerstann, K., Cardones, A. R., Finkelstein, S. E., Palmer, D. C., Antony, P. A., Hwang, S. T., Rosenberg, S. A., Waldmann, T. A. & Restifo, N. P. (2005). Central memory self/tumor-reactive CD8+ T cells confer superior antitumor immunity compared with effector memory T cells. *Proc Natl Acad Sci U S A*, 102(27): 9571-9576.

Knupfer, H. & Preiss, R. (2007). Significance of interleukin-6 (IL-6) in breast cancer (review). *Breast Cancer Res Treat*, 102(2): 129-135.

Krabbe, K. S., Pedersen, M. & Bruunsgaard, H. (2004). Inflammatory mediators in the elderly. *Exp Gerontol*, 39(5): 687-699.

Kuo, C. P., Wu, C. L., Ho, H. T., Chen, C. G., Liu, S. I. & Lu, Y. T. (2008). Detection of cytomegalovirus reactivation in cancer patients receiving chemotherapy. *Clin Microbiol Infect*, 14(3): 221-227.

Letvin, N. L. & Walker, B. D. (2003). Immunopathogenesis and immunotherapy in AIDS virus infections. *Nat Med*, 9(7): 861-866.

Limaye, A. P., Huang, M. L., Leisenring, W., Stensland, L., Corey, L. & Boeckh, M. (2001). Cytomegalovirus (CMV) DNA load in plasma for the diagnosis of CMV disease before engraftment in hematopoietic stem-cell transplant recipients. *J Infect Dis*, 183(3): 377-382.

Liu, Y. & Linsley, P. S. (1992). Costimulation of T-cell growth. *Curr Opin Immunol*, 4(3): 265-270.

Lowe, D. B., Shearer, M. H., Jumper, C. A. & Kennedy, R. C. (2007). Towards progress on DNA vaccines for cancer. *Cell Mol Life Sci*, 64(18): 2391-2403.

Mackay, C. R., Marston, W. L. & Dudler, L. (1990). Naive and memory T cells show distinct pathways of lymphocyte recirculation. *J Exp Med*, 171(3): 801-817.

Messaoudi, I., Lemaoult, J., Guevara-Patino, J. A., Metzner, B. M. & Nikolich-Zugich, J. (2004). Age-related CD8 T cell clonal expansions constrict CD8 T cell repertoire and have the potential to impair immune defense. *J Exp Med*, 200(10): 1347-1358.

Mozaffari, F., Lindemalm, C., Choudhury, A., Granstam-Bjorneklett, H., Helander, I., Lekander, M., Mikaelsson, E., Nilsson, B., Ojutkangas, M. L., Osterborg, A., Bergkvist, L. & Mellstedt, H. (2007). NK-cell and T-cell functions in patients with breast cancer: effects of surgery and adjuvant chemo- and radiotherapy. *Br J Cancer*, 97(1): 105-111.

Mueller, D. L., Jenkins, M. K. & Schwartz, R. H. (1989). Clonal expansion versus functional clonal inactivation: a costimulatory signalling pathway determines the outcome of T cell antigen receptor occupancy. *Annu Rev Immunol*, 7: 445-480.

O'Mahony, L., Holland, J., Jackson, J., Feighery, C., Hennessy, T. P. & Mealy, K. (1998). Quantitative intracellular cytokine measurement: age-related changes in proinflammatory cytokine production. *Clin Exp Immunol*, 113(2): 213-219.

Ogata, M., Satou, T., Kawano, R., Yoshikawa, T., Ikewaki, J., Kohno, K., Ando, T., Miyazaki, Y., Ohtsuka, E., Saburi, Y., Kikuchi, H., Saikawa, T. & Kadota, J. (2011). High incidence of cytomegalovirus, human herpesvirus-6, and Epstein-Barr virus reactivation in patients receiving cytotoxic chemotherapy for adult T cell leukemia. *J Med Virol*, 83(4): 702-709.

Okkenhaug, K., Wu, L., Garza, K. M., La Rose, J., Khoo, W., Odermatt, B., Mak, T. W., Ohashi, P. S. & Rottapel, R. (2001). A point mutation in CD28 distinguishes proliferative signals from survival signals. *Nat Immunol*, 2(4): 325-332.

Pantaleo, G. & Koup, R. A. (2004). Correlates of immune protection in HIV-1 infection: what we know, what we don't know, what we should know. *Nat Med*, 10(8): 806-810.

Pardoll, D. M. & Topalian, S. L. (1998). The role of CD4+ T cell responses in antitumor immunity. *Curr Opin Immunol*, 10(5): 588-594.

Park, J. H., Yu, Q., Erman, B., Appelbaum, J. S., Montoya-Durango, D., Grimes, H. L. & Singer, A. (2004). Suppression of IL7Ralpha transcription by IL-7 and other prosurvival cytokines: a novel mechanism for maximizing IL-7-dependent T cell survival. *Immunity*, 21(2): 289-302.

Pawelec, G., Akbar, A., Caruso, C., Effros, R., Grubeck-Loebenstein, B. & Wikby, A. (2004). Is immunosenescence infectious? *Trends Immunol*, 25(8): 406-410.

Pawelec, G., Akbar, A., Caruso, C., Solana, R., Grubeck-Loebenstein, B. & Wikby, A. (2005). Human immunosenescence: is it infectious? *Immunol Rev*, 205: 257-268.

Pawelec, G., Derhovanessian, E., Larbi, A., Strindhall, J. & Wikby, A. (2009). Cytomegalovirus and human immunosenescence. *Rev Med Virol*, 19(1): 47-56.

Pawelec, G., Koch, S., Franceschi, C. & Wikby, A. (2006). Human immunosenescence: does it have an infectious component? *Ann N Y Acad Sci*, 1067: 56-65.

Posnett, D. N., Edinger, J. W., Manavalan, J. S., Irwin, C. & Marodon, G. (1999). Differentiation of human CD8 T cells: implications for in vivo persistence of CD8+ CD28- cytotoxic effector clones. *Int Immunol*, 11(2): 229-241.

Rawlinson, W. D. (1999). Broadsheet. Number 50: Diagnosis of human cytomegalovirus infection and disease. *Pathology*, 31(2): 109-115.

Rehermann, B. & Nascimbeni, M. (2005). Immunology of hepatitis B virus and hepatitis C virus infection. *Nat Rev Immunol*, 5(3): 215-229.

Sallusto, F., Lenig, D., Forster, R., Lipp, M. & Lanzavecchia, A. (1999). Two subsets of memory T lymphocytes with distinct homing potentials and effector functions. *Nature*, 401(6754): 708-712.

Surh, C. D. & Sprent, J. (2008). Homeostasis of naive and memory T cells. *Immunity*, 29(6): 848-862.

Toes, R. E., Ossendorp, F., Offringa, R. & Melief, C. J. (1999). CD4 T cells and their role in antitumor immune responses. *J Exp Med*, 189(5): 753-756.

Valenzuela, H. F. & Effros, R. B. (2002). Divergent telomerase and CD28 expression patterns in human CD4 and CD8 T cells following repeated encounters with the same antigenic stimulus. *Clin Immunol*, 105(2): 117-125.

van de Berg, P. J., Griffiths, S. J., Yong, S. L., Macaulay, R., Bemelman, F. J., Jackson, S., Henson, S. M., ten Berge, I. J., Akbar, A. N. & van Lier, R. A. (2010). Cytomegalovirus infection reduces telomere length of the circulating T cell pool. *J Immunol*, 184(7): 3417-3423.

van Leeuwen, E. M., de Bree, G. J., Remmerswaal, E. B., Yong, S. L., Tesselaar, K., ten Berge, I. J. & van Lier, R. A. (2005). IL-7 receptor alpha chain expression distinguishes functional subsets of virus-specific human CD8+ T cells. *Blood*, 106(6): 2091-2098.

Viola, A., Schroeder, S., Sakakibara, Y. & Lanzavecchia, A. (1999). T lymphocyte costimulation mediated by reorganization of membrane microdomains. *Science*, 283(5402): 680-682.

Wherry, E. J., Barber, D. L., Kaech, S. M., Blattman, J. N. & Ahmed, R. (2004). Antigen-independent memory CD8 T cells do not develop during chronic viral infection. *Proc Natl Acad Sci U S A*, 101(45): 16004-16009.

Wherry, E. J., Ha, S. J., Kaech, S. M., Haining, W. N., Sarkar, S., Kalia, V., Subramaniam, S., Blattman, J. N., Barber, D. L. & Ahmed, R. (2007). Molecular signature of CD8+ T cell exhaustion during chronic viral infection. *Immunity*, 27(4): 670-684.

Wikby, A., Maxson, P., Olsson, J., Johansson, B. & Ferguson, F. G. (1998). Changes in CD8 and CD4 lymphocyte subsets, T cell proliferation responses and non-survival in the very old: the Swedish longitudinal OCTO-immune study. *Mech Ageing Dev*, 102(2-3): 187-198.

Wikby, A., Nilsson, B. O., Forsey, R., Thompson, J., Strindhall, J., Lofgren, S., Ernerudh, J., Pawelec, G., Ferguson, F. & Johansson, B. (2006). The immune risk phenotype is associated with IL-6 in the terminal decline stage: findings from the Swedish NONA immune longitudinal study of very late life functioning. *Mech Ageing Dev*, 127(8): 695-704.

8

Physical Activity and Cancer: It is Never Too Late to Get Moving!

Duclos Martine
[1]Department of Sport Medicine and Functional Explorations, University-Hospital (CHU), Hopital G. Montpied, Clermont-Ferrand
[2] INRA, UMR 1019, Clermont-Ferrand
[3]University Clermont 1, UFR Médecine, Clermont-Ferrand
[4]CRNH-Auvergne, Clermont-Ferrand
France

1. Introduction

In terms of prevalence, the most common cancers in men and women worldwide are breast cancer (3.9 million breast cancer cases) and colorectal cancers (2.4 million). Moreover, the worldwide incidence of breast and colorectal cancers is destined to increase substantially in the next few decades. Therefore, the prevention of the occurrence of these various types of cancers represents a real stake in public health for which physical activity could play an important role. Indeed, numerous studies showing an association between prevention of these cancers and physical activity have been published these last years.

The number of survivors after treatment of a cancer ("cancer survivors") is also increasing. Since last years, different studies have rocked the research community involved in cancer survivorship. These studies reported a significant protective association between increased physical activity that occurred after the diagnosis of breast or colon cancer and recurrence, cancer-related mortality, and overall mortality among breast cancer or colon cancer survivors.

This chapter will consider epidemiologic evidence regarding the association between physical activity and breast and colon cancer in primary prevention (cancer occurrence) and in tertiary prevention (cancer recurrence). The second aim of this chapter will be to discuss the type and characteristics (duration, intensity) of physical activity associated with these effects both in primary prevention of breast and colon cancer and in cancer survivors. In other words, what types of exercise are most beneficial?

Evidence for the underlying mechanistic targets of physical activity interventions on the carcinogenesis process is also emerging. Studies suggest that exercise can exert its cancer-preventive effects at many stages during the process of carcinogenesis, including both tumour initiation and progression. This will be discussed in the third part of this chapter.

In the fourth part, the barriers to prescribe physical activity in physicians will be discussed as the published work provides sufficient evidence to suggest that physical activity is safe and well-tolerated even in cancer survivors and that oncologists can recommend to their patients physical activity after the completion of primary treatment. Finally we will discuss on the current guidelines on physical activity for cancer prevention and for cancer survivors, with guidance based largely on proven associations that exist between physical activity and specific comorbid conditions (such as heart disease or osteoporosis) to which cancer survivors are especially prone, or associations between physical activity and other factors, such as quality of life, functional decline, and fatigue. Effective strategies to increase physical activity will be discussed.

2. Physical activity and colon and breast cancer prevention

2.1 Colorectal cancer

2.1.1 Review of the evidence on physical activity and colon cancer prevention

Colorectal cancer is the cancer for which there is the largest number of evidences on the beneficial effect of physical activity (Friedenreich et al., 2010;Roberts & Barnard, 2005). The overall level of scientific evidence on the beneficial effects of physical activity on the prevention of colon cancer is categorized as convincing (Friedenreich et al., 2010). This characterization is based on the definitions developed and used in the World Cancer Research Fund and American Institute for Cancer Research (the categories used are "convincing", "probable", "possible" and "insufficient"). Indeed on 51 studies conducted on colon and colorectal cancer, 43 demonstrated a reduction in cancer amongst the most physically active male and female participants with an average reduction from 20 to 30 % amongst both men and women. This protective effect of physical activity for colon cancer is not found for rectal cancer (Friedenreich et al., 2010).

A recent meta-analysis (Wolin et al., 2009) measured the magnitude of the inverse association between physical activity and risk of colon cancer restricting analyses to studies where data for colon cancer alone were available (exclusion of rectal cancer). A total of 52 studies were included, showing a 24% risk reduction overall, and generally similar risk reductions when men and women were examined separately.

Evidence for a dose-response effect exists with greater risks reductions observed for higher levels of physical activity (Friedenreich et al., 2010).

2.1.2 What type of physical activity is associated with prevention of colon cancer ?

Although each study quantified activity differently limiting the ability to draw conclusion about the amount of physical activity necessary for the 24% risk reduction observed in the meta-analysis of Wolin et al. (2009) one example provides information. In the Nurses' Health Study, women who expended more than 21.5 metabolic-equivalent task (MET) hours per week (MET-h/wk) in leisure-time physical activity had a risk ratio (RR) of colon cancer of 0.54 (95% CI, 0.33– 0.90), compared with women who expended less than 2 MET hours per week (Wolin et al., 2007). These levels are equivalent to brisk walking for some 5-6h per week in the most active and 0.5h per week in the least active. Interestingly, Wolin et al. (2009) were able to examine the effects of physical activity domain (occupational vs leisure-time) and found that the results were similar. Additional research are needed on the type, intensity and duration of physical activity that may afford the greatest risk reduction.

Overall, the results from all studies indicate a dose–response relation (higher levels of physical activity have been associated with a reduced risk of colon cancer) with risk reduction present across a wide range of physical activity frequency and intensity.

Although a physically active lifestyle might be associated with other healthful behaviours, a number of characteristics of the findings indicate that higher levels of physical activity directly prevent lower colon cancer. The association has been consistently reported in many studies of various designs, in diverse populations, for men and women, and after statistical control for a variety of other lifestyle factors. A compelling finding is that the inverse association has been observed for both leisure-time and occupational activities, for which patterns of potential confounding lifestyle characteristics are likely to differ.

The characteristics of physical activity which could have a protective effect towards colon cancer remained controversial, the data of the literature being contradictory. The categorizations and the methods of measure of physical activity which differ between studies are probably at the origin of these inconsistencies. Measuring physical activity in all its components, type, intensity and duration is complex. Although the results are heterogeneous, the available evidence suggest that at least 30-60 minutes per day of moderate to vigorous intensity for at least 5 days per week is required to significantly reduce the risk of colon cancer (Friedenreich et al., 2010).

Concerning the optimal period of life to practice physical activity to maximize its protective effect, the authors recommend a regular practice of physical activity throughout the life.

2.2 Breast cancer

2.2.1 Review of the evidence on physical activity and breast cancer prevention

More than a dozen of cohort studies and an even more important number of case-control studies have examined the relations between physical activity and risk of breast cancer. More than three quarters of these studies have observed a beneficial of physical activity on breast cancer risk with a risk reduction about 25% when comparing the most to least active subjects. These results were confirmed and specified in a review of articles published between 1994 and 2006 on the relations between risks of breast cancer and physical activity (Monninkhof et al., 2007). The methodological quality of these articles was calculated on the basis of a statistical quality score and only articles of high quality were eligible: 19 cohort studies and 29 case-control studies. The higher quality cohort studies showed a risk reduction ranging from 20 to 40%. A more recent overview of the existing evidence relating physical activity to breast cancer risk has been recently published (73 studies) (Friedenreich et al., 2010). They found a consistent reduction of about 25% of breast cancer risk when comparing the most to least active study participants (Friedenreich et al., 2010). Moreover, there is consistent evidence of a dose-response effect of decreasing risk with increasing activity levels.

2.2.2 What type of physical activity is associated with prevention of breast cancer ?

Most studies have investigated the association between breast cancer and leisure physical activity (walking, cycling, swimming, gymnastics) but few studies have included low intensity leisure physical activity such as gardening, home repair, stair climbing or housework (cleaning, washing, cooking, child care...) which probably led to an underestimation of total energy expenditure, especially among women who do not have access to a sport activity. The inclusion in the physical activity questionnaires of household activity is important because it is one of the main sources of physical activity for women in most developed countries. This is highlighted in the European cohort EPIC (The European Prospective Investigation into Cancer and Nutrition study), which showed that the risk of breast cancer was reduced in women in the top quartile of household activities (>90 MET-h/wk) compared with women in the lowest quartile activities (<28 MET-h/wk): -19% for postmenopausal women (HR: 0.81; 95%CI, 0.70-0.93) and -29% for premenopausal women (HR: 0.71; 95%CI, 0.55-0.90) (Lahmann et al., 2007). These results based on a large and heterogeneous cohort (218 169 women from nine European countries, aged 20 to 80 years at baseline followed for an average period of 6.4 years) and which used standardized data collection of physical activity and that could control for all the potential confounding factors, provide additional evidence that moderate forms of physical activity, such as household activity, may be more important than less frequent more intense recreational physical activity in reducing breast cancer risk.

Similarly, E3N French study, which is the French part of the EPIC, refers to a decrease in the relative risk of 18% when household activities are of light intensity while this decline is 38% when the activity is of high intensity (Tehard et al., 2006), a dose-response effect being also shown for these household activities. A negative trend in risk of breast cancer associated with total recreational activity (p trend <0.01) and total physical activity (p trend <0.05) was also observed.

Moreover, in review of Monninkhof et al. (2007), a trend analysis showed that the risk of developing breast cancer decreased by 6% per hour of physical activity added per week (assuming that the activity would be sustained over a long period of time) showing that this is the total amount of physical activity which is essential.

Overall, the analysis of the literature shows that at least 4 to 7 hours per week of moderate to vigorous physical activity would be required to produce a statistically significant decrease of the risk of breast cancer.

Several studies have attempted to determine the existence of a period of life in which the protective effects of physical activity would be maximum. In the absence of conclusive studies (pubertal period for some practice, adulthood for others), sustained lifetime physical activity appears as the most suitable preventive means (Friedenreich et al., 2010).

2.3 Summary of the evidence on the protective effects of physical activity on colon and breast cancer

The available evidence suggest that:

- at least 30-60 minutes per day of moderate to vigorous intensity for at least 5 days per week is required to significantly reduce the risk of colon cancer (24% risk reduction of colon cancer risk when comparing the most to least active study participants).
- at least 4 to 7 hours per week of moderate to vigorous physical activity is required to produce a statistically significant decrease of the risk of breast cancer (reduction of about 25% of breast cancer risk when comparing the most to least active study participants).

3. Effects of physical activity on colon and breast cancer survival

Length of survival after colon cancer or breast cancer diagnosis varies widely, even after accounting for stage at diagnosis and treatment, suggesting other factors may also be important. Lifestyle habit such as physical activity is a modifiable behaviour with multitude of health benefits (Haskell et al., 2007) including beneficial effect on cancer survival. Indeed, several prospective studies have shown that the level of physical activity performed after the diagnosis of cancer significantly decreased overall mortality, cancer mortality and the number of recurrences of cancer.

3.1 Physical activity and breast cancer survival

At least seven prospective studies have investigated the relations between physical activity and breast cancer survival (for a review see Barbaric et al., (2010).

The cohort of the Nurses' Health Study (121 700 women followed since 1976) has been the support of the first important study. This study focused on 2987 women with 280 breast cancer deaths and 8 years median follow-up (Holmes et al., 2005). Physical activity was measured by questionnaire every 2 years. The risk of death by breast cancer or breast cancer recurrence was reduced by 20 to 50% among women who walk 3 to 5 h per week (compared to those who walk less than 3 h per week). There was also a reduced risk of breast cancer recurrence and total mortality (Holmes et al., 2005).

The collaborative Women's Longevity Study (CWLS) of 4482 women with breast cancer followed for 6 years with 109 deaths reported a comparable decreased risk of breast cancer death and total death (Holick et al., 2008). These results were confirmed by the Women's Healthy Eating and Living Study (WHEL study) which reported a relative risk of recurrence reduced to 0.56 for women walking 30 minutes a day 6 times per week (Pierce et al., 2007).

Two smaller sized cohorts reported a decreased risk for total mortality but not breast cancer mortality with greater physical activity: the Life after Cancer Eidemiology (LACE) (Sternfeld et al., 2009) and the Health, Eating, Activity and Lifestyle (Heal) study (Irwin et al., 2008).

3.2 Physical activity and colon cancer survival

Three studies investigated the effects of exercise on cancer survival in patients diagnosed with colon (Meyerhardt et al., 2006a) or colorectal cancer (Haydon et al., 2006;Meyerhardt et al., 2006b).

Meyerhardt et al. (2006a) demonstrated that disease-free colon-cancer survival improved with increasing levels of physical activity (p trend <0.01). Based on the results of this study, it is suggested that a protective HR is observed with >18 total MET-h/wk or equivalent (HR= 0.51; 95% CI: 0.26–0.97, for 18 to 26.9 MET-h/wk); the protective HR does not improve beyond 27 MET-h/wk.

Two studies investigated the effect of physical activity on mortality in patients diagnosed with colorectal cancer. Haydon et al. (2006) demonstrated that persons who exercised at least once a week had improved disease-specific survival (HR = 0.73; 95% CI: 0.54–1.00, p = 0.05). The benefit of physical activity was largely confined to stage II–III tumours (HR = 0.49; 95% CI: 0.30–0.79, p = 0.01), while no association was seen in stage I (least severe) or stage IV (most severe) tumours. The results of the study by Meyerhardt et al. (2006b) supported the role of post-diagnosis physical activity in decreasing cancer-specific mortality (p for trend = 0.008) and overall mortality (p for trend= 0.003) (cohort of the Nurses' Health Study: 573 women whose colon cancer has been diagnosed (stage I, II or III), followed on average 9.6 years). Pre-diagnosis level of physical activity was not found to be predictive of mortality, whereas women who increased their activity level after diagnosis had an HR of 0.48 (95% CI: 0.24–0.97) for colorectal-cancer deaths and an HR of 0.51 (95% CI: 0.30–0.85) for all-cause mortality versus those with no change in activity. In contrast, among women who decreased their activity level there was a modest, though non-significant, increase in both cancer-specific and overall mortality.

All of these studies suggest that physical activity may confer additional benefits to those of the surgery, radiation therapy and/or chemotherapy for survival after treatment of breast or colon cancer. However, these results are observational and cannot formally identify a relationship of cause and effect. However the number of randomized trials testing physical activity interventions for cancer survivors is growing (Pekmezi et al., 2011). Moreover different research have started examining the impact of physical activity on surrogate/biologic markers of survival. All these studies are needed and are still ongoing.

3.3 What type of physical activity is associated with beneficial effect on survival after colon or breast cancer ?

The review of literature shows that this beneficial effect of physical activity on survival is obtained regardless of the type of training: endurance, strength, or mixed. The intensity from which effects on survival are observed is >9 MET-h/wk which is equivalent to 30 min of brisk walking 5-7 times per week and this regardless of the level of physical activity before the diagnosis.

It is necessary to take into account the state of fatigue of the patients before prescribing a program of physical activity. In all cases, the prescription must be individualized and implemented very gradually. Indeed, "the AP is well tolerated, without adverse effects and oncologists should recommend physical activity to their patients after treatment" (Irwin et al., 2008) (see paragraph 7.2.2).

3.4 Other benefits of physical activity for cancer survivors

Cancer survivors are not only at increased risk for progressive disease but also a host of comorbid conditions (other cancers, cardiovascular disease, obesity, diabetes and osteoporosis), functional decline and premature death (Demark-Wahnefried et al., 2006a). The impact of exercise is beyond the effects on cancer survival rate as exercise is also associated with other benefits for cancer survivors: exercise is consistently associated with improved quality of life, and also is effective in improving physical functioning (oxygen capacity, cardiorespiratory fitness, other fitness or strength measures, flexibility and global health), anthropometric measures (weight status, body fat, waist circumference) and health-related biomarkers (blood pressure, heart rate, circulating hormonal levels) among cancer survivors (Demark-Wahnefried, 2006b).

These effects are obtained with the levels of physical activity recommended for cancer survivors (Haskell et al., 2007) (Table 1).

4. Physical activity recommendations for colon and breast cancer prevention and for cancer survivors

Physical activity recommendations for colon and breast cancer prevention and after cancer treatment are summarized in table 1.

5. Physical activity during cancer treatment

More than 40 studies of randomised trials published since 1980 have evaluated the effects of physical activity during adjuvant cancer treatments. Despite methodological limitations and small samples sizes, all reported that physical activity (light to moderate intensity exercise using bicycle or walking program and/or structured exercise program using treadmill, various other forms aerobic equipment and strength training, at least 3 times a week for 20-30 minutes) is safe and feasible during cancer treatment. Physical activity can improve functional capacities, cardio-respiratory fitness and decrease the treatment-related symptoms (fatigue, nausea). Quality of life and sleep quality are also improved with physical activity (for a review see Kirshbaum, 2007 and Doyle et al., 2007).

Type of physical activity	Intensity	Duration of each session	Frequency per week
1) Endurance exercices *PA of moderate intensity* (exemple: brisk walking) OR *PA of high intensity* OR *Combination of both*	Moderate Vigorous	30 min 20 min	at least 5 times 3 times
2) Resistance exercises for muscle strength and endurance	8-10 exercises (with 8-12 repetitions for each exercise) on main muscle groups	20 min	2 times
3) Stretching exercise for flexibility			2-3 times

- for cancer prevention : combination of 1) + 2),
- for cancer survivor: combination of 1)+ 2) +3).

Table 1. Recommendations of physical activity (PA: physical activity):

There are few recommendations on the type, duration and intensity of physical activity to be practised during the cancer treatment (chemotherapy and/or radiotherapy). In most of the studies, the proposed physical activity was of light to moderate intensity, at the rate of 3 to 5 times a week with a duration from 20 to 30 minutes by session.
For people who were sedentary before diagnosis, low-intensity activities such as stretching and brief slow walks should be adopted and slowly advanced.

6. What biological mechanisms explain the associations between physical activity and colon and breast cancer

Evidence for the underlying mechanisms involved in the pathways between physical activity and cancer is emerging. Numerous biological mechanisms have been proposed and in some cases tested in randomized controlled trials (for a review see (Friedenreich et al., 2010;Rogers et al., 2008; Chan & Giovannucci, 2010).
In 2007 the World Cancer Research Fund examined associations for physical activity and several cancer types. They concluded that there is a statistical association between excess weight and some cancers including colon cancer and breast cancer in postmenopausal

women. These results were confirmed by a large standardized meta-analysis (Renehan et al., 2008). The authors did a systematic review and meta-analysis to assess the strength of associations between BMI and different sites of cancer and to investigate differences in these associations between sex and ethnic groups. The objective was to determine the risk of cancer associated with a 5 kg/m^2 increase in BMI (which corresponds to weight gains of about 15 kg in men and 13 kg in women who have an average BMI of 23 kg/m^2). They analyzed 141 articles, including 282 137 incident cases. In men, a 5 kg/m^2 increase in BMI was strongly associated with colon cancer (risk ratio [RR]=1.24, $p<0.0001$). In women, they recorded positive association between increased BMI and premenopausal ($p=0.009$) and postmenopausal ($p=0.06$) breast cancers. Associations were stronger in men than in women for colon ($p<0.0001$) cancer. Associations were generally similar in studies from North America, Europe and Australia, and the Asia–Pacific region.

Mechanisms that link excess weight and cancer risk are not fully understood, though three hormonal systems -the insulin and insulin-like growth factor (IGF) axis, sex steroids, and adipokines - are the most studied candidates (Renehan et al., 2008). All three systems are interlinked through insulin (Figure 1).

Obesity and a sedentary lifestyle induce insulin-resistance and a compensatory hyperinsulinism. Chronic hyperinsulinaemia decreases concentrations of IGF binding protein-1 and IGF binding protein-2, which increases bioavailable or free IGF-I with concomitant changes in the cellular environment (mitogenesis and anti-apoptosis) that favor tumour formation (Rogers et al., 2008). Circulating total IGF-1, which is a major determinant of free IGF-1 concentrations, is also associated with an increased risk of colorectal cancer, and with premenopausal rather than postmenopausal breast cancer (Renehan et al., 2008). For postmenopausal breast cancer, the increase in risk might be explained by the higher rates of conversion of androgenic precursors to oestradiol through increased aromatase enzyme activity in adipose tissue. Furthermore, chronic hyperinsulinaemia might promote tumorigenesis in oestrogen-sensitive tissues, since it reduces blood concentrations of sex-hormone-binding globulin, and in turn, increases bioavailable oestrogen (Calle & Thun, 2004).

Beyond these mechanisms, other candidate systems include obesity-related inflammatory cytokines, altered immune response, oxidative stresses, the nuclear factor κB system.

The beneficial effects of regular physical activity on the risk of cancer can be explained, among others, by their protective effect on weight gain and the reduction of abdominal adiposity. Independently of the variations of fat mass, regular physical activity decreases insulinemia by increasing peripheral insulin sensitivity (Dwyer et al., 2011). The direct effects of physical activity on IGF-1 are contradictory, some studies showing a decrease and others no variation of plasma IGF-1 levels with physical activity (Duclos et al., 2007). Regular physical activity can also reduce the risk of occurrence and/or recurrence of breast cancer by reducing the endogenous production of the estrogens but also by increasing the SHBG (Sex Hormone Binding Globulin) (Duclos 2001; Chatard et al., 2004). By binding to estradiol or testosterone, the SHBG therefore reduces their biologically active free fraction. The production of SHBG also depends on diet (normal or hypo-calorie intake, high-fibre diet, etc.), and the effects of physical activity are sometimes confused with the effects of diet (Longcope et al., 2000). Figure 1 presents an explanatory hypothesis of the pathways linking physical activity and insulin/IGF-1 /sex hormones to breast cancer development. physical activity could act by inverting these various pathways.

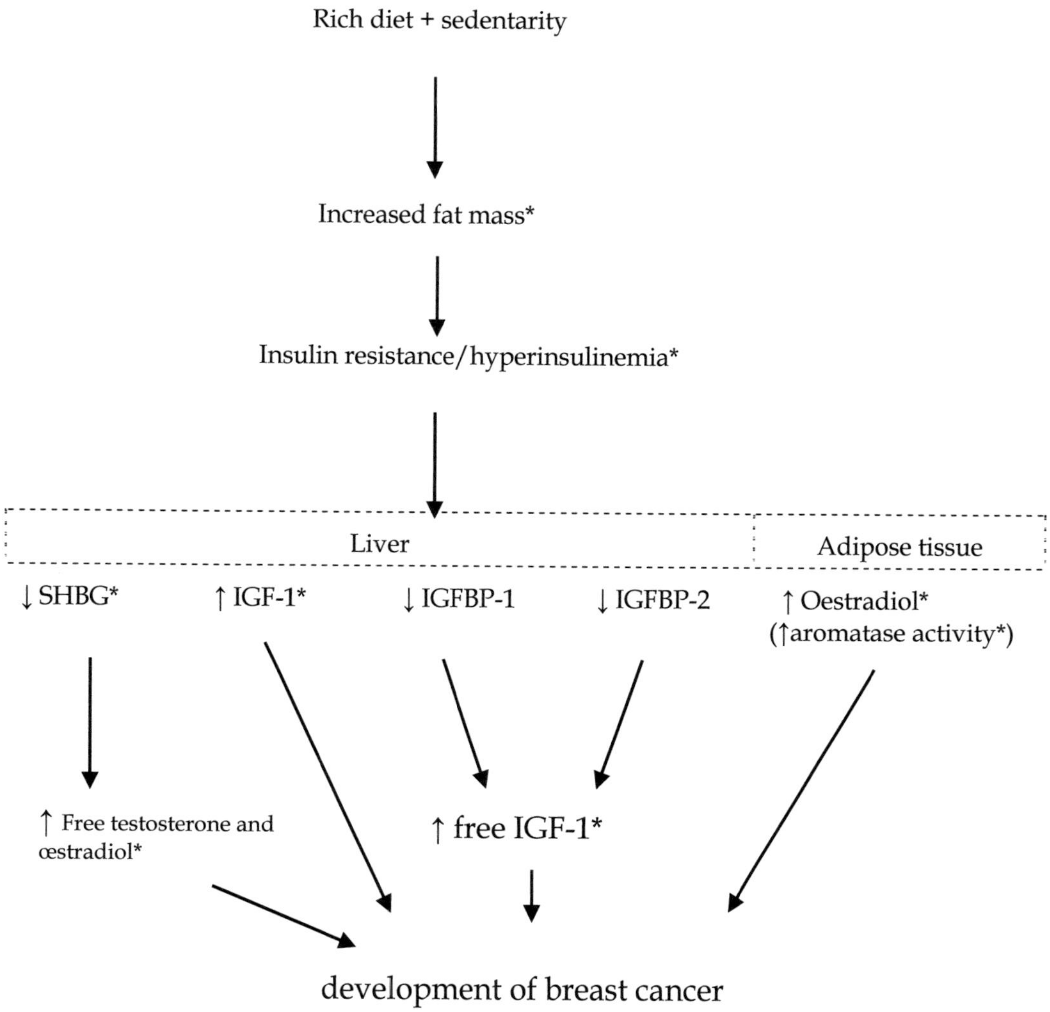

*: possible target and effects of regular physical activity
IGF-1 : Insulin like Growth Factor ; IGFBP-1 : Insulin like Growth Factor Binding Protein 1 ; IGFBP-2 : Insuline like Growth Factor Binding Protein 2 ; SHBG : Sex Hormone Binding Globulin

Fig. 1. Proposed mechanisms relating diet, physical activity and insulin to breast cancer

For colon cancer, the protective effects of regular physical activity marshal systemic effects of physical activity and local effects (Chan & Giovannucci 2010). Physical activity could also increase colonic motility, although colonic motility has not been definitely linked to colon cancer risk.

Other biological mechanisms of protective effects of physical activity have been suggested, such as the reduction of oxidative stress and effects on immunity. It is clear that the beneficial effects of physical activity depend on many inter-connected mechanisms. However, the level of scientific proof in each case is a matter of debate and further research is needed in order to determine the preventive mechanisms for each type of cancer.

In summary, exercise can alter biological processes that contribute to both anti-initiation and anti-progression events in the carcinogenesis process. However, more detailed studies are needed to examine each of the potential mechanisms contributing to an exercise-induced decrease in carcinogenesis in order to determine the minimum dose, duration and frequency of exercise needed to yield significant cancer-preventive effects, and whether exercise can be used prescriptively to reverse the sedentarity-induced and obesity-induced physiological changes that increase cancer risk (Rogers et al., 2008).
Moreover, the mechanisms of the beneficial effects of regular physical activity on survival after cancer treatment, and most importantly on the quality of life (decreased post-treatment fatigue, improved symptoms secondary to treatment) have yet to be determined (not to mention the need to know when to begin physical activity in relation to treatment, and at what dose: duration and intensity).

7. Barriers to physical activity in cancer survivor and in their physicians

Cancer survivors are not only at increased risk for progressive disease but also a host of comorbid conditions (other cancers, cardiovascular disease, obesity, diabetes and osteoporosis), functional decline and premature death (Demark-Wahnefried et al., 2006a). The impact of exercise is beyond the effects on cancer survival rate as exercise is also associated with other benefits for cancer survivors: exercise is consistently associated with improved quality of life, and also is effective in improving physical functioning (oxygen capacity, cardiorespiratory fitness, other fitness or strength measures, flexibility and global health), anthropometric measures (weight status, body fat, waist circumference) and health-related biomarkers (blood pressure, heart rate, circulating hormonal levels) among cancer survivors (Demark-Wahnefried et al., 2006a).
Therefore initiating and maintaining an exercise regimen long term should be generalized in the growing population of cancer survivors. In other words, cancer survivors should be encouraged to initiate and maintain physical activity.
However, adoption and maintenance of physical activity is a difficult challenge for healthy adults and is likely to be even more difficult after a cancer diagnosis. Concerning physical activity, cancer survivors are faced to two types of barriers:
- their own barriers to adoption and maintenance of physical activity
- barriers of their physicians to prescribe physical activity in cancer survivors.

This suggests that interventions to increase physical activity in patients should be multifactorial and multidirectional, i.e. directed towards patients and their physicians.

7.1 Cancer survivor barriers to adoption and maintenance of physical activity

As a result of the cancer diagnosis, surgery and adjuvant treatments some cancer survivors experience fatigue, depression anxiety, reduced overall quality of life (Irwin, Smith, McTiernan, Ballard-Barbash, Cronin, Gilliland, Baumgartner, Baumgartner, & Bernstein 2008). All these comorbid conditions favor sedentarity.
Patients should be informed and educated on the role of physical activity, not only to aid in the prevention of cancer but also to improve survival rates following diagnosis.
Thus, oncologists and physicians should discuss with their patients the benefits of physical activity after a diagnosis of cancer, reassure them that exercise is safe and associated with improved overall survival and quality of life, and to refer them to a certified cancer exercise trainer who will prescribe an exercise program that is tailored to them. The oncologist and

certified exercise trainer should also consider any preexisting conditions and adverse effects of treatment (Irwin et al., 2008).

It is necessary to take into account the state of fatigue of the patients before prescribing a program of physical activity. In all cases, the prescription must be individualized and implemented very gradually.

7.2 Barriers of physicians to prescribe physical activity in cancer survivors: What physicians should know, understand and explain to their patients

There is a reluctance of oncologists and of physicians to prescribe physical activity. Many elements prevent them from providing exercise advice: lack of sufficient knowledge of the benefits of being physically active after a cancer diagnosis, fear of side-effects of exercise (cardiovascular risks, lymphedema). Finally most physicians do not have the training or resources to develop individualized exercise prescription for cancer survivors.

7.2.1 Physician should know, understand and explain the wide spectrum of health benefits of physical activity

In addition to the risk of recurrence of the cancer, cancer survivors are also at risk of chronic fatigue, loss of muscle mass, weight gain. It should be noticed that the average weight gain after breast cancer treatment is 3-5 kg, and that epidemiological studies have shown that weight gain after a cancer diagnosis is associated with an increased risk for recurrence and death compared with maintaining normal weight after diagnosis (Kroenke et al., 2005). Cancer survivors also have the same risks as the general population to develop cardiovascular diseases or metabolic diseases, or even they present an increased risk of developing these as obesity and a sedentary lifestyle are highly prevalent in cancer survivors. Specifically there is evidence that cancer survivors die of noncancer causes at a higher rate than persons in the general population (deaths being primarily from cardiovascular diseases and diabetes) (Carver et al., 2007).

As detailed in paragraph 3.4, physical activity can reduce risk of other chronic diseases (cardiovascular diseases and diabetes) on one hand, and on the other hand, physical activity may help subjects with cancer avoid dying from their cancer.

7.2.2 Physician should know, understand and explain that physical activity in cancer survivor is safe and well-tolerated

The published work provides sufficient evidence to suggest that exercise is a safe and well-tolerated supportive intervention that oncologists can recommend to their patients after the completion of primary treatment.

In one of the largest studies to date, Courneya and colleagues examined the effects of aerobic exercise alone, resistance exercise alone, or usual care, on fitness, muscular strength, body composition, and quality of life in 242 breast cancer survivors initiating chemotherapy (Courneya et al., 2007). There were significant favorable effects of both aerobic and resistance exercise on multiple outcomes including self esteem, fitness, and body composition, as well as increased chemotherapy completion rates compared with usual care. Furthermore, no significant adverse events were reported; lymphedema did not increase or was not exacerbated by aerobic or resistance exercise. Recently, other clinical trials of women with breast cancer have shown no increased risk for or exacerbation of lymphedema from either aerobic and/or resistance exercise (Ahmed et al., 2006).

Courneya and colleagues also completed a similar trial of aerobic exercise vs usual care in breast cancer survivors who had completed adjuvant treatment, and observed similar favorable effects of exercise on fitness and overall quality of life (Courneya et al., 2003). Overall, these, and other, studies have demonstrated that exercise is safe in cancer survivors and produces beneficial effects on quality of life and cancer-related symptoms with no adverse side effects.

A long-term concern in breast-cancer survivors starting an exercise program is lymphoedema. The few studies that have assessed this issue clearly showed that upper body exercise does not induce or exacerbate lymphoedema, and on the contrary, it would seem that a suitable AP allow to limit this risk.

7.2.3 Physician should know and understand the influence of their beliefs on physical activity on the beliefs and physical activity of their patients

General practitioners (GP) are cited as the primary source of information influencing healthy lifestyle decisions, but few studies have evaluated whether GPs' perceived barriers towards physical activity affect physical activity uptake in their patients. In type 2 diabetes patients, Duclos et al. (2011) have assessed the associations between GPs' perceived barriers to prescribing physical activity and type 2 diabetes patients' perceived barriers to adopting physical activity. Their findings showed that GPs' physical activity and GPs' perceived barriers, are associated with type 2 diabetes patients' physical activity. An effect of GPs barriers on patients' ones towards physical activity was depicted since the higher the GP's barriers score, the higher the type 2 diabetes patient's barriers score. Examining the nature of perceived barriers to physical activity in both type 2 diabetic patients (regarding physical activity practice) and their GPs (regarding physical activity prescription), common barriers emerged with a high score: "A low fitness level", "The fear of being tired", "Their actual physical health status, excluding diabetes", "The fear of suffering a heart attack". These common barriers are inconsistent with evidence-based medicine (Haskell et al., 2007). These results are consistent with the hypothesis that the beliefs of GPs might influence the beliefs of their type 2 diabetes patients. Finally, GPs' physical activity was positively correlated with their patients' physical activity.

It has been shown that endorsement of physical activity is more credible coming from a professional who practices physical activity (Abramson et al., 2000). GPs should practise physical activity themselves, not only for their own benefit, but also as a stimulus for physical activity of their patients (Duclos et al., 2011).

It remain to determine if this proves to be the case in cancer survivors. However this suggests that identifying and working on GPs' barriers but also promoting physical activity in GPs may improve the uptake of physical activity in their patients.

7.2.4 Recommendations for physicians

As in other clinical and non-clinical populations, cancer survivors should obtain clearance from their physician or oncologist program. This clearance is especially important in cancer survivors who are at high risk for late-occurring toxic effects secondary to treatment that can increase their risk of cardiovascular disease. Thus, appropriate screening procedures for cardiac and cardiovascular disease are recommended before an exercise program is started.

The prerequisite is that patients have obtained the prior agreement of their cancer specialist and that patients should be screened for osteoporosis, bone metastasis, cardiac toxicities, and lymphedema.

Oncologist and primary care physicians should not lose sight of the fact that a substantial body of research shows the benefit of a healthy diet and regular exercise for reducing risk for many of the comorbid conditions (ie, other cancers, cardiovascular disease, diabetes, and osteoporosis) and side-effects (ie, fatigue and depression) for which cancer survivors are especially prone. Thus, oncology care providers can assist their patients by endorsing existing health guidelines for their patients and for themselves and encouraging their patients to take active roles in pursuing general preventive health strategies (Jones & Demark-Wahnefried, 2006).

8. Conclusion

There is a large body of evidence that physical activity has an important role in prevention and management of cancer: physical activity reduces risk of breast and colon cancer, during and after cancer treatment physical activity ameliorate symptom experience, ameliorate treatment side effects, improve quality of life and reduce mortality and morbidity. As such, regular physical activity should be encouraged in all populations (general population, subjects at high risk of cancer, survivors of cancer... and in physicians) throughout all life. Now, the question is not: "why should I prescribe physical activity in my patients?" but "How initiating and maintaining physical activity in patients?". Initiating exercise is important; however, maintaining an exercise regimen long term is a significant challenge. Behavioural interventions are complex and involve multidisciplinary approach (patients, physicians, scientists, government, urbanists...). Whatever, it's time to get moving and it is never too late to get moving!

9. References

Abramson, S., Stein, J., Schaufele, M., Frates, E.& Rogan S.: Personal exercise habits and counseling practices of primary care physicians: a national survey. *Clin J Sport Med* 10 (2000):40-48.

Ahmed, R.L., Thomas, W., Yee, D., & Schmitz, K.H. (2006) Randomized controlled trial of weight training and lymphedema in breast cancer survivors. *J Clin.Oncol.*, 24 (2006), 2765-2772.

Barbaric, M., Brooks, E., Moore, L., & Cheifetz, O. Effects of physical activity on cancer survival: a systematic review. *Physiother.Can.*, 62 (2010), 25-34.

Calle, E.E. & Thun, M.J. Obesity and cancer. *Oncogene*: 23 (2004), 6365-6378.

Carver, J.R., Shapiro, C.L., Ng, A., Jacobs, L., Schwartz, C., Virgo, K.S., Hagerty, K.L., Somerfield, M.R., & Vaughn, D.J. American Society of Clinical Oncology clinical evidence review on the ongoing care of adult cancer survivors: cardiac and pulmonary late effects. *J Clin.Oncol.* 25 (2007): 3991-4008.

Chan, A.T. & Giovannucci, E.L. Primary prevention of colorectal cancer. *Gastroenterology,* 138 (2010): 2029-2043.

Chatard, J.C., Duclos, M., Rossi, D.& Toutain, J. Androgens, skeletal muscle and muscle exercise. *Progress in Urology*, 14 (2004): 703-717.

Courneya, K.S. Exercise in cancer survivors: an overview of research. *Med.Sci.Sports Exerc.* 35 (2003): 1846-1852.

Courneya, K.S., Segal, R.J., Mackey, J.R., Gelmon, K., Reid, R.D., Friedenreich, C.M., Ladha, A.B., Proulx, C., Vallance, J.K., Lane, K., Yasui, Y., & McKenzie, D.C. (2007) Effects of aerobic and resistance exercise in breast cancer patients receiving adjuvant chemotherapy: a multicenter randomized controlled trial. *J Clin.Oncol.*25 (2007): 4396-4404.

Demark-Wahnefried, W., Pinto, B.M., & Gritz, E.R. Promoting health and physical function among cancer survivors: potential for prevention and questions that remain. *J Clin.Oncol.* 24 (2006a): 5125-5131.

Demark-Wahnefried, W. Cancer survival: time to get moving? Data accumulate suggesting a link between physical activity and cancer survival. *J Clin Oncol.* 24 (2006b): 3517-3518.

Doyle, C., Kushi, L. H., Byers, T., Courneya, K. S., Demark-Wahnefried, W., Grant, B., McTiernan, A., Rock, C. L., Thompson, C., Gansler, T., & Andrews, K. S. Nutrition and physical activity during and after cancer treatment: an american cancer society guide for informed choices. *CA Cancer J Clin* 56 (2007), 323-353.

Duclos, M. Impact of muscular exercise on endocrine functions. *Annales d'Endocrinologie*, 62 (2001): 19-32.

Duclos, M., Guinot, M., & LeBouc,Y. Cortisol and GH: odd and controversial ideas. *Appl.Physiol Nutr.Metab* 32 (2007): 895-903.

Duclos, M., Coudeyre, E. & Ouchchane, L. General practitioners' barriers to physical activity negatively influence type 2 diabetes mellitus patients' involvement in regular physical activity. *Diabetes Care*: in press

Dwyer, T., Ponsonby, A.L., Ukoumunne, O.C., Pezic,A., Venn,A., Dunstan,D., Barr,E., Blair,S., Cochrane,J., Zimmet,P., & Shaw,J. Association of change in daily step count over five years with insulin sensitivity and adiposity: population based cohort study. *BMJ* 342 (2011): c7249.

Friedenreich, C.M., Neilson,H.K., & Lynch,B.M. State of the epidemiological evidence on physical activity and cancer prevention. *Eur.J Cancer* 46 (2010): 2593-2604.

Haskell, W.L., Lee,I.M., Pate,R.R., Powell,K.E., Blair,S.N., Franklin,B.A., Macera,C.A., Heath,G.W., Thompson,P.D., & Bauman,A. Physical activity and public health: updated recommendation for adults from the American College of Sports Medicine and the American Heart Association. *Med.Sci.Sports Exerc.* 39 (2007): 1423-1434.

Haydon, A.M., Macinnis, R.J., English, D.R., & Giles, G.G. Effect of physical activity and body size on survival after diagnosis with colorectal cancer. *Gut* 55 (2006): 62-67.

Holick, C.N., Newcomb, P.A., Trentham-Dietz, A., Titus-Ernstoff, L., Bersch, A.J., Stampfer, M.J., Baron, J.A., Egan, K.M., & Willett, W.C. Physical activity and survival after diagnosis of invasive breast cancer. *Cancer Epidemiol.Biomarkers Prev.* 17 (2008): 379-386.

Holmes, M.D., Chen, W.Y., Feskanich, D., Kroenke, C.H., & Colditz, G.A. Physical activity and survival after breast cancer diagnosis. *JAMA* 293 (2005): 2479-2486.

Irwin, M.L., Smith, A.W., McTiernan ,A., Ballard-Barbash, R., Cronin, K., Gilliland, F.D., Baumgartner, R.N., Baumgartner, K.B., & Bernstein, L. Influence of pre- and postdiagnosis physical activity on mortality in breast cancer survivors: the health, eating, activity, and lifestyle study. *J Clin Oncol.* 26 (2008): 3958-3964.

Jones, L.W. & Demark-Wahnefried, W. Diet, exercise, and complementary therapies after primary treatment for cancer. *Lancet Oncol.* 7 (2006): 1017-1026.

Kirshbaum, M.N. A review of the benefits of whole body exercise during and after treatment for breast cancer. *J Clin Nurs.* 16 (2007): 104-121.

Kroenke, C.H., Chen, W.Y., Rosner, B., & Holmes, M.D. Weight, weight gain, and survival after breast cancer diagnosis. *J Clin Oncol.* 23 (2005): 1370-1378.

Lahmann, P.H., Friedenreich, C., Schuit, A.J., Salvini, S., Allen, N.E., Key, T.J., Khaw, K.T., Bingham, S., Peeters, P.H., Monninkhof, E., Bueno-de-Mesquita, H.B., Wirfalt, E., Manjer, J., Gonzales, C.A., Ardanaz, E., Amiano, P., Quiros, J.R., Navarro, C., Martinez, C., Berrino, F., Palli, D., Tumino, R., Panico, S., Vineis, P., Trichopoulou, A., Bamia, C., Trichopoulos, D., Boeing, H., Schulz, M., Linseisen, J., Chang-Claude, J., Chapelon, F.C., Fournier, A., Boutron-Ruault, M.C., Tjonneland, A., Fons, J.N., Overvad, K., Kaaks, R., & Riboli, E. Physical activity and breast cancer risk: the European Prospective Investigation into Cancer and Nutrition. Cancer *Epidemiol.Biomarkers Prev.* 16 (2007): 36-42.

Longcope, C., Feldman, H.A., McKinlay, J.B., & Araujo,A.B. Diet and sex hormone-binding globulin. *J.Clin.Endocrinol.Metab* 85 (200): 293-296.

McNeely, M.L., Campbell, K.L., Rowe, B.H., Klassen, T.P., Mackey, J.R., & Courneya, K.S. Effects of exercise on breast cancer patients and survivors: a systematic review and meta-analysis. *CMAJ.* 175 (2006):34-41.

Meyerhardt, J.A., Heseltine, D., Niedzwiecki, D., Hollis, D., Saltz, L.B., Mayer, R.J., Thomas, J., Nelson, H., Whittom, R., Hantel, A., Schilsky, R.L., & Fuchs, C.S. Impact of physical activity on cancer recurrence and survival in patients with stage III colon cancer: findings from CALGB 89803. *J Clin Oncol.* 24 (2006a): 3535-3541.

Meyerhardt, J.A., Giovannucci, E.L., Holmes, M.D., Chan, A.T., Chan, J.A., Colditz, G.A., & Fuchs, C.S.Physical activity and survival after colorectal cancer diagnosis. *J Clin Oncol.* 24 (2006b): 3527-3534.

Monninkhof, E.M., Elias, S.G., Vlems, F.A., van,d.T., I, Schuit, A.J., Voskuil, D.W., & van Leeuwen, F.E. Physical activity and breast cancer: a systematic review. *Epidemiology* 18 (2007): 137-157.

Pekmezi, D.W. & Demark-Wahnefried, W. Updated evidence in support of diet and exercise interventions in cancer survivors. *Acta Oncol.* 50 (2011): 167-178.

Pierce, J.P., Stefanick, M.L., Flatt, S.W., Natarajan, L., Sternfeld, B., Madlensk, L., Al-Delaimy, W.K., Thomson, C.A., Kealey, S., Hajek, R., Parker, B.A., Newman, V.A., Caan, B. & Rock, C.L. Greater survival after breast cancer in physically active women with high vegetable-fruit intake regardless of obesity. *J Clin Oncol* 25 (2007): 2345-2351.

Renehan, A.G., Tyson, M., Egger, M., Heller, R.F., & Zwahlen, M. Body-mass index and incidence of cancer: a systematic review and meta-analysis of prospective observational studies. *Lancet* 371 (2008): 569-578.

Roberts, C.K. & Barnard, R.J. Effects of exercise and diet on chronic disease . *J Appl.Physiol* 98 (2005): 3-30.

Rogers, C.J., Colbert, L.H., Greiner, J.W., Perkins, S.N., & Hursting, S.D. Physical activity and cancer prevention : pathways and targets for intervention. Sports Med. 38 (2008): 271-296.

Sternfeld, B., Weltzien, E., Quesenberry, C.P., Jr., Castillo, A.L., Kwan, M., Slattery, M.L., & Caan, B.J. Physical activity and risk of recurrence and mortality in breast cancer survivors: findings from the LACE study. *Cancer Epidemiol.Biomarkers Prev.* 18 (2009), 87-95.

Tehard, B., Friedenreich, C.M., Oppert, J.M., & Clavel-Chapelon, F. Effect of physical activity on women at increased risk of breast cancer: results from the E3N cohort study. *Cancer Epidemiol.Biomarkers Prev.* 15 (2006): 57-64.

Wolin, K.Y., Lee, I.M., Colditz, G.A., Glynn, R.J., Fuchs, C., & Giovannucci, E. Leisure-time physical activity patterns and risk of colon cancer in women. *Int.J Cancer* 121 (2007): 2776-2781.

Wolin, K.Y., Yan, Y., Colditz, G.A., & Lee, I.M. Physical activity and colon cancer prevention: a meta-analysis. *Br.J Cancer* 100 (2009): 611-616.

9

The Role of Exercise in Cancer Survivorship

Karen Y. Wonders
Wright State University, Maple Tree Cancer Alliance, Dayton,
United States of America

1. Introduction

At the turn of the 20th century, the outlook was bleak for individuals diagnosed with cancer. The pathophysiology of cancer was not well understood, and the associated treatments were as dire as the disease itself. In 1971, President Nixon declared "war" on cancer (Haran & DeVita, 2005). Since then we have seen dramatic improvements in cancer prognoses. At present, more than 11.7 million men and women are living as cancer survivors in the US, primarily due to early detection and advances in treatment options (Centers for Disease Control, 2007). However, such treatments often result in long-term physical and psychological toxicities, which negatively impact the cancer survivor's quality of life (QOL). These sequelae include, but are not limited to, decreased muscle strength, reduced cardiorespiratory fitness, reduced lean body mass, bone loss, fatigue (Pihkala et al., 1995; Lucia et al., 2003), depression, emotional distress, and anxiety (Jones et al., 2010). Thus, cancer research has shifted from its initial focus on prevention, to one that is centered on controlling or eliminating treatment-related toxicities with pharmacologic, physical, or social interventions. Now more than ever, healthy behavior choices are being promoted in attempt to limit this disease. In 2006, 42% of NIH-funded research projects contained an intervention component designed to improve the psychosocial well-being, physical status, and/or health behaviors of cancer survivors (National Institutes of Health, 2011). One such intervention, exercise rehabilitation, has been widely reported in the literature to benefit cancer patients. With more than two decades of literature examining this topic, research continues to support a link between a physically active lifestyle and improvements in mental and physical QOL in cancer survivors (Douglas, 2005; Wiggins & Simonavice, 2009). Thus, the primary aim of this chapter will be to explore the role of physical activity and exercise in cancer recovery.

2. Precautions during exercise

Cancer survivors often have disease or treatment-specific limitations that affect the exercise response. The specific effects of cancer on the exercise response are determined by the tissues affected and their level of involvement. Treatment-specific limitations arise from the type and duration of anticancer therapy employed. Surgery, chemotherapy, and radiation are the most common forms of cancer treatment, and all are associated with both acute and chronic effects that may negatively impact the exercise response. Table 1 briefly lists some of the more common treatment-related effects. In addition, most people are treated with a combination of surgery, radiation, and chemotherapy, which may cause a host of treatment-related problems. Pain, lymphedema, risk of infection, shortness of breath, neural deficits, fatigue, nausea and vomiting, cachexia, dehydration, and emotional distress are all common effects of cancer and its associated treatments on the patient's exercise tolerance.

Cancer Treatment	Potential Side Effects
Surgery	Pain Loss of flexibility
Radiation	Fatigue Skin changes Loss of flexibility Cardiac and/or lung scaring
Chemotherapy	Anemia Fatigue Nausea Myopathies Neuropathies Muscle weakness Wasting Changes in body composition that influence gait and balance.

Table 1. Potential Side Effects of Anticancer Therapy (Swartz, 2009).

2.1 Pain

Depending on the specific location of the cancer, patients may experience high levels of pain. A tumor often causes pain, particularly when it involves the musculoskeletal system, causing it to press on bones, nerves, or body organs. In addition, chronic pain is frequently reported following surgery, often when large amounts of healthy tissue are removed along with cancer tissue. Chemotherapy and radiation treatments may also cause pain resulting from such side effects as peripheral neuropathy, mucositis, and radiation injuries (American Cancer Society, 2011). In most situations, physicians can prescribe medications to alleviate pain; however the intensity, type, duration, and frequency of exercise may need to be adjusted until the pain is brought under control.

2.2 Lymphedema

Lymphedema is a swelling that results from a blockage of the lymph vessels that drain fluid from tissues. It is commonly caused by a mastectomy or the removal of underarm lymph nodes during breast cancer surgery, and is experienced by approximately 10-15% of breast cancer patients (Muss, 2007). It is characterized by a persistent swelling, typically of the arm or leg. Often, patients may be treated with compression bandages to limit swelling. It is advised that exercises be carefully designed, so as not to increase the swelling or cause infection (Kercher et al., 2008).

2.3 Risk of infection

Chemotherapy, radiation, and immunotherapy often have a substantial impact on white blood cell count. Consequently, immune function often weakens during cancer treatment.

Patients with very low blood counts are advised to avoid exercise all together, as they are at an increased risk for anemia. Frequent hand washing is advised, particularly in fitness centers, where germ count tends to be very high.

2.4 Shortness of breath

Shortness of breath is common when cancer has affected the lungs. It also may result when the bone marrow is affected, causing low red blood cell counts. Red blood cells carry oxygen throughout the body. Their ability to carry oxygen is measured by the amount of hemoglobin present in the blood. A low level of hemoglobin is indicative of anemia. With anemia, the body must work harder to supply oxygen to the tissues, causing the patient to feel fatigued and short of breath. Thus, anemic patients often have a limited aerobic performance because of the reduced oxygen-carrying capacity (Swartz, 2009).

2.5 Neural deficits

Neural deficits are common when tumors involve the central nervous system and brain. Problems with neural repair and decreased neurotransmitter activity may also arise as a side effect of anticancer therapy, related to the ability of chemotherapy to cross the blood-brain barrier and cause DNA damage and shortened telomere length (Klein, 2009). Neurological deficits can impact memory and emotion in cancer patients and may influence their motivation to adhere to an exercise program.

2.6 Fatigue

Fatigue is the most frequently reported symptom of cancer treatment (Schneider et al., 2003), affecting up to 96% of patients (Douglas, 2005). It is a whole-body tiredness that interferes with normal functioning and leaves the patient feeling irritable and unmotivated. Chronic fatigue has a negative impact on activities of daily life, social reintegration, and overall quality of life (Hartvig et al., 2006). In some patients, this fatigue is so debilitating to the individual that treatment must be discontinued or limited (Schneider et al., 2003).

2.7 Nausea and vomiting

Nausea, vomiting, and diarrhea are common effects of radiation and chemotherapy, leaving the patient feeling weak and at risk for electrolyte imbalances and dehydration. Cancer patients should avoid exercise for 24-hours after bouts of vomiting and diarrhea (Young-McCaughan, 2006). As a result, it is important that exercise schedules be flexible to accommodate these bouts of irritation. Research indicates that in some instances, exercise will reduce feelings of nausea. However, if nausea persists upon initiation of exercise, activity should be stopped (Young-McCaughan, 2006).

2.8 Cachexia

Cachexia is a physical wasting syndrome accompanied by loss of muscle mass, fat mass, overall weight, and appetite. It affects up to 75% of cancer patients, especially those who are in the advanced stages of pancreas, esophagus, and stomach cancer. It is a metabolic disturbance that can result in electrolyte imbalances, weakness, fatigue, and reduced strength. Often, treatment with nutrient supplementation is ineffective (Martingnoni et al., 2003). Patients suffering from cachexia often lack the energy to exercise, so little is known about the impact of exercise on this condition.

2.9 Dehydration

Dehydration is often experienced during chemotherapy, either as a side effect of frequent vomiting and diarrhea, or as a direct effect on the kidneys. Large quantities of water are necessary to help the kidneys filter chemotherapy medication. Fatigue and dizziness are symptoms of dehydration, both of which will impact the exercise response. It is important to ensure adequate fluid intake before, during, and after each exercise session.

2.10 Emotional distress

Cancer survivors will face a multitude of emotions as they battle cancer, creating a strain on interpersonal relationships. These emotions may include anger, depression, anxiety, and elation. This emotional distress can significantly impact a cancer patient's desire to participate in an exercise program.

3. Benefits of exercise

3.1 Risk factors

Not all risk factors that predispose an individual to cancer can be controlled (i.e., age, gender, race, genetic factors). However, healthy behaviors and lifestyle choices, along with environmental exposure risk reduction, can help reduce cancer development. Fifty to 75% of cancer deaths in the US are related to risk factors such as smoking, poor dietary choices, and physical inactivity (National Cancer Institute, 2009). Specifically, obesity and physical inactivity are associated with approximately 25-30% of colon, breast, endometrial, kidney, and esophageal cancers in the US (National Cancer Institute, 2009). The World Health Organization lists physical activity among the nine modifiable risk factors for cancer (World Health Organization, 2009). In addition, recent research supports the assertion that physical activity helps to prevent certain forms of cancer (Kruk, 2007; Miles, 2007), including cancer of the colon (Courneya & Friedenreich, 2007), breast (Courneya & Friedenreich, 2007), endometrium (Courneya & Friedenreich, 2007), prostate (Courneya & Friedenreich, 2007; Friedenreich & Orenstein, 2002), lung (Courneya & Friedenreich, 2007; Friedenreich & Orenstein, 2002), kidney (Friedenreich & Orenstein, 2002), rectus (Friedenreich & Orenstein, 2002), and esophagus (Friedenreich & Orenstein, 2002) cancer. The average risk reduction for each of these cancers varies from approximately 10-40% (Wiggins & Simonavice, 2010). Moderate physical activity (>4.5 METs) appears to be associated with a greater protective effect than activities of lower intensity (Lee, 2003).

3.1.1 Cancer survivorship

In addition to reducing the risk of developing certain forms of cancer, physical activity has also been suggested to increase cancer survivorship by decreasing the risk of cancer recurrence, slowing the progression of cancer, and reducing the risk of secondary life-threatening diseases (Courneya & Friedenreich, 2007; Holmes et al., 2005; Haydon et al., 2005). One investigation (Holmes et al., 2005), revealed a reduction of 26-40% in the relative risk of breast cancer-related death and recurrence among the most active women compared with the least active. Similarly, higher levels of physical activity pre- and post-diagnosis of colon cancer and post-diagnosis of colorectal cancer were associated with a decrease in cancer-related mortality (Haydon et al., 2006; Meyerhardt et al., 2006a, 2006b). As such, the American Cancer Society recommends that exercise serve as an important part of an individual's cancer care plan, asserting that exercise will decrease feelings of fatigue both during and after treatment, and improve an individual's feeling of control and hope (American Cancer Society, 2011). In addition, the 2008 US Department of Health and Human Services (US DHHS) Physical Activity Guidelines for Americans indicate that individuals with chronic conditions, such as cancer, should be "as physically active as their abilities and conditions allow" (Physical Activities Guidelines Advisory Committee, 2008).

3.2 General health benefits of exercise

The general health benefits associated with participating in an exercise program are numerous, and include: improved cardiac output, increased ventilation; improved flexibility and range of motion; increased muscular strength and endurance; decreased resting heart rate; improved stroke volume, vasodilation, perfusion; improved metabolic efficiency; and improved blood counts (Wilmore et al., 2008). Likewise, there are several positive physiological and psychological changes for cancer survivors associated with moderate levels of physical activity and structured exercise.

3.2.1 Aerobic capacity

Research indicates that individuals being treated for cancer have the potential to significantly increase their aerobic capacity by engaging both home-based and structured exercise programs. Young-McCaughan et al (2003) reported an increase in VO_{2max} in cancer survivors following a 12-week exercise program. Thorsen et al (2005) found a significant increase in VO_{2max} for cancer survivors following a 14-week home training program. Wiggins and Simonavice (2008) reported an increase in VO_{2max} in breast cancer survivors after 3 months of resistance and aerobic training. Improvements in VO_{2max} will enhance heart and lung functioning, thereby promoting healthy a blood pressure, blood volume, and gas exchange (Swartz, 2009). In addition, beneficial effects on energy balance, body mass, intestinal transit time, hormone concentrations, and antioxidant enzyme levels have been observed following improvements in aerobic capacity. Research also indicates an inverse relationship between fatigue and aerobic capacity, in that the higher an individual's aerobic capacity, the lower their levels of fatigue, which translates into a positive influence on QOL (DeVita et al., 2008).

3.2.2 Muscular strength and endurance

Several studies report improvements in muscular strength and endurance as a result of participating in an exercise program. In one study, muscular strength increased by approximately 41% in patients who participated in a 6-week resistance training program (Quist et al., 2006). Likewise, a 12-month exercise program resulted in increases in upper body muscular strength and lower body endurance in breast cancer survivors (Wiggins & Simonavice, 2008). Finally, Cheema and Gual (2006) reported improvements in upper and lower body muscular endurance in previously trained breast cancer survivors following an 8-week exercise program. Increased levels of muscular strength and endurance have a positive effect on body composition, and is therefore associated with lower cancer mortality risk (American Heart Association, 2011).

3.2.3 Psychosocial measures

A favorable link between exercise and fatigue, psychosocial measures, and QOL has been reported in the literature. Historically, rest was the most common medical advice given for the treatment of fatigue (Courneya et al., 2000; Coon & Coleman, 2004; Meyerowitz et al., 1983). Unfortunately, this can lead to even more fatigue (Schneider et al., 2003), as well as to aerobic de-conditioning and a lower functional capacity (Courneya et al., 2005). Conversely, several investigations have found that exercise is beneficial in reducing the fatigue experienced by individuals undergoing cancer treatment (Dimeo et al., 1996; Mock et al., 2007; Schwartz et al., 2001; Segal et al., 2001). In general, fatigue tends to subside within the first 5-10 minutes of activity. In terms of long-term improvement, research indicates that regular aerobic exercise over a period of 6 months improved endurance in breast cancer survivors (Damush et al., 2005) and decreased fatigue in patients with prostate and Hodgkin Disease (Watson & Mock, 2004).

Improvements in QOL (Wiggins & Simonavice, 2008, 2009; Courneya et al., 2009), anxiety (Courneya et al., 2003, 2000), depression (Courneya et al., 2003, 2000; Pirl & Roth, 1999), body image (Pinto et al., 2003), immune function (Galvo & Newton, 2005), and emotional well-being (Courneya et al., 2003) have also been reported following structured exercise programs. This holds true, even when cancer treatment has failed. It is believed that feelings of self-confidence and hope are directly related to the restored energy levels obtained through improved cardiorespiratory functioning. In addition, chronic exercise leads to a reduction in obesity and improved gastrointestinal functioning, both of which improve self-image and overall outlook on life (Harriss et al., 2007).

3.2.4 Cancer-specific benefits

A concern with cancer survivors is that they often have comorbid conditions that will influence exercise prescription and management. More often than not, these comorbidities result from the very medications that are used to fight cancer. The good news, however, is that in most cases, exercise has been found to exert a positive effect on these toxicities. An outline of some of these conditions and the associated benefits of exercise is presented in Table 2. It should be noted that, for these adverse effects of cancer treatment, there may be predisposing factors which will influence the severity of the treatment effects.

4. Components of an exercise program

As demonstrated above, exercise is safe and effective both during and after most types of cancer treatment, and should therefore be included as an integral part of an individual's cancer care plan. The American Cancer Society recommends that exercise be part of a continuum of cancer survival care, spanning from treatment to recovery, as well as after-recovery maintenance and living-with-advanced-cancer (Doyle et al., 2006). At present, exercise and cancer recovery programs specifically designed for survivors are being implemented all over the country. The following protocols for exercise training with cancer patients are those employed by the Maple Tree Cancer Alliance® (MTCA®), a cancer rehabilitation center in southwest Ohio dedicated to improving the quality of life of individuals afflicted with cancer by focusing on their physical and spiritual needs. All procedures used by MTCA® follow the guidelines set forth by the American College of Sports Medicine (ACSM). Typically, the training sessions resemble that of a general exercise program, in that they often involve an aerobic component, resistance training, and flexibility exercises. However, given the unique challenges imposed by working with cancer survivors, ACSM recommends that fitness professionals working with cancer patients obtain a specialized training certification prior to training this group of individuals (Schneider & Carter, 2003).

Cancer Treatment Toxicity	Effect of Exercise
Muscular Degeneration: Cancer treatments damage muscle tissue. Muscle damage may be severe enough to cause weakness and fatigue.	Exercise increases the integrity of muscle tissue and protein synthesis, stimulates the release of numerous hormones that increase muscle cell growth and development, and improves metabolism (DeVita et al., 2001; Fischer et al., 2003).
Neurotoxicity: Cancer treatments cause a decrease in motor function.	Exercise can enhance motor unit recruitment and improve neurochemical availability at the cellular and tissue levels (Fischer et al., 2003; Snyder, 1986).
Cardiotoxicity: Cancer treatments cause: decreased left ventricular dysfunction, reduced ejection fraction, diminished contractility, reduced cardiac output and stroke volume, decreased nutrient and oxygen delivery to tissues	Exercise can improve cardiovascular efficiency by strengthening the myocardium, increasing cardiac output and stroke volume, and decreasing resting heart rate and lowering exercise heart rate (DeVita et al., 2001; Fischer et al., 2003).
Pulmonary Toxicity: Cancer treatments cause a disruption in the structural integrity of the airways	Exercise can improve ventilation and transport of oxygen from the environment to the cellular level (Chabner & Longo 2010; Wilson, 1978).

Table 2. Persistent Effects of Cancer Treatments Relative to Exercise Training.

4.1 Phase 1: Exercise during treatment

The following procedures will assist the fitness trainer to design a safe and effective exercise program for patients who are currently undergoing cancer treatment.

4.1.1 Prescreening

Given that cancer survivors often have limitations that pose challenges to exercise, it is necessary that the exercise intervention be individualized according to the needs of each patient. Current health status, cancer treatments, and anticipated disease trajectory must all be taken into consideration by the fitness trainer before designing an exercise program (Schmitz et al., 2010). Therefore, it is important that fitness professionals work closely with physicians and understand the specifics of the cancer survivor's diagnosis and treatments received, including existing health conditions and fitness level prior to cancer diagnosis. This is best obtained through comprehensive prescreening paperwork, which should include information regarding health history, cancer history, and psychological status, along with a medical examination and physician referral (Schneider et al., 2003).

4.1.2 Fitness assessment

Once the prescreening paperwork is completed and reviewed, the patient's current level of fitness should be evaluated through a comprehensive fitness assessment. A comprehensive fitness assessment is one that measures body composition, cardiorespiratory fitness, muscular strength and endurance, flexibility, balance, and range of motion. Specifically, ACSM recommends a graded treadmill or bicycle ergometer test to assess cardiovascular function, a spirometer test for pulmonary function, dumbbells or resistance machines for muscular strength and endurance tests, and the modified sit and reach for flexibility assessment (Schneider & Carter, 2003). In most cases, cancer patients can tolerate the standardized assessment protocols (Swartz, 2009); however, adaptations for certain exercise tests may be necessary if the patient has limited mobility or impaired functioning. Pictures of standard assessments are shown below (Figures 1-5).

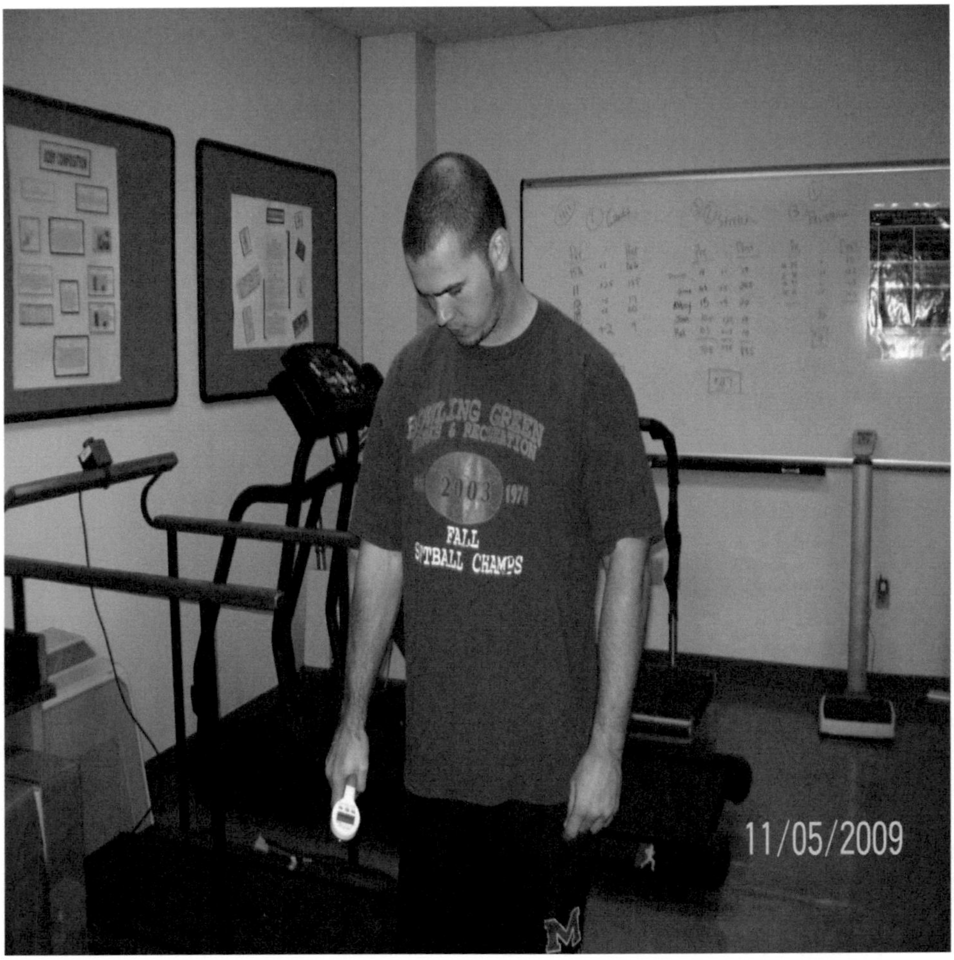

Fig. 1. Muscular Strength Assessment.

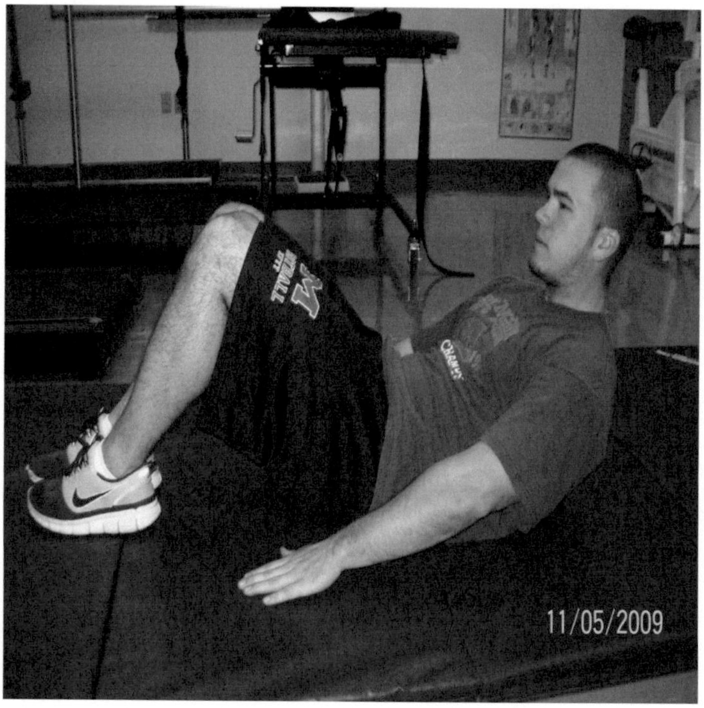

Fig. 2. Muscular Endurance Assessment.

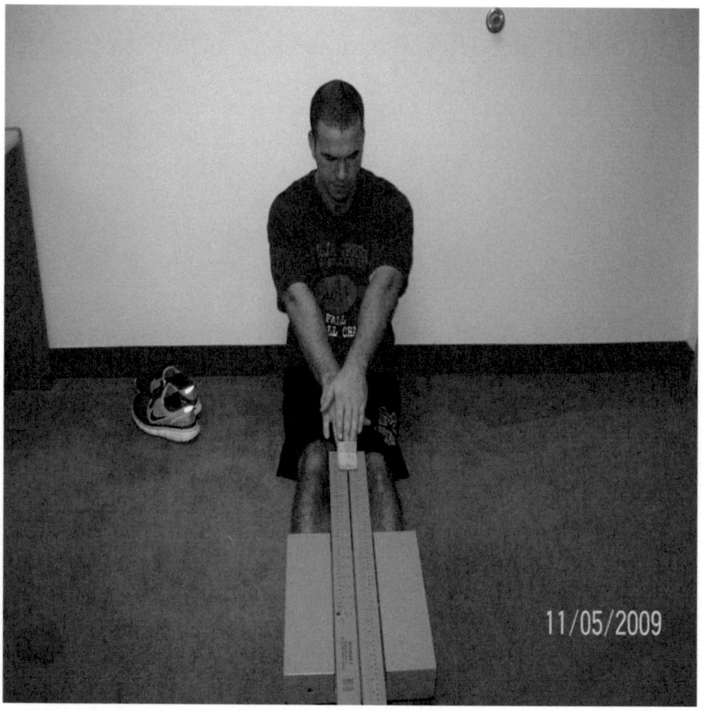

Fig. 3. Flexibility Assessment.

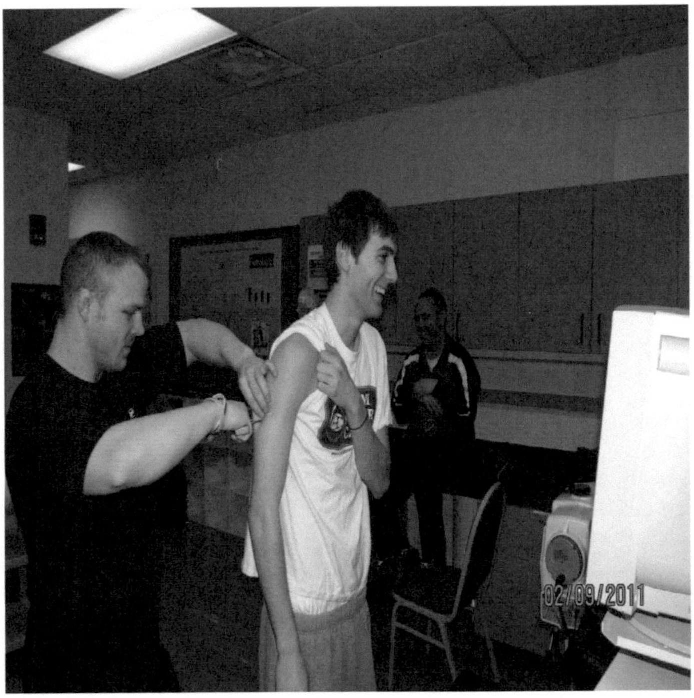

Fig. 4. Body Composition Assessment.

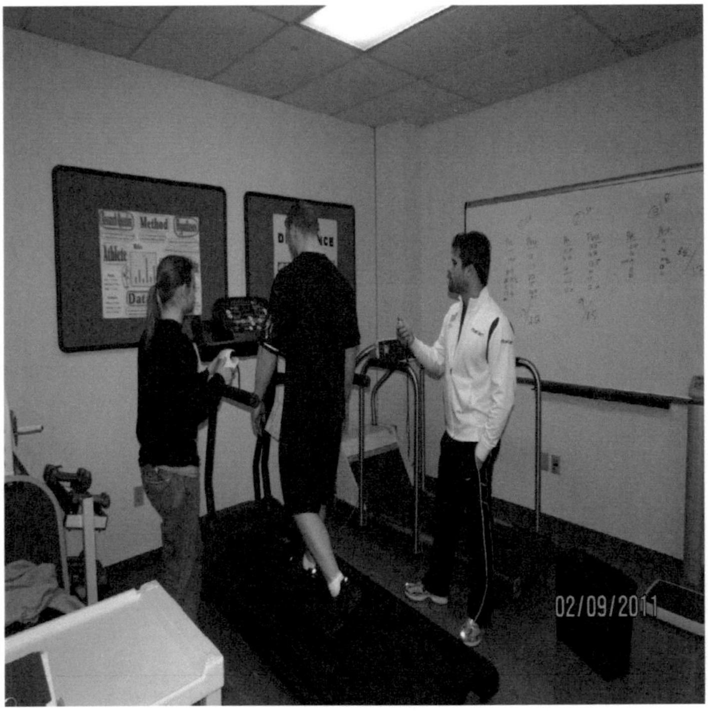

Fig. 5. Cardiovascular Endurance Assessment.

Fitness assessments are useful to quantitatively monitor progress during exercise training. Of note, however, is the fact that cancer-specific norms have not yet been developed. Therefore, the scores received by the cancer patient during his/her fitness assessment are compared to norm charts from a healthy population. This must be taken into consideration during goal setting, particularly for those individuals who are currently undergoing treatment. Typically, for these individuals, as well as patients with recurrent disease, the goal of the exercise program should be simply to preserve function. It is important to have realistic expectations for the exercise intervention so that the patient does not become discouraged, as research indicates that adherence to an exercise intervention is a challenging task (Markes et al., 2006).

4.1.3 Exercise prescription

Once the fitness assessment has been completed and reviewed, the fitness trainer may design an individualized exercise prescription for the patient. An exercise prescription is a plan of fitness-related activities designed for a specific purpose. In other words, an exercise prescription is a prescription for exercise. Recommendations pertaining to the frequency, intensity, duration, mode, and progression of exercise must be addressed. Ideally, for an individual undergoing cancer treatment, the prescription will include a whole-body workout that targets all the major muscle groups. The overall goal of the exercise program should be to minimize the general de-conditioning that often results from cancer treatment so that the cancer treatments are better tolerated. In general, the exercise prescription should include a slow progression and demonstrate adaptability to changes in the patient's health status, which frequently will change from day-to-day during treatment. According to ACSM (Schmitz et al., 2010), the general objectives for exercise training among cancer survivors are as follows:

1. To regain and improve physical function, aerobic capacity, strength, and flexibility.
2. To improve body image and QOL.
3. To improve body composition.
4. To improve cardiorespiratory, endocrine, neurological, muscular, cognitive, and psychosocial outcomes.
5. Potentially, to reduce or delay recurrence or a second primary tumor.
6. To improve the ability to physically and psychologically withstand the ongoing anxiety regarding recurrence or a second primary cancer.
7. To reduce, attenuate, and prevent long-term and late effects of cancer treatment.
8. To improve the physiologic and psychological ability to withstand any current or future cancer treatments.

At present, the optimal frequency, duration, and time course of adaptation to aerobic and resistance exercise training in cancer patients are not known, although research indicates that individuals undergoing cancer therapy benefit from low-to-moderate intensity aerobic and resistance exercise (Swartz, 2009). Based on available data, Table 3 presents some general guidelines a fitness professional may follow when designing an exercise program (Schmitz et al., 2010; Physical Activities Guidelines Advisory Committee, 2008; Haskell et al., 2007; Schneider & Carter, 2003).

Initially, intensity will depend on the patient's functional status and exercise history prior to cancer diagnosis. Typically, previously active cancer patients may continue their exercise regimen, although intensity may need to be decreased during treatment. Progression should consist of increases in frequency and duration rather than in intensity (Physical Activities

Guidelines Committee, 2008; Schneider & Carter, 2003). To assist in progression, patients should be reassessed approximately every 6 months (Schneider & Carter, 2003).

	Aerobic Training	Strength Training	Flexibility Training
Frequency	3-5 days/wk	2-3 days/wk	2-7 days/wk
Intensity	40-60% HRR*	40-60% HRR*	Stretch to the point of mild discomfort
Duration	20-60 min/session	1-3 sets, 8-12 reps per exercise	10-30 seconds per stretch
Mode	Walking, cycling, cross trainers, swimming	Free weights, machines, resistance bands, resistance balls	Static stretching

*HRR = Heart Rate Reserve
HRR = [(Maximum Heart Rate - Resting Heart Rate) x % Intensity] + Resting Heart Rate

Table 3. Guidelines for Designing an Exercise Prescription for Individuals Undergoing Cancer Treatment.

4.1.4 Supervised exercise sessions

Once the individualized exercise prescription has been created, the patient may begin supervised training sessions with the fitness professional. Prior to each exercise session, it is advisable to assess the patient's readiness to exercise. Resting heart rate and blood pressure should be measured, and general information regarding the patient's overall health status should be obtained. Contraindications to exercise are listed in Table 4. Depending on the information attained, the exercise intervention may need to be adjusted for that day.

Onset of nausea following exercise initiation
Vomiting within the last 24 hours
Leg pain
Decreased heart rate and blood pressure with increased workload
Chest pain
Difficult or shallow breathing
Unusual muscle weakness
Numbness in the extremities
Chemotherapy treatment within the last 24-hours
Irregular pulse during exertion
Disorientation and confusion
Dizziness

Table 4. Contraindications to exercise in cancer patients.

Each session should begin with a 5- to 10-minute warm-up that stimulates blood flow to the working muscles. The warm-up should involve some mild stretching and light aerobic activity. During the aerobic component of exercise, it is important to frequently monitor blood pressure and heart rate. If the patient is on a medication that affects heart rate, the Borg Scale of Exertion (Borg, 1973) (Figure 6) may be used to monitor intensity. Based on this scale, a light-to-moderate intensity (RPE of 11 to 14) should be encouraged. If dizziness, nausea, or chest pain occurs, all exercise should be stopped. Frequent short breaks are sometimes encouraged to accommodate therapy-related fatigue. Aerobic exercise should be followed up by static stretching and range of motion exercises for all major muscle groups.

The Borg Scale

6	No exertion at all
7	Extremely light
8	
9	Very light
10	
11	Light
12	
13	Somewhat hard
14	
15	Hard (heavy)
16	
17	Very hard
18	
19	Extremely hard
20	Maximal exertion

Fig. 6. The Borg Scale Rating Perception of Effort (RPE).

The type of resistance exercise performed will depend on the patient's range of motion, tissue removal, and wound healing. ACSM recommends at least 48 hours of rest between each resistance training session (Schneider & Carter, 2003). Therefore, it may be advisable to plan a whole body approach to resistance training, where all major muscle groups are targeted in one day. If the patient is unwilling or unable to participate in traditional modes of strength training, Yoga or Pilates may serve as an alternative form of strength exercise. Sample exercises are shown in pictures below (Figures 7-10).

At the conclusion of the exercise session, the patient should perform a 5-10 minute cool down along with some mild stretching. Sample stretches are shown in the pictures below (Figures 11 and 12). A proper cool down will reduce the potential for muscle soreness, decrease post-exercise dizziness, and allow the heart rate to return to its resting state.

4.2 Phase 2: Exercise after cancer recovery

For patients who have completed cancer therapy, exercise is important to maintain or improve function and prevent the development of diseases associated with inactivity (i.e. diabetes, cardiovascular disease, obesity) (Swartz, 2009). The objective of exercise training during cancer recovery should be to return the patient to their former level of physical function and make exercise an integral part of everyday life. Some side effects of anticancer medications do not appear for months or years after the discontinuation of treatment, therefore it is advised to maintain contact with the patient's physician, in order to monitor any changes in health status. The fitness professional should follow the same general guidelines and procedures listed above when working with a cancer survivor.

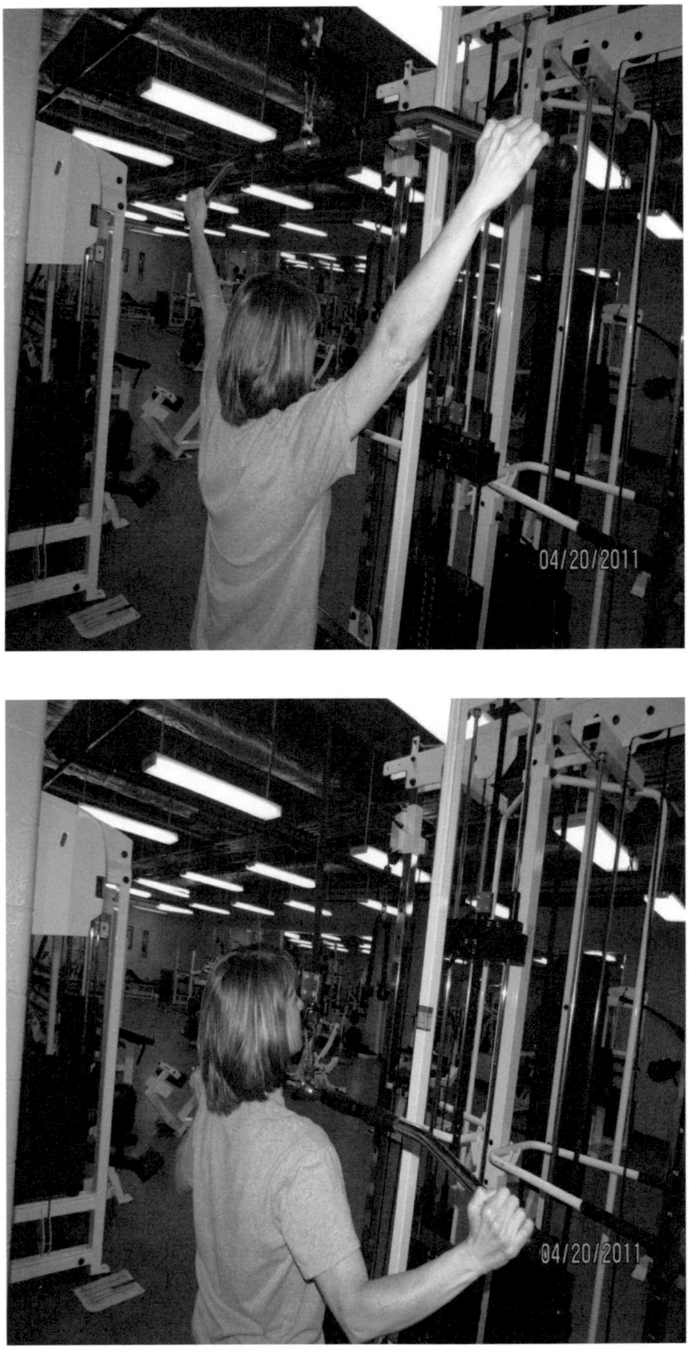

Fig. 7. Lat Pull Down.

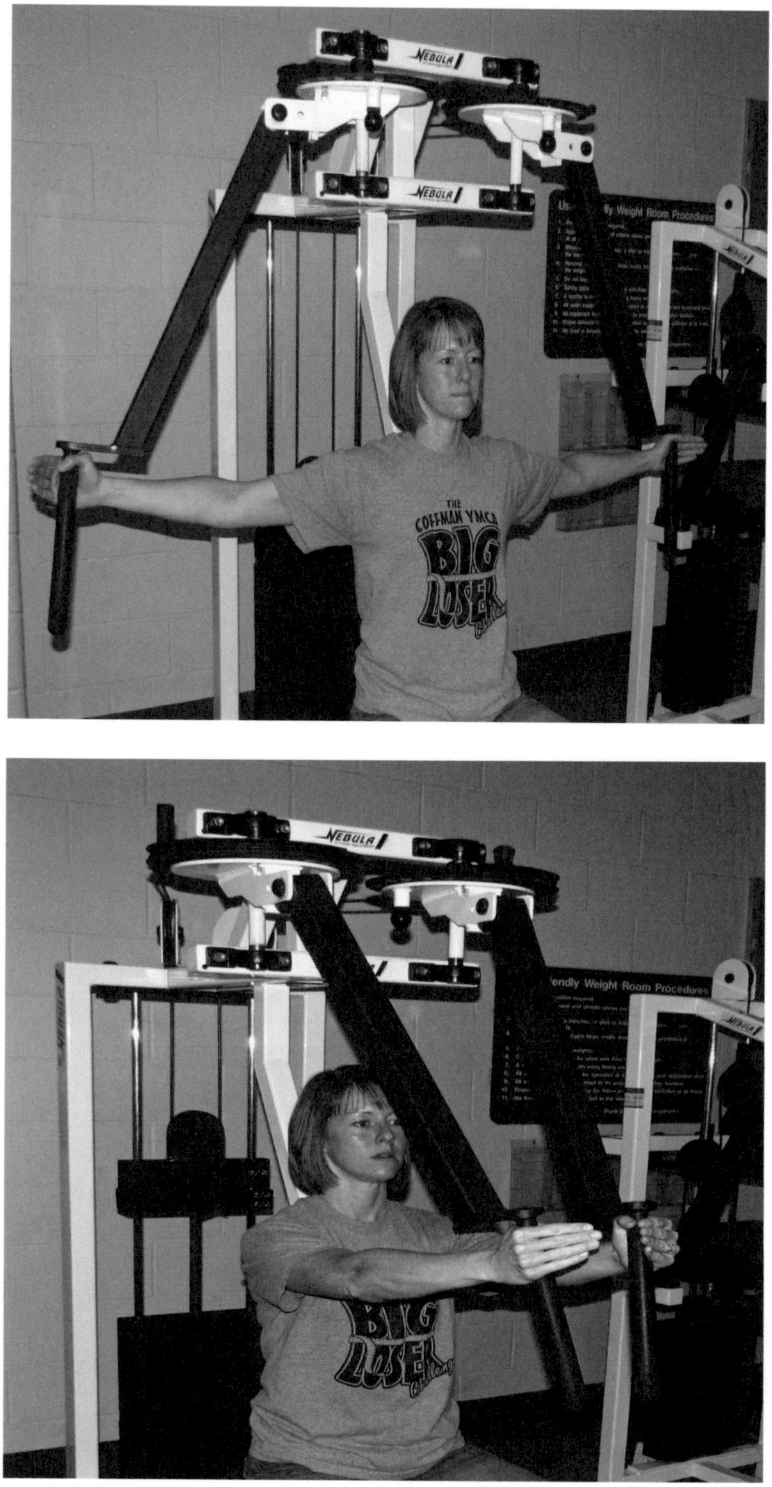

Fig. 8. Lateral Chest Press.

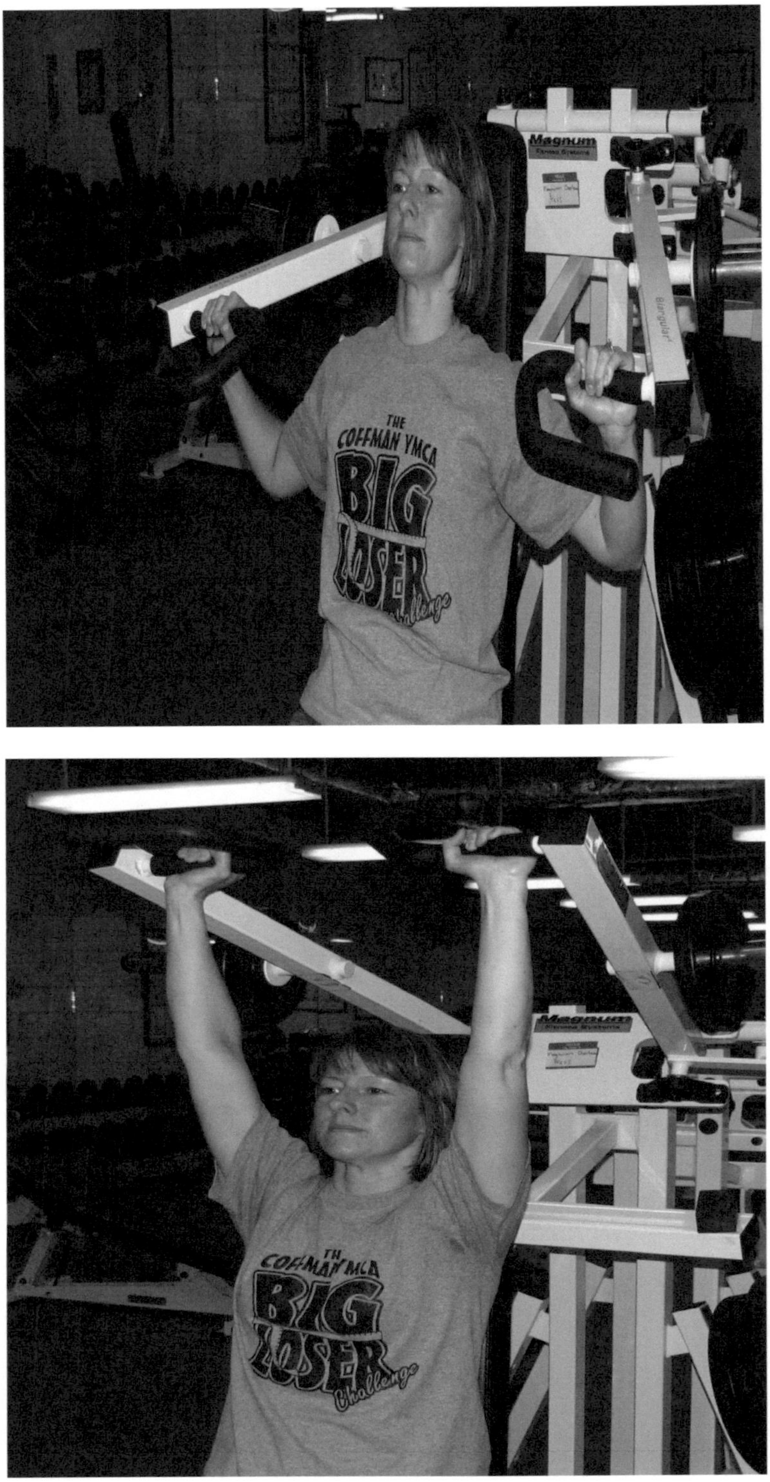

Fig. 9. Shoulder Press.

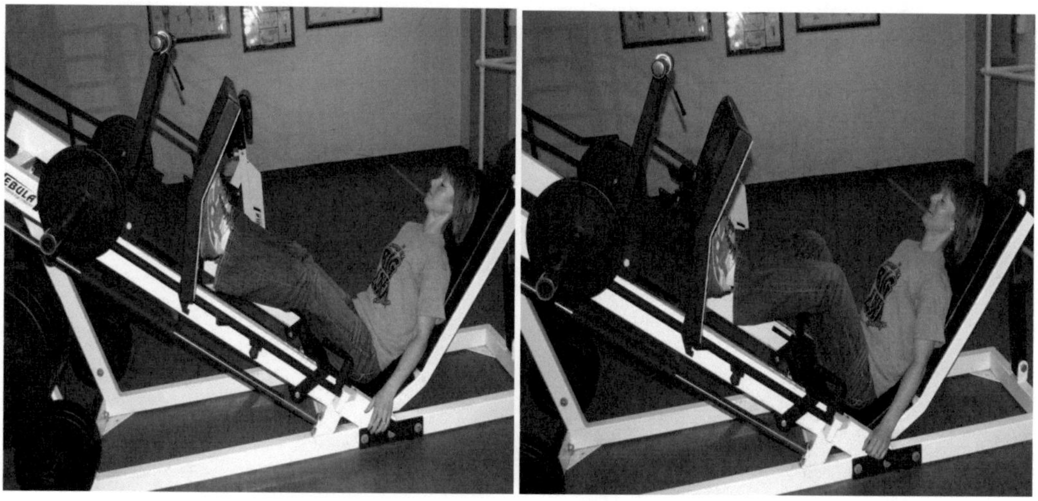

Fig. 10. Leg Press.

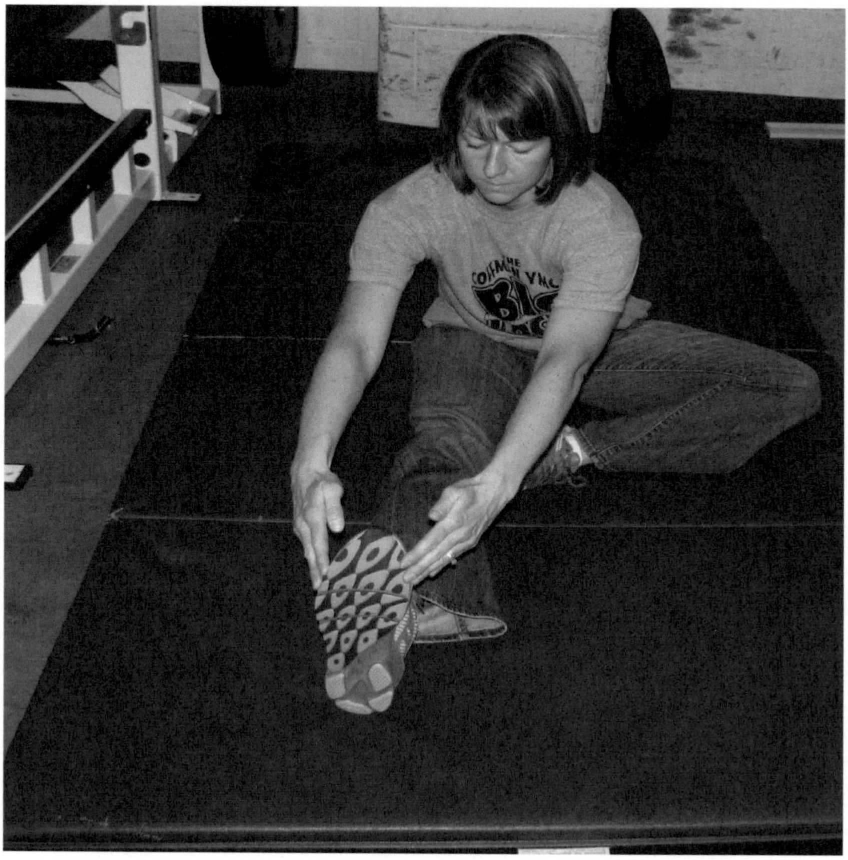

Fig. 11. Lower body stretch.

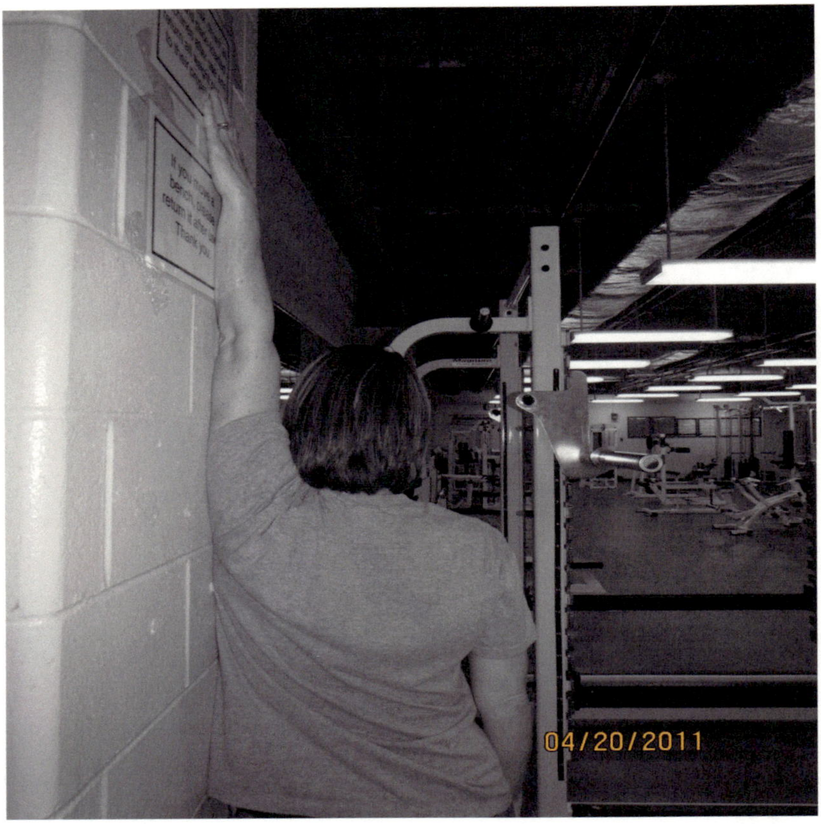

Fig. 12. Upper body stretch.

5. Conclusion

Two decades of research support the assertion that exercise is both safe and beneficial during cancer treatment. Most standard exercise protocols are well tolerated by patients. However, it is important that the fitness professional be aware of the specific effects of cancer and its treatments on the exercise response. Exercise prescriptions must be individualized according to the specific needs and health status of each patient. During each exercise session, modifications may need to be made to ensure patient safety, depending on the changing health of each patient. With the right program, remaining physically active during and after cancer treatment will improve the patient's muscular strength and aerobic functioning, decrease fatigue, improve QOL and have a favorable effect on anxiety.

6. References

Activities Guidelines Advisory Committee. (2008). *Physical Activity Guidelines Advisory Committee Report*. US Department of Health and Human Services, Philadelphia, PA.

American Cancer Society. (2010). Pain Control. Date of access: April 13, 2011. Available from: http://www.cancer.org/Treatment/TreatmentsandSideEffects/PhysicalSideEffects/Pain/PainDiary/pain-control-causes-of-cancer-pain

American Cancer Society. (2011). Stay Healthy. Healthy living information to help you stay well. Date of access: March 24, 2011. Available from: http://www.cancer.org/Healthy/EatHealthyGetActive/GetActive/index

American Heart Association. (2011). Physical Activity. Date of Access: April 14, 2011. Available from: http://www.americanheart.org/presenter.jhtml?identifier=4563

Borg, G.A.V. (1973). *Rating Perception of Effort*. Lippincott, Williams, & Wilkins, Philadelphia, PA.

Cella, D., Lai, J.S., Chang, C.H., Peterman, A., & Slavin, M. (2002). Fatigue in cancer patients compared with fatigue in the general United States population. *Cancer,* 94, No. 2, pp. 528-38.

Centers for Disease Control and Prevention. (2007). Cancer survivors—United States, 2007. *MMWR. Recommendations and reports : Morbidity and mortality weekly report. Recommendations and reports / Centers for Disease Control,* 60,9, pp. 269–272.

Chabner, B.A., & Longo D.L. (2010). *Cancer Chemotherapy and Biotherapy* (5th ed.). Lippincott Williams & Wilkins, ISBN-10: 1605474312, Philadelphia, PA.

Cheema, B.S.B, & Gual, C.A. (2006). Full-body exercise training improves fitness and quality of life in survivors of breast cancer. *Journal of Strength and Conditioning Research,* 20, No. 1, pp.14-21.

Coon, S.K. & Coleman, E.A. (2004). Keep moving: Patients with myeloma talk about exercise and fatigue. *Oncology Nursing Forum.* 31, No. 6, pp. 1127-35.

Courneya, K.S. & Friedenreich, C.M. (2007). Physical activity and cancer control. *Seminars in Oncology Nursing,* 23, pp. 242-52.

Courneya, K.S., Friedenreich, C.M., Quinney, H.A., Fields, A.L.A, Jones, L.W., & Fairey A,S. (2003) A randomized trial of exercise and quality of life in colorectal cancer survivors. *European Journal of Pharmacology,* 12, 347-57.

Courneya, K.S., Keats, M.R., & Turner, A.R. (2000). Physical exercise and quality of life in cancer patients following a high dose chemotherapy and autologous bone marrow transplatation. *Psycho-oncology.* 9, No. 2, pp. 127-36.

Courneya, K.S., Stellar, C.M., Stevinson, C., McNeely, M.L., Peddle, C.J., Friedenreich, C.M., Tankel, K., Basi, S., Chua, N., & Mazurek, A. (2009). Randomized controlled trial of the effects of aerobic exercise on physical functioning and quality of life in lymphoma patients. *Journal of Clinical Oncology,* 27, No. 27, pp. 4605-12.

Courneya, K.S., Vallance, J.K.H., Jones, L.W., & Reiman, T. (2005). Correlates of exercise interventions in non-Hodgkin's lymphoma survivors: An application of the Theory of Planned Behavior. *Journal of Sport and Exercise Psychology,* 27, pp. 335-49.

Damush, T., Perkins, A., & Miller, K. (2006). The implementation of an oncologist referred, exercise self-management program for older breast cancer survivors. *Psycho-oncology* 15, No. 10, pp. 884-90.

DeVita, V.T., Hellman, S., & Rosenberg, S.A. (2001). *Cancer: Principles and Practice of Oncology* (6th ed.). Vols. 1 and 2. Lippincott-Williams & Wilkins, ISBN-10: 0781722292, Philadelphia, PA.

DeVita, V.T., Lawrence, T.S., & Rosenberg, S.A. (2008). Supportive Care and Quality of Life. In: *Cancer: Principles & Practice of Oncology.* Vol. 2. (8th ed.). pp. 2796. Lippincott Williams & Wilkins, ISBN-10: 9780781772075, Philadelphia, PA.

Dimeo, F., Bertz, H., Finde, J., Fetscher, S., Mertelsmann, R., & Kuel, J. (1996). An aerobic exercise program for patients with haematological malignancies after bone marrow transplantation. *Bone Marrow Transplantation*, 18, No. 6, pp. 1157-60.

Douglas, E. (2005). Exercise in cancer patients. *The Physical Therapy Review*, 10, pp. 71-88.

Doyle, C., Kushi, L., Byers, T., Courneya, K.S., Denmark-Wahnefried, W., Grant, B., McTiernan, A., Rock, C.L., Thompson, C., Gansler, T., & Andrews, K.S. (2006). Nutrition and physical activity during and after cancer treatment: an American Cancer Society guide for informed choices. *Cancer Journal for Clinicians*, 56, No. 6, pp. 323-53.

Fischer,D.S., Knobf, M.T., & Durivage, H.J. (2003). *The Cancer Chemotherapy Handbook* (6th ed.). Mosby, ISBN-10: 0323018904, St. Louis.

Friedenreich, C.M. & Orenstein, M.R. (2002). Physical activity and cancer prevention: Etiologic evidence and biological mechanisms. *The Journal of Nutrition*, 132, pp. 5456-64.

Galvo, D.A. & Newton, R.U. (2005). Review of exercise intervention studies in cancer patients. *Journal of Clinical Oncology*, 23, No. 4, 899-909.

Haran, C. & DeVita, V. (2005). The view from the top. *Cancer World*, 6 (June, 2005), pp. 38–43.

Harriss, D., Cable, T., George, K., Reilly, T., Renenan, A.G., & Haboubi, N. (2007). Physical activity before and after diagnosis of colorectal cancer. *Sports Medicine*, 37, No. 11, pp. 947-60.

Hartvig, P., Aulin, J., Hugerth, M., Wallenberg, S., & Wagenius, G. (2006). Fatigue in cancer patients treatedwith cytotoxic drugs. *Journal of Oncology Pharmacy Practice*, 12, No. 3, pp. 155-164.

Haskell, W.L., Lee, I.M., Pate, R.R., Powell, K.E., Blair, S.N., Franklin, B.A., Macera, C.A., Heath, G.W., Thompson, P.D., & Bauman, A. (2007). Physical activity and public health: Updated recommendation for adults from the American College of Sports Medicine and the American Heart Association. *Medicine and Science in Sports and Exercise*, 39, No. 8, pp. 1423-34.

Haydon, A.M., Macinnis, R, English, D, & Giles G.G. (2006). The effect of physical activity and body size on survival after diagnosis with colorectal cancer. *Gut*, 55, No. 1, pp. 62-7.

Holmes, M.D., Chen, W.Y., Feskanich, D, Kroenke, C.H., & Colditz, G.A. (2005). Physical activity and survival after breast cancer diagnosis. *JAMA*, 293, No. 20, pp. 2479-86.

Jones, J.M., Cheng, T., Jackman, M., Rodin, G., Walton, T., & Catton, P. (2010). Self-efficacy, perceived preparedness, and psychological distress in women completing primary treatment for breast cancer. *Journal of Psychosocial Oncology*, 28, No. 3, pp. 269-90.

Kercher, K., Fleischer, A., & Yosipovitch, G. (2008). Lower extremity lymphedema update: pathophysiology, diagnosis, and treatment guidelines. *Journal of the American Academy of Dermatology*, 59, No. 2, 324-31.

Klein, M. (2009). Immunobiological and neural substrates of cancer-related neurocognitive deficits. *The Neuroimmunological Basis of Behavior and Mental Disorders*, 3, pp. 327-40.

Kruk, J. (2007). Physical activity in the prevention of the most frequent chronicdiseases: An analysis of the recent evidence. *Asian Pacific Journal of Cancer Prevention*, 8, pp.325-38.

Lee, I.M. (2003). Physical activity and cancer prevention - data from epidemiologic studies. *Medicine and Science in Sports and Exercise*, 35, No. 11, pp. 1823-7.

Lucia, A., Earnest, C., & Perez M. (2003). Cancer-related fatigue: Can exercise physiology assist oncologists? The *Lancet Oncology*, 4, No. 10, pp. 616-25.

Markes, M., Brockow, T., & Resch, K.L. (2006). Exercise for women receiving adjuvant therapy for breast cancer. *Cochrane Database of Systematic Reviews (Online)*, 18, No. 4, pp. CD005001.

Martingnoni, M., Kunze, P., & Friess, H. (2003). Cancer Cachexia. *Molecular Cancer*, 2, pp. 36.

Meyerhardt, J.A., Giovannucci, E.L., Holmes, M.D., Chan, A.T., Chan, J.A., Colditz, G.A., & Fuchs C.S. (2006). Physical activity and survival after colorectal cancer diagnosis. *Journal of Clinical Oncology*, 24, No. 22, pp. 3527-34.

Meyerhardt, J.A., Heseltine, D., Niedzwiecki, D., Hollis, D., Saltz, L.B., Mayer, R.J., Thomas, J., Nelson, H., Whittom, R., Hantel, A., Schilsky, R.L., & Fuchs, C.S. (2006). Impact of physical activity on cancer recurrence and survival in patients with stage III colon cancer: Findings from CALGB 89803. *Journal of Clinical Oncology*, 24, No. 22, pp. 3535-41.

Meyerowitz, B.E., Watkins, I.K., & Sparks, F.C. (1983). Quality of life for breast cancer patients receiving adjuvant chemotherapy. *The American Journal of Nursing*, 83, No. 2, pp. 232-35.

Miles, L. (2007). Physical activity and the prevention of cancer: A review of recent findings. *Nutrition Bulletin*, 32, pp. 250-82.

Mock, V., Dow, K.H., Meares, C.J., Grimm, P.M., Dienemann, J.A., Haisfield-Wolfe, M.E., Quitasol, W.,

Mitchell, S., Chakravorthy, A., & Gage, I. (2007). Effects of exercise on fatigue, physical functioning, and emotional distress during radiation therapy for breast cancer. *Oncology Nursing Forum*, 24, No. 6, pp. 991-1000.

Muss, H.B. (2007) Breast cancer and differential diagnosis of benign lesions. In *Cecil Medicine* (23rd ed.), Goldman. L., Ausiello, D., eds. Pp. 1501-1509, Saunders Elsevier, ISBN-10: 1416028056, Philadelphia, PA.

National Cancer Institute. (2009) Cancer Trends Progress Report - 2007. Date of access: March 28, 2011. Available from http://progressreport.cancer.gov/doc.asp?pid=1&did=2007&mid=vcol&chid=71

National Institutes of Health. (2011). Estimates of Funding for Various Research,Condition, and Disease Categories. Date of access: March 24, 2011. Available from: http://report.nih.gov/rcdc/categories/

Pihkala, J., Happonen, J.M., Virtanen, K., Souijarvi, A., Simes, M.A., Pesonen, E., & Saarinen U.M. (1995). Cardiopulmonary evaluation of exercise tolerance after chest irradiation and anticancer chemotherapy in children and adolescents. *Pediatrics*. 95, No. 5, pp. 722-26.

Pinto, B., Clark, M., Maruyama, N., & Feder, F. (2003). Psychological and fitness changes associated with exercise participation among women with breast cancer. *Psycho-oncology*. 12, No. 2, pp. 118-26.

Pirl W.F. & Roth, A.J. (1999). Diagnosis and treatment of depression in cancer patients. *Oncology* 13, No. 9, pp. 1293-1301.

Quist, M., Rorth, M., Zacho, M., Andersen, C., Moeller, T., Midtgaard, J., Adamsen, L. (2006). High-intensity resistance and cardiovascular training improve physical capacity in cancer patients undergoing chemotherapy. *Scandinavian Journal of Medicine & Science in Sports*, 16, No. 5, pp. 349-57.

Schneider, C.M., Carter, S. (2003). The role of exercise in recovery from cancer treatment. Rocky Mountain Cancer Rehabilitation Institute. *ACSM Fit Society Page,* 6, pp. 9.

Schneider, C.M., Dennehy, C.A., & Carter, S.D. (2003). *Exercise and Cancer Recovery.* Human Kinetics, ISBN-10: 736036458, Champaign, IL.

Schmitz, K.H., Courneya, K.S., Matthews, C., Demark-Wahnefried, W., Galval, D.A., Pinto, B.M., Irwin, M.L., Wolin, K.Y., Segal, R.J., Lucia, A., Schneider, C.M., von *Gruenigen, V.E.,* & Schwartz, A.L. (2010). *American College of Sports Medicine Roundtable on Exercise Guidelines for Cancer Survivors. Medicine and Science in Sports and Exercise, 42, No. 7, 1409-26.*

Schwartz, A.I., Mori, M., Gao, R., Nail, L.M., & King, M.E. (2001). Exercise reduced daily fatigue in women with breast cancer receiving chemotherapy. *Medicine and Science in Sports and Exercise,* 33, No. 5, pp. 718-23.

Segal, R., Evans, W., Johnson, D., Smith, J., Colletta, S., Gayton, J., Woodard, S., Walls, G., & Reid, R. (2001). Structured exercise improves physical functioning in women with stages I and II breast cancer: Results of a randomized controlled trial. *Journal of Clinical Oncology,* 19, No. 3, pp. 657-65.

Snyder, C.C. (1986). *Oncology Nursing.* Little Brown, Boston.

Swartz, A.L. (2009). Cancer, In: *ACSM's Exercise Management for Persons with Chronic Diseases and Disabilities* (3rd ed.). Durstine, J.L., Moore, G.E., Painter, P.L., Roberts, S.O., (Eds.). pp. 211-218, Human Kinetics, ISBN-10: 0736074333, Champaign, IL.

Thorsen, L., Skovlund, E., Stromme, S.B., Hornslien, K., Dahl, A.A., & Fossa, S.D. (2005). Effectiveness of physical activity on cardiorespiratory fitness and health-Related quality of life in young and middle-aged cancer patients after chemotherapy. *Journal of Clinical Oncology,* 23, No. 10, pp. 2378-88.

Watson, T. & Mock, V. (2004). Exercise as an intervention for cancer-related fatigue. *Physical Therapy,* 84, No. 8, pp. 736-43.

Wiggins, M.S. & Simonavice, E.M. (2008). Quality of life benefits: A 12-month exercise cancer recovery casestudy. KAHPERD Journal. 44, pp.16-9.

Wiggins, M.S. & Simonavice, E.M. (2009). Quality of life benefits in cancer survivorship with supervisedexercise. *Physiological Reports,* 104, No. 2, 421-24.

Wiggins, M.S. & Simonavice, E.M. (2010). Cancer prevention, aerobic capacity, and physical functioning in survivors related to physical activity: A recent review. *Cancer Management and Research,* 2, pp. 157-64.

Wilmore, J.H., Costill, D.L., & Kenney, W.L. (2008). *Physiology of Sport and Exercise.* (4th ed.). Human Kinetics. ISBN-10: 9780736055833, Champaign, IL.

Wilson, J.K.V. (1978). Pulmonary toxicity of antineoplastic drugs. *Cancer Treatment Reports,* 62, No. 12, pp. 2003-8.

World Health Organization. (2009). Geneva: The Organization; 2009. Fact sheet no. 297: Cancer. Date of Access: March 28, 2011. Available from: http://who.int/mediacentre/factsheets/fs297/en/index.html

Young-McCaughan, S., Mays, M.Z., Arzola, S.M., Yoder, LH., Dramiga, S.A., Leclerc K.M., Caton, J.R., Sheffler, R.L., & Nowlin M.U. (2003). Change in exercise tolerance, activity and sleep patterns, and quality of life in patients with cancer participating in a structured exercise program. *Oncology Nursing Forum,* 30, No. 3, pp. 441-52.

Young-McCaughan, S. (2006). Exercise in the rehabilitation from cancer. *Medsurg Nursing,* 15, No. 6, pp. 384-88.

10

Nutritional Supplements for Cancer-Associated Fatigue and Cancer Therapy – A Molecular Basis for Restoring Mitochondrial Function

Garth L. Nicolson
Department of Molecular Pathology, The Institute for Molecular Medicine, Huntington Beach, California, USA

1. Introduction

Cancer patients routinely take multiple - dietary supplements to prevent recurrence or chronic disease, to improve quality of life and overall health, or to reduce the adverse effects of cancer therapy (Gansler et al., 2008; Miller et al., 2009; Ströhle et al., 2010; Velicer & Ulrich, 2008). In fact, one of the most common behavior changes among cancer patients is the use of dietary supplements (Miller et al., 2009).

Although cancer patients routinely use dietary supplements, there is often little consideration as to their safety, efficacy and potential negative effects (Cassileth et al., 2009; Giovannucci & Chan, 2010). In fact, some data suggest that higher than recommended doses of some vitamins and minerals might result in enhancement of carcinogenesis, changes in survival in some cancers and interference with therapy or prescription medications (Cassileth et al., 2009; Giovannucci & Chan, 2010). Nonetheless, several potentially beneficial effects of dietary supplements have been recorded, including reductions in the risk of cancer carcinogenesis and tumor progression, enhancement of immune responses against cancers or immune systems in general, improvements in nutrition and general health, and reductions in the adverse effects of cancer therapy (Cassileth et al., 2009; Doyle et al., 2006; Isenring et all, 2010; Miller et al., 2009; Conklin, 2000; Nicolson & Conklin, 2008; Nicolson, 2010; Ströhle et al., 2010),

This review will concentrate on one particularly troublesome aspect of cancer and cancer therapy—cancer-associated fatigue.

2. The importance of cancer-associated fatigue

Cancer-associated fatigue adds considerably to cancer morbidity (Brown & Kroenke, 2009; Hofman et al., 2007). It exists in all types of cancers from the least to the most progressed cancers (Brown & Kroenke, 2009; Hofman et al., 2007). Along with pain and nausea, it is one of the most common and troublesome symptoms of cancer (Hofman et al., 2007; Prue et al., 2006), especially in advanced cancers (Curt et al., 2000; Prue et al., 2006; Respini et al., 2003).

In patients receiving adjuvant therapies the prevalence of cancer-associated fatigue is reported to be as high as 95% (Sood & Moynihan, 2005). Thus cancer-associated fatigue is a problem before, during and after therapy and can continue to be a problem years after cancer treatment (Curt et al., 2000; Hofman et al., 2007). Cancer-associated fatigue has a very strong negative effect on quality of life; therefore, addressing and reducing cancer-associated fatigue should be an important consideration in the treatment of cancer (Curt et al., 2000; Nicolson, 2010).

Although not well understood, cancer-associated fatigue is thought to be a combination of the effects of having cancer plus the effects of cancer treatments (Curt et al., 2000; Hofman et al., 2007). Unfortunately, cancer-associated fatigue is rarely treated, and is often thought to be an unavoidable symptom (Brown & Kroenke, 2009; Hofman et al., 2007).

Cancer-associated fatigue can be considered to be the product of a variety of contributing factors (Ahlberg et al., 2003). In addition to a decrease in the availability of cellular energy, there are psychological factors, such as the presence of depression, anxiety, sleep disturbances, among others, as well as anemia, endocrine changes, poor nutritional status, release of inflammatory cytokines and cancer therapy that can all contribute to cancer-associated fatigue (Ahlberg et al., 2003; Gutstein, 2001; Manzullo & Escalante, 2002; Sood & Moynihan, 2005). Thus cancer-associated fatigue does not occur as an isolated symptom; rather, it occurs as one of multiple symptoms that are present in cancer patients. Similar to some other symptoms in cancer patients, the severity of cancer-associated fatigue correlates with decreased functional abilities (Given et al., 2001).

Cancer therapy also contributes to cancer-associated fatigue (Sood & Moynihan, 2005). In fact, the most commonly found and disabling effect of cancer therapy is fatigue (Given et al., 2001; Sood & Moynihan, 2005; Vogelzang et al., 1997). During cancer therapy fatigue problems can vary, from mild to severe, and excess fatigue during cancer therapy is a significant reason why patients discontinue therapy (Liu et al., 2005). Reviewing articles on the effects of cancer therapy on fatigue, it was noted that 80-96% of patients receiving chemotherapy and 60-93% receiving radiotherapy experienced moderate to severe fatigue, and fatigue continued for months to years after cancer therapy ended (Manzullo & Escalante, 2002). Therefore, in cancer patients controlling cancer-associated fatigue as well as therapy-induced fatigue are both important strategies (Marrow, 2007).

There have been efforts at understanding and treating cancer-associated fatigue as well as developing ways to distinguish between depression and cancer-associated fatigue (Brown & Kroenke, 2009). Both cancer-associated fatigue and depression have multidimensional and heterogeneous qualities, possessing physical, cognitive and emotional dimensions and a certain degree of overlap across these dimensions (Brown & Kroenke, 2009; Sood & Moynihan, 2005). In cancer patients fatigue or loss of energy is a core aspect of diagnosing depression—thus both fatigue and depression are often diagnosed together. This is usually accomplished by self-assessment, where fatigue and depression are considered to be part of a clinical symptom cluster, co-morbitity or syndrome (Arnold, 2008; Bender et al., 2008). There are techniques, moreover, that can distinguish between these two different symptoms by removal of fatigue-associated assessments from an analysis of depression (Smets et al., 1996; Stone et al., 2000). When assessing fatigue or cancer-associated fatigue, criteria have been established that take depression into consideration, and these two symptoms can thus be separated out by considering unshared properties (Cella et al., 2001).

Chronic or intractable fatigue lasting more than 6 months that is not reversed by normal sleep is the most common complaint of patients seeking general medical care (Kroenke et al., 1988; Morrison, 1980). It occurs naturally during aging and is also an important secondary condition in many clinical diagnoses (Kroenke et al., 1988; McDonald et al., 1993).

Most fatigued patients understand fatigue as a loss of energy and inability to perform even simple tasks without exertion. Many medical conditions are associated with fatigue, including respiratory, coronary, musculoskeletal, and bowel conditions as well as infections (Kroenke et al., 1988; McDonald et al., 1993; Morrison, 1980). However, this symptom is especially important in the overwhelming majority of cancer patients (Ahlberg et al., 2003; Curt et al., 2000; Hofman et al., 2007; Sood, & Moynihan, 2005).

3. Oxidative stress and damage to mitochondrial membranes – Relationship to fatigue

Another phenomenon associated with cancer and its progression as well as aging and age-related degenerative diseases is oxidative stress (Dreher & Junod,1996; Halliwell, 1996; Kehrer, 1993). Oxidative stress is caused by an intracellular excess of reactive oxygen (ROS) and nitrogen (RNS) free radical species over intracellular antioxidants. When this imbalance occurs, it results in oxidation of cellular structures, such as membrane lipids and proteins, and mutation of mitochondrial and nuclear DNA (Abidi & Ali, 1999; Bartsch & Nair, 2004; Marnett, 2000; Stadtman, 2002). ROS and RNS are naturally occurring cellular free radical oxidants that are usually present in low concentrations and are involved in gene expression, intracellular signaling, cell proliferation, antimicrobial defense and other normal cellular processes (Castro & Freeman, 2001; Ghaffari, 2008; Johnson et al., 1996). However, when ROS/RNS are in excess over cellular antioxidants, damage can occur to cellular structures (Abidi & Ali, 1999; Castro & Freeman, 2001; Ghaffari, 2008; Maes & Twisk, 2009). Recently Maes (2009) has proposed a link between excess oxidative stress (and activation of ROS/RNS pathways and fatigue and fatiguing illnesses.

Under normal physiological conditions our cellular antioxidant defenses usually maintain ROS/RNS at appropriate concentrations that prevent excess oxidation of cellular structures (Barber & Harris, 1994; Fridovich,1995; Sun, 1990). Endogenous cellular antioxidant defenses include glutathione peroxidase, catalase and superoxide dismutase, among other enzymes (Jagetia et al., 2003; Seifried et al., 2003), and low molecular weight dietary antioxidants (Aeschbach et al., 1994; Schwartz,1996). Some of these dietary antioxidants have been used as natural chemopreventive agents to shift the excess concentrations of oxidative molecules towards more physiological levels (Prasad et al., 200; Tanaka, 1994).

Excess oxidative stress (or primarily its mediators—excess ROS/RNS) within cancer cells has been linked to promotion and progression of malignancy of cancers (Brown & Bicknell, 2001; Klaunig & Kamendulis, 2004; Ray et al., 2000; Tas et al., 2005; Toyokuni et al., 1995). Thus oxidative stress and antioxidant status have been examined in various malignant cancers, such as breast (Brown & Bicknell, 2001; Kang, 2002; Ray et al., 2000; Tas et al., 2005), prostate (Aydin et al., 2006; Sikka, 2003), colorectal (Otamiri & Sjodahl,1989; Oxdemirler et al., 1989), renal (Asal et al., 1990; Gago-Dominguez et al., 2002), and other malignancies (Batcioglu et al., 2006; Manoharan et al., 2005; Seril et al., 2003). In all of these cancers ROS/RNS were in excess of antioxidant concentrations, resulting in cellular oxidative stress. Thus these cancers could possibly have been induced as a consequence of excess ROS/RNS and oxidative damage to the genetic apparatus (Abidi & Ali, 1999; Dreher & Junod, 1996; Jaruga et al., 1992). Even more likely than carcinogenesis is the promotion of progression of tumors that might not evolve to malignancy in the absence of excess oxidative stress (Nicolson, 2010; Nicolson & Conklin, 2008).

4. Cancer therapy causes excess oxidative stress and severe fatigue

The most common therapies used against cancers, such as chemotherapy, can result in the generation of excess ROS/RNS (Conklin, 2000; 2004). Thus cancer therapy and the resulting production of excess oxidative stress can damage biological systems other than tumors (Conklin, 2004; Nicolson, 2010; Nicolson & Conklin, 2008). During chemotherapy the highest known levels of oxidative stress are generated by anthracycline antibiotics, followed (in no particular order) by alkylating agents, platinum-coordination complexes, epipodophyllotoxins, and camptothecins (Conklin, 2004). The primary site of ROS/RNS generation during cancer chemotherapy is the cytochrome P450 monooxygenase system within liver microsomes. Enzyme systems such as the xanthine-xanthine oxidase system, and non-enzymatic mechanisms (Fenton and Haber-Weiss reactions) also play a role in creating excess oxidative stress during chemotherapy. The very high levels of oxidative stress caused by anthracyclines are also related to their ability to displace coenzyme Q_{10} (CoQ_{10}) from the electron transport system of cardiac mitochondria, resulting in diversion of electrons directly to molecular oxygen with the formation of superoxide radicals (Conklin, 2000; 2004).

Although anthracyclines and other chemotherapeutic agents cause generation of high levels of ROS/RNS, not all chemotherapeutic agents generate excess oxidative stress. Some agents generate only modest amounts of ROS/RNS. Examples of this are: platinum-coordination complexes and camptothecins, taxanes, vinca alkaloids, anti-metabolites, such as the antifolates, and nucleoside and nucleotide analogues (Conklin, 2000; 2004; Nicolson & Conklin, 2008). Most chemotherapeutic agents do, however, generate some oxidative stress, as do all anti-neoplastic agents when they induce apoptosis in cancer cells. Drug-induced apoptosis is usually triggered by the release of cytochrome c from the mitochondrial electron transport chain. When this occurs, electrons are diverted from NADH dehydrogenase and reduced CoQ_{10} to oxygen, resulting in the formation of superoxide radicals (Betteridge, 2000; Conklin, 2000).

Use of chemotherapeutic agents to treat cancer causes oxidative stress that produces side effects, including fatigue. This can reduce the efficacy of therapy (Nicolson & Conklin, 2008; Nicolson, 2010). Many anti-neoplastic agents have clearly established mechanisms of action that are not dependent upon the generation of ROS/RNS; however, these drugs can only mediate their anticancer effects on cancer cells that exhibit unrestricted progression through the cell cycle and have intact apoptotic pathways. Oxidative stress interferes with cell cycle progression by inhibiting the transition of cells from the G_0 to G_1 phase, slowing progression through S phase by inhibition of DNA synthesis, inhibiting cell cycle progression of G_1 to S phase, and by checkpoint arrest (Balin et al., 1978; Gonzalez, 1992; Hauptlorenz et al., 1985; Kurata, 2000; Schackelford et al., 2000).

Chemotherapeutic agents can also activate DNA repair systems. DNA repair of damage caused by alkylating agents and platinum complexes results in resistance to these drugs, and checkpoint arrest during oxidative stress can enhance the repair processes and diminish the efficacy of treatment (Fojo, 2001; Wei et al., 2000; Zhen et al., 1992). Abolishing checkpoint arrest produces the opposite effect and enhances the cytotoxicity of antineoplastic agents. By reducing oxidative stress, antioxidants counteract the effects of chemotherapy-induced oxidative stress on the cell cycle and enhance the cytotoxicity of antineoplastic agents (Conklin, 2004).

Oxidative stress can affect important intracellular signal transduction pathways that are necessary for the action of some antineoplastic agents (Conklin, 2004; Hampton et al., 1998;

Shacter et al., 2000). There are two major pathways of drug-induced apoptosis following cellular damage by antineoplastic agents: the mitochondrial pathway, initiated by release of cytochrome c, and the CD95 death receptor pathway, initiated by CD95L binding to its death receptor (Fojo, 2001). Oxidative stress during chemotherapy results in the generation of highly electrophilic aldehydes that have the ability to bind to the nucleophilic active sites of caspases as well as the extracellular domain of the CD95 death receptor. This inhibits caspase activity and the binding of CD96L ligand, and this results in the impairment of the ability of antineoplastic agents to initiate apoptosis (Chandra et al., 2000; Hampton et al., 1998; Shacter et al., 2000).

In addition to chemotherapy, radiotherapy also results in generation of oxidative stress and excess ROS/RNS (Feinendegen et al., 2007; Greenberger et al., 2001). The principal target of radiation is tumor cell DNA, and this can be directly damaged by radiation. However, genetic damage is also mediated by excess ROS/RNS (Epperly et al., 2003; Feinendegen et al., 2007). Recently the principal source of excess ROS/RNS during radiotherapy has been shown to be the mitochondria (Epperly et al., 2003; Sabbarova & Kanai, 2007). The initial cytotoxicity of radiation is now thought to be due to excess ROS/RNS triggering of apoptosis via alteration of mitochondrial metabolism. This causes transiently opening of mitochondrial permeability transition pores, which increases the influx of calcium ions into the matrix. The influx of calcium ions stimulates mitochondrial nitric oxide synthase and generation of nitric oxide, which inhibits the respiratory chain and eventually stimulates excess ROS/RNS free radicals that initiate apoptosis (Leach et al., 2002; Sabbarova & Kanai, 2007).

5. Cancer therapy and mitochondrial damage

Cancer therapy is associated with several adverse side effects. One of the most difficult side effects is caused by chemotherapeutic drug damage to mitochondria (Conklin, 2000; Nicolson & Conklin, 2008). Cardiac mitochondria are especially sensitive to certain chemotherapy agents, such as anthracycline antibiotics (Conklin, 2004). Anthracycline-induced cardiac toxicity is characterized by acute, reversible toxicity that causes electrocardiographic changes and depressed myocardial contractility and by chronic, irreversible, dose-related cardiomyopathy (Conklin, 2004; 2005). The selective anthracycline-induced toxicity to cardiac cells is due to damage of cardiac mitochondria. The sensitivity of cardiac cells to anthracyclines, such as doxorubicin, has been found to be due to the unique properties of cardiac mitochondria in that they possess a Complex I-associated NADH dehydrogenase in the inner mitochondrial membrane facing the cytosol (Lehninger, 1951; Rasumssen & Rasmussen, 1985).

Doxorubicin is a relatively small molecule, and because of this property it readily penetrates the outer mitochondrial membrane. However, because it is hydrophilic and cannot partition into the lipid membrane matrix, it cannot penetrate the inner mitochondrial membrane (Conklin, 2005; Nohl, 1987). Thus, it cannot participate in oxidation-reduction reactions with the type of inner matrix-facing, electron transport chain dehydrogenases found in most types of cells, including most tumor cells (Conklin, 2005; Nohl, 1987). But in heart cells doxorubicin can interact with the mitochondrial cytosolic-facing NADH dehydrogenase that is unique to this tissue (Davies & Doroshow, 1986; Doroshow & Davies, 1986). This interaction produces doxorubicin aglycones, which are highly lipid soluble and readily penetrate the inner mitochondrial membrane (Conklin, 2005; Gille & Nohl, 1997). At this location they can displace CoQ_{10} from the electron transport chain (Conklin, 2005; Davies & Doroshow, 1986).

The displacement of CoQ_{10} from the electron transport chain during doxorubicin treatment results in decreases of CoQ_{10} in cardiac muscle (Karlsson et al., 1986) as the plasma concentration of CoQ_{10} increases (Eaton et al., 2000). CoQ_{10} normally accepts electrons from Complexes I and II and transfers them down the electron transport chain, resulting in the formation of water. However, the presence of aglycones in the inner mitochondrial membrane and inner matrix results in the transfer the electrons directly to molecular oxygen, resulting in the formation of superoxide radicals (Papadopoulou & Tsiftsoglou, 1996). Thus, doxorubicin generates a high level of oxidative stress in cardiac mitochondria, causing acute cardiac toxicity and damage to mitochondrial DNA (Conklin, 2005; Doroshow & Davies, 1986; Palmeira et al., 1991).

Anthracycline-damaged cardiac cell mitochondria cannot sustain their function, and changes in their structure results in disruption of mitochondria and eventually apoptosis (Serrano et al., 1999; Conklin, 2005; Gille & Nohl, 1997). This produces cardiac insufficiency and an inability to respond to pharmacological interventions, resulting ultimately in cardiac failure. However, if CoQ_{10} is administered during anthracycline chemotherapy, damage to the heart is prevented by decreasing anthracycline metabolism within cardiac mitochondria and by competing with aglycones for the CoQ_{10} sites within the electron transport chain (Conklin, 2005). Thus, CoQ_{10} administered concurrently with anthracyclines can maintain the integrity of cardiac mitochondria and prevent damage to the heart, and at the same time enhancing the anti-cancer activity of anthracyclines (Conklin, 2000; 2005).

In addition to chemotherapy, radiotherapy also produces damage to tissues other than cancerous tissues. Agents that protect tissues against radiation effects have been used to reduce unwanted damage (Brizel, 2007; Sabbarova & Kanai, 2007).

Radioprotective agents that have been used to decrease the adverse effects of radiotherapy are: antioxidants, free radical scavengers, inhibitors of nitric oxide synthase and anti-inflammatory and immunomodulatory agents (Brizel, 2007; Sabbarova & Kanai, 2007). The most effective of these under development target mitochondria, such as proteins and peptides that can be transported into mitochondria and plasmids or nucleotide sequences, for example, agents that target and stimulate mitochondrial manganese superoxide dismutase genes to produce this important dismutase have been used as radioprotective agents (Sabbarova & Kanai, 2007).

6. Molecular replacement of mitochondrial components during cancer therapy

As discussed in Section 5, chemotherapy can displace important mitochondrial cofactors, such as CoQ_{10} (Conklin, 2000; 2005). During chemotherapy replacement of CoQ_{10} dramatically prevents development of anthracycline-induced cardiomyopathy and histopathological changes. It can also prevent changes in electrocardiograms (EKG) characteristic of anthracycline-induced heart damage (Domae et al., 1981). Indeed, the administration of CoQ_{10} to animals resulted in increased survival, improvement in the EKG patterns, and reduced heart histopathological changes (Usui et al., 1982). These preclinical data, along with clinical data (discussed in Conklin, 2004 and Nicolson & Conklin, 2008) support the contention that CoQ_{10} protects the heart tssue from anthracycline-induced damage.

During chemotherapy of cancer, patients have received concurrent administration of CoQ_{10}. This can affect both acute and chronic cardiotoxicity caused by anthracyclines (Conklin, 2004; 2005; Nicolson & Conklin, 2008). For example, Judy et al. (1984) studied the importance of administering CoQ_{10} on the development of doxorubicin-induced cardiotoxicity in patients with lung cancer. Doxorubicin given alone without CoQ_{10} caused marked impairment of cardiac function with a significant increase in heart rate and a substantial decrease in ejection fraction, stroke index and cardiac index. In contrast, doxorubicin administered along with CoQ_{10}, did not cause cardiotoxicity—cardiac function remained unchanged. Other studies have confirmed these results and have shown that CoQ_{10} can reduce the cardiac toxicity of doxorubicin in adults (Buckingham et al., 1997; Cortes et al., 1978) and children (Iarussi et al., 1994; Loke et al., 2006).

Thus in preclinical and clinical studies the data indicate that CoQ_{10} protects the heart from the cardiotoxicity of anthracyclines. The impact of CoQ_{10} on the anti-neoplastic efficacy of anthracycline-based chemotherapy, however, was not studied in these reports (Buckingham et al., 1997; Cortes et al., 1978; Iarussi et al., 1994; Loke et al., 2006).

7. Cancer-associated fatigue and other cancer-associated conditions

The most common complaint of patients undergoing anti-neoplastic therapy is fatigue, but there are also other complaints that include: pain, nausea, vomiting, malaise, diarrhea, headaches, rashes and infections (Buckingham et al., 1997; Loke et al., 2006; Manzullo & Escalante, 2002). Other more serious problems can also occur, such as cardiomyopathy, peripheral neuropathy, hepatotoxicity, pulmonary fibrosis, mucositis and other effects (Buckingham et al., 1997; Liu et al., 2005; Loke et al., 2006; Manzullo & Escalante, 2002). Due to misconceptions among patients and their physicians, most patients feel that cancer therapy-associated fatigue is an untreatable symptom (Vogelzang et al., 1997). Although fatigue is usually the most commonly reported adverse symptom during cancer therapy, up until recently there was little effort directed at reducing fatigue before, during or after cancer therapy (Von Roenn & Paice, 2005). This has changed recently (Nicolson, 2010; Nicolson & Conklin, 2008).

Reducing cancer-associated fatigue and fatigue associated with cancer therapy are now considered important therapeutic goals. Psychological, physical, pharmaceutical and nutraceutical methods have been undertaken to reduce fatigue and improve the quality of life of cancer patients (Borneman et al., 2007; Escalante et al., 2011; Nicolson, 2010). These treatments are based on suppressing fatigue but also on controlling co-morbid or related symptoms, such as pain, anemia, cachexia, sleep disorders, depression and other symptoms (Escalante et al., 2011; Mustian et al., 2007; Nicolson, 2010; Ryan et al., 2007; Watson & Mock, 2004; Zee & Acoli-Isreal, 2009).

Unfortunately, there is no standard protocol related to treating cancer-associated fatigue and related symptoms. In reviewing the types of supportive measures used to control fatigue and related symptoms, the data suggest that graded exercise, nutritional support, treatment of psychological problems (such as depression with certain anti-depressants or psycostimulants), treatment of anemia with hematopoetic growth factors and control of insomnia with cognitive behavioral therapy or pharmacological and nonpharmacological therapies all have a role to various degrees in controlling cancer-associated fatigue

(Escalante et al., 2011; Mustian et al., 2007; Nicolson, 2010; Ryan et al., 2007; Watson & Mock, 2004; Zee & Acoli-Isreal, 2009). Some of these approaches using pharmacological drugs and growth factors have been systematically analyzed in 27 studies (meta-analysis) by Milton et al. (2008). In this limited analysis, only a psycostimulant (methylphenidate) and hematopoetic growth factors (erythropoietin and darbopeitin) were more effective than placebo treatments. Other treatments were no better than placebo in the treatment of cancer-related fatigue (Milton et al., 2008).

8. Cancer-associated fatigue, aging and oxidative mitochondrial damage

Cancer-associated fatigue has been defined as a multidimensional sensation (McDonald et al., 1993; Milton et al., 2008; Mustian et al., 2007; Ryan et al., 2007). Most patients understand fatigue as a loss of energy and inability to perform even simple tasks without exertion (Levy, 2008; Milton et al., 2008). Cancer-associated fatigue has been described as the dysregulation of several interrelated physiological, biochemical and psychological systems (Mustian et al., 2007; Ryan et al., 2007), but at the tissue and cellular levels fatigue is related to reductions in the efficiency of cellular energy systems, mainly found in mitochondria (Agadjanyan et al., 2003; Nicolson, 2003; 2005). Damage to mitochondrial components, mainly by ROS/RNS oxidation, can impair mitochondrial function, and this can also result in oxidative damage (reviewed in Bartsch & Nair, 2004; Castro & Freeman, 2001; Kehrer, 1993). Mitochondrial membranes and DNA are major targets of oxidative stress, and with aging ROS/RNS mitochondrial damage can accumulate (Huang & Manton, 2004; Wei & Lee, 2002).

During aging and in certain medical conditions oxidative damage to mitochondrial membranes impairs mitochondrial function (Huang & Manton, 2004; Logan & Wong, 2001; Wei & Lee, 2002). For example, in chronic fatigue syndrome patients there is evidence of oxidative damage to DNA and lipids (Logan & Wong, 2001; Manuel y Keenoy et al., 2001) as well as oxidized blood markers (Richards et al., 2000) and muscle membrane lipids (Felle et al., 2000) that are indicative of excess oxidative stress (Dianzani, 1993). In chronic fatigue syndrome patients also have sustained elevated levels of peroxynitrite due to excess nitric oxide, which can result in lipid peroxidation and loss of mitochondrial function as well as changes in cytokine levels that exert a positive feedback on nitric oxide production, increasing the rate of membrane damage (Pall, 2000).

9. Molecular replacement of oxidized membrane components and its effect on fatigue

In cancer patients mitochondrial membranes as well as other cellular membranes are especially sensitive to oxidative damage by ROS/RNS, which occurs at high rates in cancer (Batcioglu et al., 2006; Dianzani, 1993; Gago-Dominguez et al., 2002; Manoharan et al., 2005; Otamiri & Sjodahl, 1989; Oxdemirler et al., 1989; Seril et al., 2003). Oxidation of membrane phospholipids alters their structure, affecting lipid fluidity, permeability and membrane function (Dianzani, 1993; Nicolson et al., 1977; Subczynski & Wisniewska, 2000). One of the most important events caused by ROS/RNS damage is loss of electron transport function, and this appears to be related to mitochondrial membrane lipid peroxidation. Membrane oxidation induces permeability changes in mitochondria, and this can cause loss of mitochondrial transmembrane potential, an essential requirement of oxidative phosphorylation (Kanno et al., 2004; Radi et al., 1994).

Lipid Replacement Therapy (Nicolson, 2003; 2005; 2010) has been used to reverse the accumulation of damaged lipids in mitochondria and other cellular membranes. Lipid Replacement Therapy plus antioxidants can reverse ROS/RNS damage and increase mitochondrial function in certain fatiguing disorders, such as chronic fatigue, chronic fatigue syndrome and fibromyalgia syndrome. Lipid Replacement Therapy has been found to be effective in preventing ROS/RNS-associated changes and reversing mitochondrial damage and loss of function (reviewed in Nicolson, 2010; Nicolson & Ellithrope, 2006).

Lipid Replacement Therapy with unoxidized lipid and antioxidant supplements has been effective in replacement of damaged cellular and mitochondrial membrane phospholipids and other lipids that are essential structural and functional components of all biological membranes (reviewed in Nicolson, 2010; Nicolson & Ellithrope, 2003). NTFactor, a Lipid Replacement oral supplement containing phospholipids, phosphoglycolipids, cardiolipid precursors and other membrane lipids, has been used successfully in animal and clinical lipid replacement studies (Agadjanyan et al., 2003; Ellithorpe et al., 2003; Nicolson & Ellithorpe, 2006; Nicolson et al., 2010). NTFactor's encapsulated lipids are protected from oxidation in the gut and can be absorbed and transported into tissues via lipid carriers without oxidation. Once inside cells the membrane lipids naturally replace oxidized, damaged membrane lipids by natural diffusion, and carrier proteins pick up the damaged lipids for degradation, transport and excretion (Mansbach & Dowell, 2000).

In preclinical studies NTFactor has been used to reduce age-related functional damage. Using rodents Seidman et al. (2002) found that NTFactor prevented hearing loss associated with aging and shifted the threshold hearing from 35-40 dB in control, aged rodents to 13-17 dB. They also found that NTFactor preserved cochlear mitochondrial function and prevented aging-related mitochondrial DNA deletions found in the cochlear. Thus NTFactor was successful in preventing age-associated hearing loss and reducing mitochondrial damage and DNA deletions in rodents (Seidman et al. 2002).

In clinical studies Lipid Replacement Therapy has been used to reduce fatigue and protect cellular and mitochondrial membranes from oxidative damage by ROS/RNS (reviewed in Nicolson, 2003; 2005; 2010). A vitamin supplement mixture containing NTFactor was by used by Ellithorpe et al. (2003) in a study of patients with severe chronic fatigue and was found to reduce their fatigue by approximately 40.5% in 8 weeks. In these studies fatigue was monitored by use of the Piper Fatigue Scale to measure clinical fatigue and quality of life (Piper et al., 1987). In addition, in a subsequent study we examined the effects of NTFactor on fatigue and mitochondrial function in patients with chronic fatigue (Agadjanyan et al., 2003). Oral administration of NTFactor for 12 weeks resulted in a 35.5% reduction in fatigue and 26.8% increase in mitochondrial function; whereas after a 12-week wash-out period fatigue increased and mitochondrial function decreased back towards control levels (Agadjanyan et al., 2003). Thus in fatigued subjects dietary Lipid Replacement Therapy can significantly improve and even restore mitochondrial function and significantly decrease fatigue. Similar findings were observed in chronic fatigue syndrome and fibromyalgia syndrome patients (Nicolson & Ellithorpe, 2003). Recently a new formulation of NTFactor plus vitamins, minerals and other supplements resulted in a 36.8% reduction in fatigue within one week (Nicolson et al., 2010) (Table 1).

Subjects/patients	n	age	Average Time on NTFactor	Piper Fatigue Scale fatigue reduction (%)	Reference
Chronic fatigue	34	50.3	8 wks	40.5**	Ellithorpe et al., 2003
Aging, chronic fatigue	20	68.9	12 wks	35.5*	Agadjanyan et al., 2003
Chronic fatigue syndrome (and/or fibromyalgia syndrome#)	15	44.8	8 wks	43.1*	Nicolson & Ellithorpe, 2003
Aging, chronic fatigue	67	57.3	1 wk	36.8*	Nicolson et al., 2010

Modified from Nicolson (2010)
**P<0.0001, *P<0.001 compared to without NTFactor
#5/15 fibromyalgia syndrome; 3/15 chronic fatigue syndrome plus fibromyalgia syndrome
Ad

Table 1. Effects of dietary Lipid Replacement supplement NTFactor on Piper Fatigue Scale scores.

10. Lipid replacement therapy in conjunction with cancer therapy

Lipid Replacement Therapy has been used to reduce the adverse effects of chemotherapy in cancer patients (Nicolson, 2010). For example, a vitamin-mineral mixture with NTFactor has been used in cancer patients to reduce some of most common adverse effects of cancer therapy, such as chemotherapy-induced fatigue, nausea, vomiting, malaise, diarrhea, headaches and other side effects (Colodny et al., 2000). In two studies on patients with advanced metastatic colon, pancreatic or rectal cancers receiving a 12-week chemotherapy treatment schedule of 5-florouracil/methotrexate/leukovorin Lipid Replacement Therapy was used to reduce adverse effects of chemotherapy.

In the first unblinded part of the clinical study the effectiveness of NTFactor in a vitamin-mineral mixture administered before and during chemotherapy was determined by examining signs and symptoms, and in particular, the side effects of therapy. A quality of life evaluation was conducted by a research nurse, and it was determined that patients on NTFactor supplementation experienced significantly fewer episodes of fatigue, nausea, diarrhea, constipation, skin changes, insomnia and other side effects (Colodny et al., 2000). In this open label trial 81% of patients demonstrated an overall improvement in quality of life parameters while on chemotherapy with Lipid Replacement Therapy (Colodny et al., 2000).

In the double-blinded, cross-over, placebo-controlled, randomized part of the study on advanced cancers the patients on chemotherapy plus Lipid Replacement Therapy showed improvements in signs/symptoms associated with the adverse effects of chemotherapy (Colodny et al., 2000). Adding Lipid Replacement resulted in improvements in the incidence of fatigue, nausea, diarrhea, impaired taste, constipation, insomnia and other quality of life indicators. Following cross-over from the placebo arm to the Lipid Replacement Therapy arm, 57-70% of patients on chemotherapy reported improvements in nausea, impaired taste, tiredness, appetite, sick feeling and other quality of life indicators (Colodny et al., 2000) (Table 2). This clinical trial and other data clearly demonstrated the usefulness of Lipid Replacement Therapy given during chemotherapy to reduce the adverse effects of cancer therapy (Nicolson, 2010).

First arm	Second arm	Average % patients on test arm# improvement	no change	worsening
placebo	Propax(+NTFactor)	57	22	21
Propax(+NTFactor)	placebo	70	6	24

Table modified from Nicolson (2010).
* The same regimen of 5-flurouracil/methotrexate/leukovoran was used for colon, pancreatic or rectal cancers.
#The percent of patients' self-reporting adverse effects was averaged with the percent of patients with adverse effects reported by a research nurse.

Table 2. Effects of Propax with NTFactor on the adverse effects of chemotherapy in a cross-over trial.

11. Summary – Cancer-sssociated fatigue and its treatment

Nutritional supplements have been used in a variety of diseases to provide patients with a natural, safe alternative to pharmacological drugs. In patients with cancer nutritional supplements are often used for specific purposes or to improve quality of life. For example, cancer-associated fatigue is one of the most common symptoms in all forms and stages of cancer, but few patients receive assistance for their fatigue. Cancer-associated fatigue is associated with cellular oxidative stress, and during cancer therapy excess drug-induced oxidative stress can cause a number of adverse effects, including: fatigue, nausea, vomiting and more serious effects. Cancer-associated fatigue and the adverse effects of cancer therapy can be reduced with Lipid Replacement Therapy, a natural lipid supplement formulation that replaces damaged membrane lipids along with providing antioxidants and enzymatic cofactors. Administering dietary Lipid Replacement Therapy can reduce oxidative membrane damage and restore mitochondrial and other cellular functions. Recent clinical trials using cancer and non-cancer patients with chronic fatigue have shown the benefits of specific Lipid Replacement Therapy nutritional lipid supplements in reducing fatigue and restoring mitochondrial function.

12. References

Abidi, S. & Ali, A. (1999). Role of oxygen free radicals in the pathogenesis and etiology of cancer, *Cancer Letters* 142: 1-9.

Aeschbach, R., Loliger, J., Scott, B. C., et al. (1994). Antioxidant actions of thymol, carvacrol, 6-gingerol, zingerone and hydroxytyrosol, *Food Chemistry and Toxicology* 32: 31-36.

Agadjanyan, M., Vasilevko, V., Ghochikyan, A., et al. (2003). Nutritional supplement (NTFactor) restores mitochondrial function and reduces moderately severe fatigue in aged subjects, *Journal of Chronic Fatigue Syndrome* 11(3): 23-26.

Ahlberg, K., Ekman, T., Gaston-Johansson, F. & Mock, V. (2003). Assessment and management of cancer-related fatigue in adults, *The Lancet* 362 (9384): 640–650.

Arnold, L. M. (2008). Understanding fatigue in major depressive disorder and other medical disorders, *Psychosomatics* 49: 185–190.

Asal, N. R., Risser, D. R., Kadamani, S., et al. (1990). Risk factors in renal cell carcinoma. I. Methodology, demographics, tobacco beverage use and obesity, *Cancer Detection and Prevention* 11: 359-377.

Aydin, A., Arsova-Sarafinovska, Z., Sayal, A., et al. (2006). Oxidative stress and antioxidant status in non-metastatic prostate cancer and benign prostate hyperplasia, *Clinical Biochemistry* 39: 176-179.

Balin, A. K., Goodman, D. B. P., Rasmussen, H., et al. (1978). Oxygen-sensitive stages of the cell cycle of human diploid cells, *Journal of Cell Biology* 78: 390-400.

Barber, D. A. & Harris, S. R. (1994). Oxygen free radicals and antioxidants: a review, *American Pharmacology* 34: 26-35.

Bartsch, H. & Nair, J. (2004). Oxidative stress and lipid peroxidation-driven DNA-lesions in inflammation driven carcinogenesis, *Cancer Detection and Prevention* 28: 385-391.

Batcioglu, K., Mehmet, N., Ozturk, I. C., et al. (2006). Lipid peroxidation and antioxidant status in stomach cancer, *Cancer Investigation* 24: 18-21.

Bender, C. M., Engberg, S. J., Donovan, H. S., et al. (2008). Symptom clusters in adults with chronic health problems and cancer as a co-morbidity, *Oncology Nursing Forum* 35: E1-E11.

Betteridge, D. J. (2000). What is oxidative stress? *Metabolism* 49(suppl 1): 3-8.

Borneman, T., Piper, B. F., Sun, V. C., et al. (2007). Implementing the fatigue guidelines at one NCCN member institution: process and outcomes, *Journal of the National Comprehensive Cancer Network* 5: 1092-1101.

Brizel, D. M. (2007). Pharmacologic approaches to radiation protection, *Journal of Clinical Oncology* 25: 4084–4089.

Brown, L. F. & Kroenke, K. (2009). Cancer-related fatigue and its association with depression and anxiety: a systematic review, *Psychosomatics* 50: 440-447.

Brown, N. S. & Bicknell, R. (2001). Hypoxia and oxidative stress in breast cancer. Oxidative stress: its effects on the growth, metastatic potential and response to therapy of breast cancer, *Breast Cancer Research* 3: 323-327.

Buckingham, R., Fitt, J. & Sitzia, J. (1997). Patients' experience of chemotherapy: side-effects of carboplatin in the treatment of carcinoma of the ovary, *European Journal of Cancer Care* 6: 59-71.

Cassileth, B. R., Heitzer, M. & Wesa, K. (2009). The public health impact of herbs and nutritional supplements, *Pharmaceutical Biology* 47: 761-767.

Castro, L. & Freeman, B. A. (2001). Reactive oxygen species in human health and disease, *Nutrition* 17: 295-307.

Cella, D., Davis, K., Breitbart, W., et al. (2001). Cancer-related fatigue: prevalence of proposed diagnostic criteria in a United States sample of cancer survivors, *Journal of Clinical Oncology* 19: 3385–3391.

Chandra, J., Samali, A. & Orrenius, S. (2000). Triggering and modulation of apoptosis by oxidative stress. *Free Radical Biology and Medicine* 29: 323-333.

Colodny, L., Lynch, K., Farber, C., et al. (2000). Results of a study to evaluate the use of Propax to reduce adverse effects of chemotherapy, *Journal of the American Nutraceutical Association* 2(1): 17-25.

Conklin, K. A. (2000). Dietary antioxidants during cancer chemotherapy: impact on chemotherapeutic effectiveness and development of side effects, *Nutrition and Cancer* 37: 1-18.

Conklin, K. A. (2004). Chemotherapy-associated oxidative stress: impact on chemotherapeutic effectiveness, *Integrated Cancer Therapies* 3: 294-300.

Conklin, K. A. (2005). Coenzyme Q_{10} for prevention of anthracycline-induced cardiotoxicity, *Integrated Cancer Therapies* 4: 110-130.

Cortes, E. P., Gupta, M., Chou, C., et al. (1978). Adriamycin cardiotoxicity: early detection by systolic time interval and possible prevention by coenzyme Q_{10}, *Cancer Treatment Reports* 62: 887-891.

Curt, G. A., Breitbart, W., Cella, D., et al. (2000). Impact of cancer-related fatigue on the lives of patients: new findings from The Fatigue Coalition, *The Oncologist* 5: 353–360.

Davies, K. J. A. & Doroshow, J. H, (1986). Redox cycling of anthracyclines by cardiac mitochondria. I. Anthracycline radical formation by NADH dehydrogenase, *Journal of Biological Chemistry* 261: 3060-3067.

Dianzani, M. U. (1993). Lipid peroxidation and cancer, *Critical Reviews in Oncology and Hematology* 15: 125-147.

Domae, N., Sawada, H., Matsuyama, E., et al. (1981). Cardiomyopathy and other chronic toxic effects induced in rabbits by doxorubicin and possible prevention by coenzyme Q_{10}, *Cancer Treatment Reports* 65: 79-91.

Doroshow, J. H., Davies, K. J. A. (1986). Redox cycling of anthracyclines by cardiac mitochondria. II. Formation of superoxide anion, hydrogen peroxide, and hydroxyl radical, *Journal of Biological Chemistry* 261: 3068-3074.

Doyle, C., Kushi, L. H., Byers, T., et al. (2006). Nutrition ad physical activity during and after cancer treatment: an American Cancer Society guide for informed choices, *CA Cancer Journal* 56: 323-353.

Dreher, D. & Junod, A. F. (1996). Role of oxygen free radicals in cancer development, *European Journal of Cancer* 32A: 30-38.

Eaton, S., Skinner, R., Hale, J. P., et al. (2000). Plasma coenzyme Q_{10} in children and adolescents undergoing doxorubicin therapy, *Clinica Chimica Acta* 302: 1-9.

Ellithorpe, R. R., Settineri, R. & Nicolson, G. L. (2003). Reduction of fatigue by use of a dietary supplement containing glycophospholipids, *Journal of the American Nutraceutical Association* 6(1): 23-28.

Epperly, M. W., Gretton, J. E., Sikora, C. A., et al. (2003). Mitochondrial localization of superoxide dismutase is required for decreasing radiation-induced cellular damage, *Radiation Research* 160: 568–578.

Escalante, C. P., Kallen, M. A., Valdres, R. U., et al. (2011). Outcomes of a cancer-related fatigue clinic in a comprehensive cancer center, *Journal of Pain and Symptom Mangement* in press.

Feinendegen, L. E., Pollycove, M., & Neumann, R. D. (2007). Whole-body responses to low-level radiation exposure: New concepts in mammalian radiobiology, *Experimental Hematology* 35: 37–46.

Felle, S., Mecocci, P., Fano, G., et al. (2000). Specific oxidative alterations in vastus lateralis muscle of patients with the diagnosis of chronic fatigue syndrome, *Free Radical Biology and Medicine* 29: 1252-1259.

Fojo, T. (2001). Cancer, DNA repair mechanisms, and resistance to chemotherapy, *Journal of the National Cancer Institute* 93: 1434-1436.

Fridovich, I. (1995). Superoxide radical and superoxide dismutases, *Annual Review of Biochemistry* 64: 97-112.

Gago-Dominguez, M., Castelao, J. E., Yuan, J. M., et al. (2002). Lipid peroxidation: a novel and unifying concept of the etiology of renal cell carcinoma, *Cancer Causes and Control* 13: 287-293.
Gansler, T., Kaw, C., Crammer, C. & Smith, T. (2008). A population-based study of prevalence of complementary methods use by cancer survivors, *Cancer* 113: 1048-1057.
Ghaffari, S. (2008). Oxidative stress in the regulation of normal and neoplastic hematopoiesis, *Antioxidation and Redox Signaling* 10: 1923-1940.
Gille, L. & Nohl, H. (1997). Analyses of the molecular mechanism of Adriamycin-induced cardiotoxicity, *Free Radical Biology and Medicine* 23: 775-782.
Giovannucci, E. & Chan, A. T. (2010). Role of vitamin and mineral supplementation and aspirin use in cancer survivors, *Journal of Clinical Oncology* 28: 4081-4085.
Given, B., Given, C., Azzouz, F. & Stommel, M. (2001). Physical functioning of elderly cancer patients prior to diagnosis and following initial treatment, *Nursing Research* 50: 222–232.
Gonzalez, M. J. (1992). Lipid peroxidation and tumor growth: an inverse relationship, *Medical Hypotheses* 38: 106-110.
Greenberger, J. S., Kagan, V. E., Pearce, L., et al. (2001). Modulation of redox signal transduction pathways in the treatment of cancer, *Antioxidants and Redox Signaling* 3: 347–359.
Gutstein, H. B. (2001). The biological basis for fatigue. *Cancer* 92: 1678–1683.
Halliwell, B. (1996). Oxidative stress, nutrition and health, *Free Radical Research* 25: 57-74.
Hampton, M. B., Fadeel, B. & Orrenius, S. (1998). Redox regulation of the caspases during apoptosis, *Annals of the New York Academy of Science* 854: 328-335.
Hauptlorenz, S., Esterbauer, H., Moll, W., et al. (1985). Effects of the lipid peroxidation product 4-hydroxynonenal and related aldehydes on proliferation and viability of cultured Ehrlich ascites tumor cells, *Biochemical Pharmacology* 34: 3803-3809.
Hofman, M., Ryan, J. L., Figueroa-Moseley, C. D., et al. (2007). Cancer-related fatigue: the scale of the problem, *The Oncologist* 12: 4–10.
Huang, H. & Manton, K. G. (2004). The role of oxidative damage in mitochondria during aging: a review, *Frontiers in Bioscience* 9: 1100-1117.
Iarussi, D., Auricchio, U., Agretto, A., et al. (1994). Protective effect of coenzyme Q_{10} on anthracyclines cardiotoxicity: control study in children with acute lymphoblastic leukemia and non-Hodgkin lymphoma, *Molecular Aspects of Medicine* 15: S207-S212.
Isenring, E., Cross, G., Kellett, E. & Koczwara, B. (2010). Nutritional status and iformation needs of medical oncology patients receiving treatment at an Australian public hospital, *Nutrition and Cancer* 62: 220-228.
Jagetia, G. C., Rajanikant, G. K., Rao, S. K., et al. (2003). Alteration in the glutathione, glutathione peroxidase, superoxide dismutase and lipid peroxidation by ascorbic acid in the skin of mice exposed to fractionated gamma radiation, *Clinica Chimica Acta* 332: 111-121.
Jaruga, P., Zastawny, T. H., Skokowski, J., et al. (1992). Oxidative DNA base damage and antioxidant enzyme activities in human lung cancer, *FEBS Letters* 341: 59-64.
Johnson, T. M., Yu, Z. X., Ferrans, V. J., et al. (1996). Reactive oxygen species are downstream mediators of p53-dependent apoptosis, *Proceedings of the National Academy of Science USA* 93: 11848-11852.
Judy, W. V., Hall, J. H., Dugan, W., et al. (1984). Coenzyme Q_{10} reduction of Adriamycin cardiotoxicity, *in* Folkers, K. & Yamamura, Y. (eds). *Biomedical and Clinical Aspects of*

Coenzyme Q, Vol. 4, Amsterdam:Elsevier/North-Holland Biomedical Press, pp. 231-241.

Kang, D. H. (2002). Oxidative stress, DNA damage and breast cancer, *AACN Clinical Issues* 13: 540-549.

Kanno, T., Sato, E. E., Muranaka, S., et al. (2004). Oxidative stress underlies the mechanism for Ca(2+)-induced permeability transition of mitochondria, *Free Radical Research* 38: 27-35.

Karlsson, J., Folkers, K., Astrom, H., et al. (1986). Effect of Adriamycin on heart and skeletal muscle coenzyme Q_{10} (CoQ_{10}) in man, *in* Folkers, K. & Yamamura, Y. (eds), *Biomedical and Clinical Aspects of Coenzyme Q*, Vol. 5, Amsterdam:Elsevier/North-Holland Biomedical Press, pp. 241-245.

Kehrer, J. P. (1993). Free radicals and mediators of tissue injury and disease, *Critical Reviews in Toxicology* 23: 21-48.

Klaunig, J. E. & Kamendulis, L. M. (2004). The role of oxidative stress in carcinogenesis, *Annual Review of Pharmacology and Toxicology* 44: 239-267.

Kroenke, K., Wood, D. R., Mangelsdorff, A. D., et al. (1988). Chronic fatigue in primary care. Prevalence, patient characteristics, and outcome, *JAMA* 260: 929-934.

Kurata, S. (2000). Selective activation of p38 MAPK cascade and mitotic arrest caused by low level oxidative stress, *Journal of Biological Chemistry* 275: 23413-23416.

Leach, J. K., Black, S. M., Schmidt-Ullrich, R. K. & Mikkelsen, R. B. (2002). Activation of constitutive nitric-oxide synthase activity is an early signaling event induced by ionizing radiation. *Journal of Biological Chemistry* 277: 15400–15406.

Lehninger, A. L. (1951). Phosphorylation coupled to oxidation of dihydrodiphosphopyridine nucleotide, *Journal of Biological Chemistry* 190: 345-359.

Levy, M. (2008). Cancer fatigue: a review for psychiatrists, *General Hospital Psychiatry* 30: 233-244.

Liu, L., Marler, M. R., Parker, B. A., et al. (2005). The relationship between fatigue and light exposure during chemotherapy, *Supportive Care in Cancer* 13: 1010-1017.

Logan, A. C. & Wong, C, (2001). Chronic fatigue syndrome: oxidative stress and dietary modifications, *Alternative Medicine Reviews* 6: 450-459.

Loke, Y. K., Price, D., Derry, S., et al. (2006). Case reports of suspected adverse drug reactions—systematic literature survey of follow-up, *British Medical Journal* 232: 335-339.

Maes, M. & Twisk, F. N. (2009). Why myalgic encephalomyelitis/chronic fatigue syndrome (ME/CFS) may kill you: disorders in the inflammatory and oxidative and nitrosative stress (IO&NS) pathways may explain cardiovascular disorders in ME/CFS, *NeuroEndocrinology Letters* 30: 677-693.

Maes, M. (2009). Inflammatory and oxidative and nitrosative stress pathways underpinning chronic fatigue, somatization and psychosomatic symptoms, *Current Opinions in Psychiatry* 22: 75-83.

Manoharan, S., Kolanjiappan, K., Suresh, K., et al. (2005). Lipid peroxidation and antioxidants status in patients with oral squamous cell carcinoma, *Indian Journal of Medical Research* 122: 529-534.

Mansbach, C. M. & Dowell, R. (2000). Effect of increasing lipid loads on the ability of the endoplasmic reticulum to transport lipid to the Golgi, *Journal of Lipid Research* 41: 605-612.

Manuel y Keenoy, B., Moorkens, G., Vertommen, J. & De Leeuw, I. (2001). Antioxidant status and lipoprotein peroxidation in chronic fatigue syndrome, *Life Science* 68: 2037-2049.

Manzullo, E. F. & Escalante, C. P. (2002). Research into fatigue, *Hematology Oncology Clinics of North America* 16: 619-628.

Marnett, L.J. (2000). Oxyradicals and DNA damage, *Carcinogenesis* 21: 361-370.

Marrow, G. R. (2007). Cancer-related fatigue: causes, consequences and management, *The Oncologist* 12(suppl 1): 1-3.

McDonald, E., David, A. S., Pelosi, A. J. & Mann, A. H. (1993). Chronic fatigue in primary care attendees, *Psycholgical Medicine* 23: 987-998.

Miller, P. E., Vasey, J. J., Short, P. F. & Hartman, T. J. (2009). Dietary supplement use in adult cancer survivors, *Oncology Nursing Forum* 36(1): 61-68.

Milton, O., Richardson, A., Sharpe, M., et al. (2008). A systematic review and meta-analysis of the pharmacological treatment of cancer-related fatigue, *Journal of the National Cancer Institute* 100: 1-12.

Morrison, J. D. (1980). Fatigue as a presenting complaint in family practice, *Journal of Family Practice* 10: 795-801.

Mustian, K. M., Morrow, G. R., Carroll, J. K., et al. (2007). Integrative nonpharmacological behavioral interventions for the management of cancer-related fatigue, *The Oncologist* 12(Suppl. 1): 52-67.

Nicolson, G. L. & Conklin, K. A. (2008). Reversing mitochondrial dysfunction, fatigue and the adverse effects of chemotherapy of metastatic disease by Molecular Replacement Therapy, *Clinical and Experimental Metastasis* 25: 161-169.

Nicolson, G. L. & Ellithrope, R. (2006). Lipid replacement and antioxidant nutritional therapy for restoring mitochondrial function and reducing fatigue in chronic fatigue syndrome and other fatiguing illnesses, *Journal of Chronic Fatigue Syndrome* 13(1): 57-68.

Nicolson, G. L. (2003). Lipid replacement as an adjunct to therapy for chronic fatigue, anti-aging and restoration of mitochondrial function, *Journal of the American Nutraceutical Association* 6(3): 22-28.

Nicolson, G. L. (2005). Lipid replacement/antioxidant therapy as an adjunct supplement to reduce the adverse effects of cancer therapy and restore mitochondrial function, *Pathology and Oncology Research* 11: 139-144.

Nicolson, G. L. (2010). Lipid replacement therapy: a nutraceutical approach for reducing cancer-associated fatigue and the adverse effects of cancer therapy while restoring mitochondrial function. *Cancer & Metastasis Reviews* 29: 543-552.

Nicolson, G. L., Ellithorpe, R. R., Ayson-Mitchell, C., et al. (2010). Lipid Replacement Therapy with a glycophospholipid-antioxidant-vitamin formulation significantly reduces fatigue within one week, *Journal of the American Nutraceutical Association* 13(1): 11-15.

Nicolson, G. L., Poste, G. & Ji, T. (1977). Dynamic aspects of cell membrane organization, *Cell Surface Reviews* 3: 1-73.

Nohl, H. (1987). Demonstration of the existence of an organo-specific NADH dehydrogenase in heart mitochondria, *European Journal of Biochemistry* 169: 585-591.

Otamiri, T. & Sjodahl, R. (1989). Increased lipid peroxidation in malignant tissues of patients with colorectal cancer, *Cancer* 64: 422-425.

Oxdemirler, G., Pabuççoglu, H., Bulut, T., et al. (1989). Increased lipoperoxide levels and antioxidant system in colorectal cancer, *Journal of Cancer Research and Clinical Oncology* 124: 555-559.

Pall, M. L. (2000). Elevated, sustained peroxynitrite levels as the cause of chronic fatigue syndrome, *Medical Hypotheses* 54: 115-125.

Palmeira, C. M., Serrano, J., Kuehl, D.W., et al. (1997). Preferential oxidation of cardiac mitochondrial DNA following acute intoxication with doxorubicin, *Biochimica et Biophysica Acta* 1321: 101-106.

Papadopoulou, L. C. & Tsiftsoglou, A. S. (1996). Effects of hemin on apoptosis, suppression of cytochrome C oxidase gene expression, and bone-marrow toxicity induced by doxorubicin, *Biochemical Pharmacology* 52: 713-722.

Piper, B. F., Linsey, A. M. & Dodd, M. J. (1987). Fatigue mechanism in cancer, *Oncology Nursing Forum* 14: 17-23.

Prasad, K. N., Cole, W. C., Kumar, B. et al. (2001). Scientific rationale for using high-dose multiple micronutrients as an adjunct to standard and experimental cancer therapies, *Journal of the American College of Nutrition* 20: 450S-453S.

Prue, G., Rankin, J., Allen, J., et al. (2006). Cancer-related fatigue: a critical appraisal, *European Journal of Cancer* 42: 846-863.

Radi, R., Rodriguez, M., Castro, L., et al. (1994). Inhibition of mitochondrial electronic transport by peroxynitrite, *Archives of Biochemistry and Biophysics* 308: 89-95.

Rasmussen, U. F. & Rasmussen, H. N. (1985). The NADH oxidase system (external) of muscle mitochondria and its role in the oxidation of cytoplasmic NADH, *Biochemical Journal* 229: 632-641.

Ray, G., Batra, S., Shukla, N. K., et al. (2000). Lipid peroxidation, free radical production and antioxidant status in breast cancer, *Breast Cancer Research and Treatment* 59: 163-170.

Respini, D., Jacobsen, P. B., Thors, C., et al. (2003). The prevalence and correlates of fatigue in older cancer patients, *Critical Reviews in Oncology and Hematology* 47: 273–279.

Richards, R. S., Roberts, T. K., McGregor, N. R., et al. (2000). Blood parameters indicative of oxidative stress are associated with symptom expression in chronic fatigue syndrome, *Redox Reports* 5: 35-41.

Ryan, J. L., Carroll, J. K., Ryan, E. P., et al. (2007). Mechanisms of cancer-related fatigue, *The Oncologist* 12(Supp. 1): 22-34.

Sabbarova, I. & Kanai, A. (2007). Targeted delivery of radioprotective agents to mitochondria, *Molecular Interventions* 8: 295-302.

Schackelford, R. E., Kaufmann, W. K & Paules, R. S. (2000). Oxidative stress and cell cycle checkpoint function, *Free Radical Biology and Medicine* 28: 1387-1404.

Schwartz, J. L. (1996). The dual roles of nutrients as antioxidants and prooxidants: their effects on tumor cell growth, *Journal of Nutrition* 126: 1221S-1227S.

Seidman, M., Khan, M. J., Tang, W. X., et al. (2002). Influence of lecithin on mitochondrial DNA and age-related hearing loss, *Otolaryngology and Head and Neck Surgery* 127: 138-144.

Seifried, H. E., McDonald, S. S., Anderson, D. E., et al. (2003). The antioxidant conundrum in cancer, *Cancer Research* 61: 4295-4298.

Seril, D. N., Liao, J., Yang, G. Y., et al. (2003). Oxidative stress and ulcerative colitis-associated carcinogenesis: studies in humans and animal models, *Carcinogenesis* 34: 353-362.

Serrano, J., Palmeira, C. M., Kuehl, D. W., et al. (1999). Cardioselective and cumulative oxidation of mitochondrial DNA following subchronic doxorubicin administration, *Biochimica et Biophysica Acta* 1411: 201-205.

Shacter, E., Williams, J. A., Hinson, R. M., et al. (2000). Oxidative stress interferes with cancer chemotherapy: inhibition of lymphoma cell apoptosis and phagocytosis, *Blood* 96: 307-313.

Sikka, S. C. (2003). Role of oxidative stress response elements and antioxidants in prostate cancer pathobiology and chemoprevention—a mechanistic approach, *Current Medicinal Chemistry* 10: 2679-2692.

Smets, E. M. A., Garssen, B., Cull, A., et al, (1996). Applications of the Multidimensional Fatigue Inventory (MFI-20) in cancer patients receiving radiotherapy, *British Journal of Cancer* 73: 241–245.

Sood, A. & Moynihan, T. J. (2005). Cancer-related fatigue: an update, *Current Oncology Reports* 7: 277-282.

Stadtman, E. (2002). Introduction to serial reviews on oxidatively modified proteins in aging and disease, *Free Radical Biology and Medicine* 32: 789.

Stone, P., Hardy, J., Huddart, R., et al. (2000). Fatigue in patients with prostate cancer receiving hormone therapy, *European Journal of Cancer* 36: 1134–1141.

Ströhle, A., Zänker, K. & Hahn, A. (2010). Nutrition in oncology: the case of micronutrients, *Oncology Reports* 24: 815-828.

Subczynski, W. K. & Wisniewska, A. (2000). Physical properties of lipid bilayer membranes: relevance to membrane biological functions, *Acta Biochimica Polonica* 47: 613-625.

Sun, Y. (1990). Free radicals, antioxidant enzymes and carcinogenesis, *Free Radical Biology and Medicine* 8: 583-599.

Tanaka, T. (1994). Cancer chemoprevention by natural products, *Oncology Reports* 1: 1139-1155.

Tas, F., Hansel, H., Belce, A., et al. (2005). Oxidative stress in breast cancer, *Medical Oncology* 22: 11-15.

Toyokuni, S., Okamoto, K., Yodio, J., et al. (1995). Persistent oxidative stress in cancer, *FEBS Letters* 358: 1-3.

Usui, T., Ishikura, H., Izumi, Y., et al. (1982). Possible prevention from the progression of cardiotoxicity in Adriamycin-treated rabbits by coenzyme Q_{10}, *Toxicology Letters* 12: 75-82.

Velicer, C. M. & Ulrich, C. M. (2008). Vitamin and mineral supplement use among U.S. adults after cancer diagnosis: a systematic review, *Journal of Clinical Oncology* 26: 665-673.

Vogelzang, N., Breitbart, W., Cella, D., et al. (1997). Patient caregiver and oncologist perceptions of cancer-related fatigue: results of a tripart assessment survey, *Seminars in Hematology* 34(Suppl. 2): 4-12.

Von Roenn, J. H. & Paice, J. A. (2005). Control of common, non-pain cancer symptoms, *Seminars in Oncology* 32: 200-210.

Watson, T. & Mock, V. (2004). Exercise as an intervention for cancer-related fatigue, *Physical Therapy* 84: 736-743.

Wei, Q., Frazier, M. L. & Levin, B. (2000). DNA repair: a double edge sword, *Journal of the National Cancer Institute* 92: 440-441.

Wei, Y. H. & Lee, H. C. (2002). Oxidative stress, mitochondrial DNA mutation and impairment of antioxidant enzymes in aging, *Experimental Biology and Medicine* 227: 671-682.

Zee, P. C. & Acoli-Isreal, S. (2009). Does effective management of sleep disorders reduce cancer-related fatigue? *Drugs* 69(Suppl. 2): 29-41.

Zhen, W., Link, C. J., O'Connor, P. M., et al. (1992). Increased gene-specific repair of cisplatin interstrand cross-links in cisplatin-resistant human ovarian cancer cell lines, *Molecular and Cellular Biology* 12: 3689-3698.

11

The Relationships Between Stress Reduction Induced by Bedside Mindfulness Program and Mental Health Status

Ando Michiyo, Kira Haruko and Ito Sayoko
St. Mary's College, Kurume University,
Okinawa Junior College,
Japan

1. Introduction

Patients receiving anti-cancer treatment experience physical problems such as pain, fatigue and nausea, and psychological problems such as anxiety, depression, distress (Speca, et al., 2006) and spiritual pain. A mindfulness approach is one of the most effective interventions to alleviate these problems. The Mindfulness-Based Stress Reduction (MBSR) program was modeled on the work of Kabat-Zinn (Kabat-Zin, 1990; Kat-Zinn, et al., 1998) and colleagues at the Center for Mindfulness-Massachusetts Medical Center. The program is based on the principal of mindfulness, defined as moment-to-moment, present-centered, purposive non-judgmental awareness. The goal of the MBSR program is to guide participants to achieve greater awareness of themselves, their thoughts, and their bodies through class discussion, meditation, and yoga exercises (Garland, et al., 2007).

For cancer patients, the MBSR have effects on mood disturbance stress symptoms (Speca, et al. 2000), or on QOL and the immune profile (Carlson, et al., 2004). The Mindfulness-Based Art-Therapy (MBAT), which includes mindfulness and art therapy, also produces a significant decrease in symptoms of distress and improvements in key aspects of health-related QOL (Monti, et al., 2006). Moreover, the MBSR affects stress symptoms, mood, post-trauma growth, and spirituality (Garland, et al., 2007; Matchim, et al., 2011).

However, since the duration of the program in these studies are from at least 4 weeks to 8 weeks, patients were sometimes hard to continue to participate. And they were easily to be tired because of chemotherapy or radiation therapy. Then we developed a mindfulness cyclic meditation program, in which participants could participate in the program even sitting on chair. After this program, anxiety and depression improved (Ando, et al., 2009).

However, some of patients with advanced cancer stage were hard to participate, because their physical strength was very low and they could not sit or walk. Thus we needed to develop a new program for cancer patient with advanced cancer stage, and we developed a novel mindfulness program, a Bedside Mindfulness program (Figure 1). A yoga instructor and a clinical psychologist discussed about program, and made the leaflet with drawing by an illustrator.

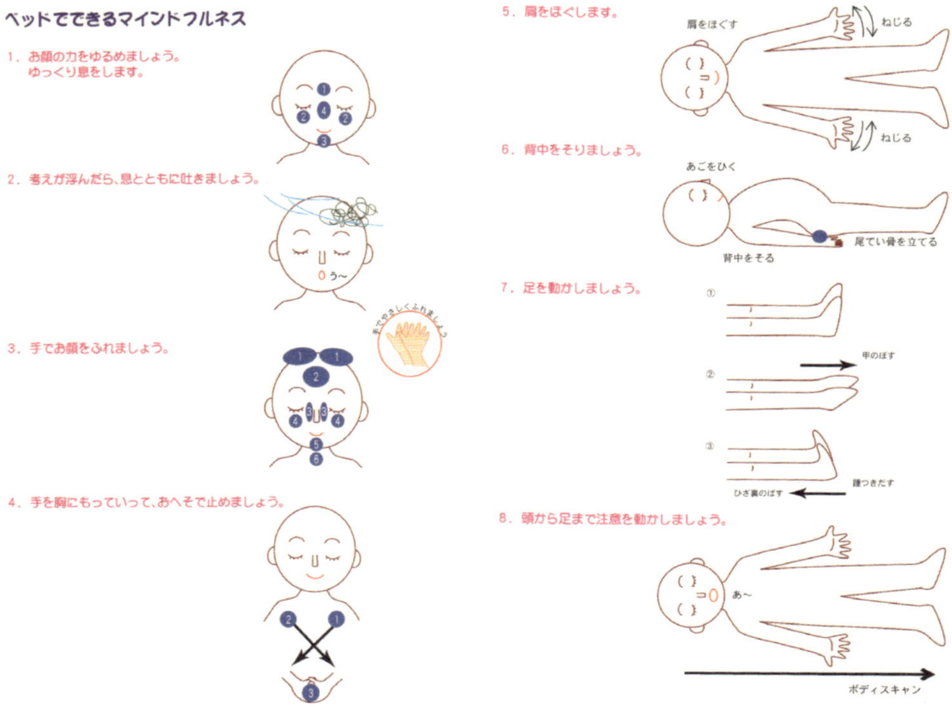

Fig. 1. The Bed-side Mindfulness Program

2. Study 1 – Efficacy of Bedside Mindfulness Program on mood related with mental health status

Firstly, we examined the efficacy of this program for college students, because we could obtained both subjective and objective data. Some previous studies examined efficacy of mindfulness including objective data.

Participants with alcohol use disorders received mindfulness program or cognitive behavior therapy. Psychological and physiological indices like **Galvanic Skin Response** of stress reduced in mindfulness program much more than cognitive behavior therapy (Brewer, et al., 2009). Or through mindfulness program, psychological distress like anxiety or depression reduced and also skin conductance level of women with chronic pain of fibromyalgia reduced (Lush, et al., 2009). These studies show that mindfulness reduced the skin conductance level which shows the stress level. Oppositely, healthy adults assigned a mindfulness group or a no mindfulness group. All participants viewed positive or negative films. Participants in the mindfulness group reported significantly greater positive affect in response to the positive film than those in the no mindfulness group. However, there was no significance between conditions on Galvanic Skin Response (GSR) or heart rate (Erisman & Roemer, 2010). That is, results of efficacy of mindfulness on skin conductance level are inconsistence.

About salivary cortisol as an indicator, for breast cancer outpatients MBSR program participants was associated with enhanced quality of life and decreased stress symptoms (Matchimy, et al., 2011), altered cortisol and immune patterns consistented with less stress and mood disturbance (Carlson, et al., 2007). In the above studies, skin conductance or salivary level was used as indicators. Moreover, we thought that effects of a mindfulness program might be different by a level of mental health states, and we predicted that the Bedside Mindfulness Program might be more effective for people or patients with mental problems.

Thus, in this study, we examined mental health and mood as psychological indicator. Mood consists of the tense arousal and the energetic arousal (Matthews, et al., 1990). Tense arousals show a level of tension and it is uncomfortable. Energetic arousal shows a level of activity. As physiological indicator, we used Galvanic Skin Response and the salivary level of amylase which measure level of stress.

Participants and methods

The participants were Japanese college students in Western Japan consist of 4 males and 16 females; mean age 22.7±4.8. As questionnaires, we used the Japanese UWIST Mood Adjective Check List : JUMACLE (Shirasawa, et al. 1999). There are 20 items (10 each for Tense Arousal and Energetic Arousal). Items for Tense Arousal were [I am] "tense," "jittery," "nervous," and so on. Items about Energetic Arousal were [I am] "active," "vigorous," "energetic," and so on. Participants answered on a 4-point Likert scale ranging from 1= not at all to 4=exactly so. The range of scores for Tense Arousal and Energetic Arousal was from 10 to 40. To measure mental state, we used the Japanese version of the General Health Questionnare-30 (Goldberg & Hillier, 1979) which was developed from the original one by Nakagawa and Daibo (1985). We separated participants into a non-risk group and a high-risk group by the cut-off point. The Bedside Mindful Program BMP included meditation, moving their hands or legs to focus their attention on bed (Figure 1). The BMP takes about 30 to 60 minutes per session and was conducted by nurses or a clinical psychologist who received training for at least 3 hours. The training included basic communication skills and Yoga skills learned directly from a Yoga specialist or using a CD. In the class, students received this program and complete questionnaires pre- and post-intervention. The study was approved by the appropriate institutional ethics committees and was performed in accordance with the ethical standards laid down in the Declaration of Helsinki. Statistical analysis, we separated participants into two groups, high risk group and non-risk group by cut off points of General Health Questionnaire. The t-test and the effects size test were performed on the scores of JUMACL, GSR, and salivary level of amylase.

Results

The Tense Arousal of the non-risk group significantly decreased from 18.4±21.6 to 14.5 ±22.3 (t=3.1, p<0.01) (Figure 2) . The effect size was large (Table 1). The Tense Arousal of the high risk group also significantly decreased from 20.0±29.1 to 14±26 (t=4.68, p<0.001)(Figure 3) and the effect size was large. The Energetic Arousal of the non-risk group significantly decreased from 29.7±39.1 to 26.6±43.6 (t=3.31, p<0.01) (Figure 4) and the effect size was large. However, that of the high risk group increased from 27.9±37.4 to 28.5±52.7 (t=-0.27, p=0.79) (Figure 5), though it was not significant and there was no effect.

The salivary level of amylase of the non-risk group decreased from 99.8 to 73.9 (t=1.01, p=0.34) and the effects size was medium (Table 2). The salivary level of amylase of the high risk group significantly decreased from 71.7 to 45.2 (t=2.27, p=0.05) and the effect size was large.

	TA		EA	
	Effect size r	Level	Effect size r	Level
Non-risk group	0.72	Large	0.74	Large
High-risk group	0.84	Large	0.09	None

Table 1. Effect Sizes in Tense Arousal (TA) and Energetic Arousal (EA) after the Bedside Mindfulness Program

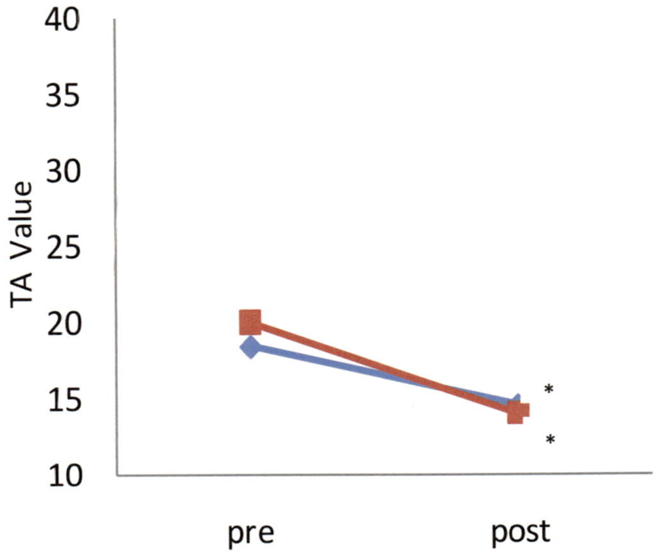

Fig. 2. Changes of Tense Arousal scores

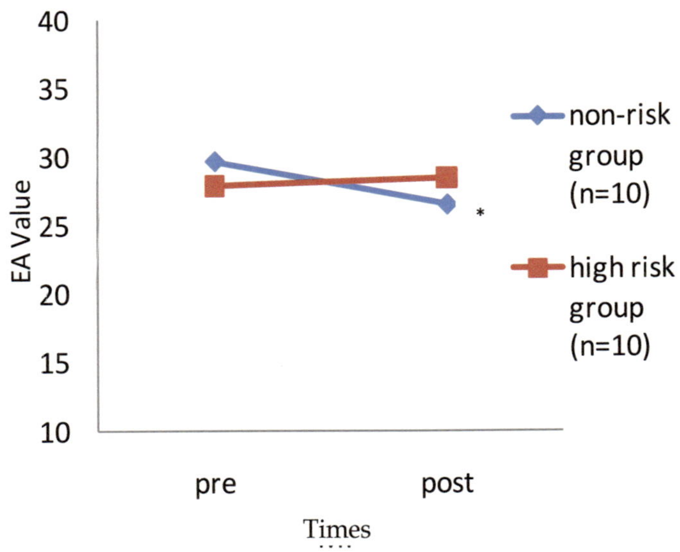

Fig. 3. Changes of Energetic Arousal scores

The GSR of the non risk group decreased a very little from 241.9 to 240 and there was no effect. Oppositely the GSR of the risk group increased from 301 to 386.2 (t=-1.21, p=0.26) and the effect size was medium.

	GSR		Amylase	
	Effect size r	Level	Effect size r	Level
Non-risk group	0.02	None	0.32	Medium
High-risk group	0.38	Medium	0.60	Large

Table 2. Effect Sizes in GSR and Amylase changes after the Bedside Mindfulness Program

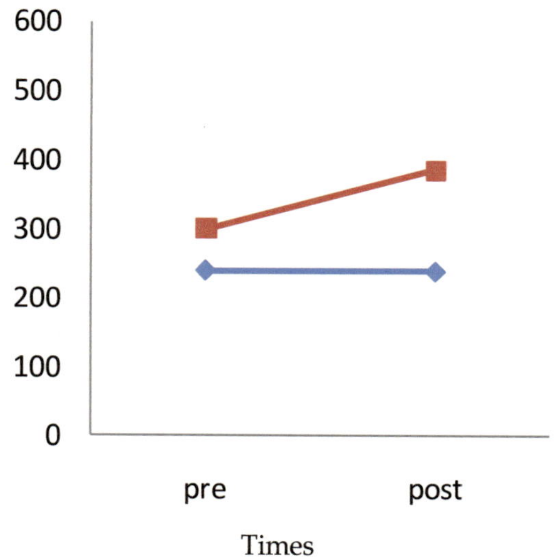

Fig. 4. Changes of GSR scores

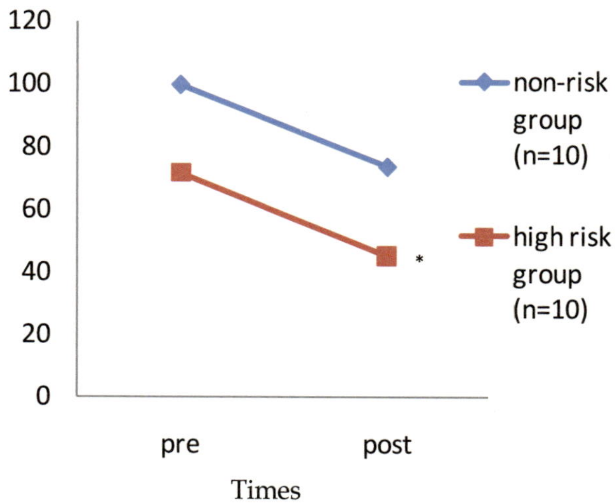

Fig. 5. Changes of Salivary level of Amylase

Discussion

The Tense Arousal significantly decreased both in the non-risk group and the hight-risk group. The effects size was large in both groups. These results show that the BMP decrease tension or anxiety, regardless the mental health status. It is because that breathing and meditation leads people to focus attention on themselves, and attention moves from things with tension or anxiety to themselves. The effects of decrease of tension by mindfulness agree with the previous studies (Garland, et al., 2007; Matchim & Armer, 2007).

The Energetic Arousal of the non-risk group significantly decreased after the therapy and showed middle effect size. It shows that BMP decrease of activity and sedate their feelings for good mental health. This result is different from Ogasawara, et al. (2006) in which the Energetic Arousal of college healthy students did not significantly change by relaxation of aroma hand massage. Ditto, et al. (2006) shows that mindfulness meditation produced different cardiovasucular and autonomic effects that relaxation, giving weight to the criticism against the conceptualization of mindfulness practice as a mere relaxation technique (Bishop, 2002).

In the high-risk group, the score did not change, showing no effect size. This result suggests that the BMP did not decrease activities for non- risk persons. The reasons of this phenomenon were that this therapy is useful to maintain energy for high-risk persons.

As for the salivary level of amylase, the high score demonstrates high level of negative stress. The scores of amylase significantly decreased in the high-risk group, but it did not change in non-risk group. It means that the BMP is more effective to reduce stress for high risk persons than non risk persons to reduce negative stress. In the previous study, the efficacy of mindfulness like decrease cortisol level which shows stress level as the physiological indicator (Carlson, et al., 2007) agreed with the present study for high risk persons. Carlson et al. (2007) demonstrated that breast cancer patients felt much psychological stress than healthy women, but the level of the salivary cortisol as the physiological indicator did not differ between patients and healthy women. Their studies suggest that physiological level was the same between patients and healthy women. However, from the present study, the effects of mindfulness program may be different by mental health level.

About GSR scores, a low score means high tension or stress. The GSR scores did not change in no-risk group, however, those of the high-risk group increased with middle effects size. It shows that the BMP has much more effects to reduce tension or stress for high risk persons than non-risk persons. Erisman & Roemer (2010) showed that the level of skin conductance was not differ between the mindfulness group and the non-mindfulness group. Though the present study design is different from Erisman & Roemer, contents of program or health level might affect people differently. The effects of mindfulness to physiological aspect will be needed to examine further more.

2.1 The efficacy of the Bedside Mindfulness Program on mood of cancer patients

We investigated the effects of the Bedside Mindfulness Program on mood by a level of mental status of cancer patients. We hypothesized that effects of the program on tension arousal may be the same regardless of mental status, however, effects of the program on energetic arousal may be differently.

Participants and methods

Four cancer patients participated in the study. Table 3 shows patients' back ground. We used the same questionnaire to patients as college students. The primary physician selected participants. A pastoral care worker conducted the BMP, in which she conducted the program about from 30 to 60 minutes. Before the program, patients completed the General Health Questionnare-30 and the Japanese UWIST Mood Adjective Check List (JUMACL), and after the program, they completed the JUMACL.

	Age	Gender	Disease	Stage
Patient A	64	Female	Breast	IV
Patient B	45	Female	Lung	IV
Patient C	50	Female	Breast	IV
Patient D	34	Female	Breast	IV

Table 3. Back ground of cancer patients.

Results

Table 4 shows the results. We reviewed each patient, patient A, Patient B, Patient C, and patient D. The score of GHQ was low and under the cut-off point. The scores of Patient A and Patient D was 1 and they had no mental problems. The scores of Patient B and Patient C show a little mental problem. The score 10 of TA was the lowest in the JUMACL, thus, patients had originally low tense arousal except patient C. As for EA, the score of Patient A and patient D who had no mental problems decreased (from 39 to 36, from 39 to 31), however, those of patient B and Patient C who had a little mental problem increased (from 30 to 40, from 34 to 39).

	GHQ	TA range	(10-40)		EA range	(10-40)	
		Pre	post	change	Pre	post	changes
Patient A	1	10	10	⇒	39	36	⇩
Patient B	3	10	10	⇒	37	40	⇧
Patient C	6	14	10	⇩	34	39	⇧
Patient D	1	10	10	⇒	39	31	⇩

Table 4. Score of GHQ (pre), Tense Arousal (TA) and Energetic Arousal (EA)

Discussion

Although patients in this study felt no mental problems originally, the decrease of TA of patient C suggests that BMP affects to decrease tense arousal. This facts support the results of college students. As for EA, the scores of Patient B and Patient C with a little mental problems increased, oppositely patient A and Patient C with no mental problem decreased. This facts also are the same of those of college students who received the same progrm, such that the EA score of the high-risk group increased, but that of the non-risk group decreased. Patients reflected the process of the program.
There were 2 patters. Some patients reflected that they were very calm before the program and they felt much more calm after the program. Other patients reflected that they had some problems before the program and they felt some energy to active something after the program. That is, this program affects on energy to elevate, particular for persons with some mental problems. In near future, we need to investigate further more.

2.2 The efficacy of the Bedside Mindfulness Program on anxiety or depression

We assess the efficacy of the Bedside Mindfulness Program (BMP) on anxiety or depression of cancer patients, because most of cancer patients feel anxiety or depression about treatments, future, works, economy, or recurrence. It seemed to be important for us to examine the efficacy of the Bedside Mindfulness Program on anxiety or depression.

Purpose

The aim of this study was to examine the efficacy of the BMP on anxiety of depression of cancer patients.

Participants and methods

Participants were cancer patients who received treatments like chemotherapy or radiation. The primary physicians selected patients. Table 5 shows the background of patients. The interviewer was a pastoral care worker. There were two sessions. In the first session, a patient received the BMP. The duration was about 60 minutes. Patients completed the questionnaires pre and post the intervention. Participants completed the Hospital Anxiety and Depression Scale.

	Basic Data
Mean age	56
Gender	Male:1 Female:13
Stage	II : 2 III : 1 IV: 12
Performance stage	0:7 1:3 2:1 3:1 4:1
Metastasis	Yes:10 No:1 Unclear:3

Table 5. Basic data of participants.

Results

The scores of HADS decreased from 9.57±7.1 to 6.86±6.9 after the program (t=1.49, p=0.161). The score of Anderson symptoms increased from 18.4±18.3 to 21.3±26.4 (t=-0.43, p=0.67). The Peason's correlation coefficient was 0.84 (p=0.00).

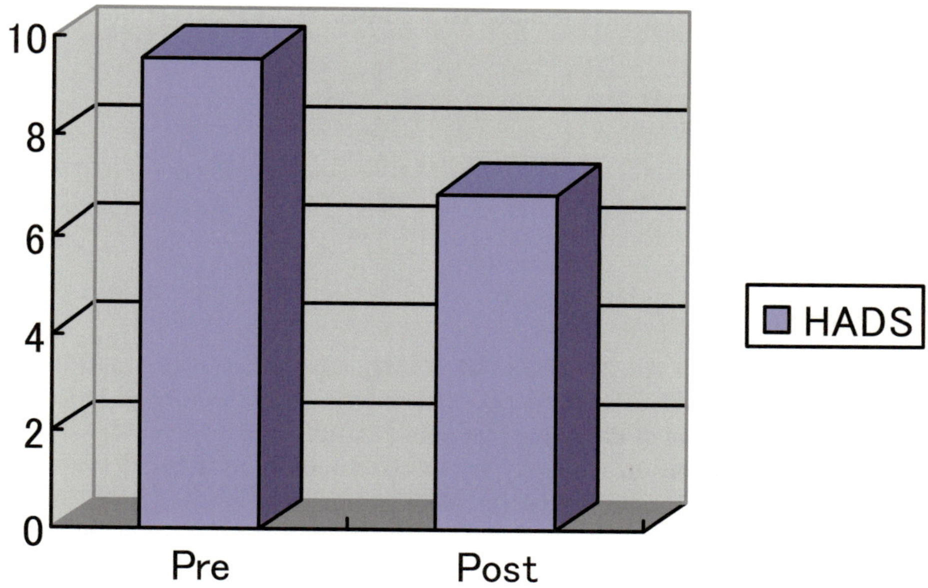

Fig. 6. Changes of HADS score

Discussion

The HADS score decreased in 10 % significance. It suggests that the BMP affects to decrease patients' anxiety or depression. Like the cyclic meditation therapy which alleviated patients' anxiety or depression (Ando, Morita, Akechi, et al., 2009), our mindfulness program for cancer patient affects on anxiety or depression. Since the cut-off points of the HADS score was 19/20, the patients in the present study did not have serious problems. It might be because the primary physician in the present study supported patients' mental aspect.

The Anderson symptom score increased a little, though it was not significant. It might be because patients under treatments were easily affected by the treatment process and the physical states were changeable. Since anxiety or depression of patients decreased regardless of the increase of symptom, this program may be useful to alleviate anxiety or depression, even though patients have symptoms.

As the co-relation coefficient between HADS score and Anderson scores was significantly high (r=0.84), patients who had much physical symptoms feel much more anxiety or depression. In the present study, since the duration was only one week, and session times were only two times, we could not assess the efficacy of this program in details. In future, we need to investigate much more.

3. Conclusion

The Bedside Mindfulness Program decreases tension and maintains energy of mood, and it is supported by the results of Galvanic Skin Response level and amylase. For cancer patients, this program may be useful to reduce anxiety and depression. Since anxiety and depression related with physical symptoms, we assess the efficacy of this program from long term perspective.

4. Acknowledgments

This research was supported by a Grant-in-Aid for Scientific Research (C). We specially thanks for all participants and staffs in hospitals, and for an illustrator, Mrs. Yukio Matsuo.

5. References

Ando, M.,; Morita, T.; Akechi, T.; et al. (2009). The efficacy of mindfulness-based meditation therapy on anxiety, depression and spirituality in Japanese cancer patients. Journal of Palliative Medicine, 12, pp. 1091-1094.

Bishop, S.R. (2002). What do we really know about mindfulness based stress reduction? *Psychosomatic Medicine*, Vol.64, pp. 71-83.

Brewer, J.A.; Sinha, R.; Chen, J.A., et al. (2009). Mindfulness training and stress reactivity in substance abuse: results from a randomized, controlled stage 1 pilot study. Substance abuse: Official publication of the association for Medical Education and Research in substance abuse, Vol.30, pp.306-317.

Carlson, L.E.; Cambell, T.S.; Garland, S.N. et al. (2007). Associations among salivary cortiso, melatonin, catecholamines, sleep quality and stress in women with breast cancer and healthy controls. *J Behavioral Medicine*, Vol. 30, pp. 45-58.

Carlson, L.; Speca, M.; Faris, et al. (2007). One year pre-post intervention follow-up of psychological, immune, endocrine and blood pressure outcomes of mindfulness-based stress reduction (MBSR) in breast and prostate cancer outpatients. *Brain, Behavior, and Immunity*, Vol.21, pp.1038-1049.

Carlson, L.E.; Speca, M.; Patel, K.D. et al. (2004). Mindfulness based stress reduction in relation to quality of life, mood, symptom, of stress and levels of cortisol, dehydroepiandrosterone sulfate (DHEAS) and melatonin in breast and prostate cancer outpatients. *Psychoneuroendocrinology*, Vol. 29, pp.448-474.

Ditto, B.; Eclache, M.; Goldman. (2006). Short-term autonomic and cardiovascular effects of mindfulness body scan meditation. *Ann of Behavioral Medicine*, Vol. 32, pp. 227-234.

Erisman, S.M. & Roemer, L. (2010). A preliminary investigation of the effects of experimentally induced mindfulness on emotional responding to film clips. *Emotion*, Vol. 10, pp.72-82.

Garland, E.L.; Gaylord, S.A.; Fredricson, B.L. (2011). Positive reappraisal mediates the stress-reductive effects of mindfulness: an upward spiral process. *Mindfulness*, Vol.2, pp. 59-67.

Garland, S.N.; Carson, L.E.; Cook, S, et al. (2007). A non-randomized comparison of mindfulness-based stress reduction and healing arts programs for facilitating post-traumatic growth and spirituality in cancer outpatients. *Support Care Cancer* Vol.15, pp.949-961.

Goldberg, D.P.; Hillier, V.E. (1979). A scaled version of the General Health Questionnaire. *Psychological Medicine*, Vol.9, pp.139-145.

Kabat-Zinn, J. (1990). Full catastrophe living: using the wisdom of your body and mind to face stress, pain and illness. Delacourt, New York.

Lampic, C.; Wennberg, A.; Schill, J.E., et al. (1994). Coping, psychosocial well-being and anxiety in cancer patients at follow-up visits. *Acta Oncologica,* Vol.33, pp.887-894.

Lush, E.; Salmon, P.; Floyd, A. (2007). Mindfulness meditation for symptom reduction in fibromylalgia: psycholophysiological correlates. Journal of Clinical psychology in Medical settings, Vol.16, pp. 200-207.

Matchim, Y.; Armer, J. (2007). Measuring the psychological impact of mindfulness meditation on health among patients with cancer. *Oncology Nursing Form,* Vol.34, pp.1059-1066.

Matchim, Y.; Armer, J.M.; Stewart, B.R. (2011). Mindfulness-based stress reduction among breast cancer survivors: a literature review and discussion. *Oncology Nursing-Forum,* Vol. 38, pp.61-71.

Matthew, G.; Jones, D.M.; Chamberlain, A.G. (1990). Refining the measurement of mood: the UWIST Mood Adjective Checklist. *British journal of Psychology,* Vol.81, pp.17-42.

Monti, D.A.; Peterson, C.; Kunkel, S. (2006). A randomized, controlled trial of mindfulness-based art therapy (MBAT) for women with cancer. *Psycho-Oncology,* Vol. 15, 363-373.

Nakagawa Y, Daibo I. The General Health Questionnaire. Tokyo: Nihon Bunka Kagakusya, 1985.

Ott, M.J.; Norris, R.L.; Bauer-Wu, S.M. (2006). Mindfulness meditation for oncology patients: a discussion and critical review. *Integrative Cancer Therapies,* Vol.5, pp. 98-108.

Ogasawara, E.; Shiihara, Y.; Koitabashi, K., et al. (2007). The relaxation and refreshing effects of aromatherapieutic massage using citrus fruit essential oil-evaluation using skin conductance and a mood adjective check list, *Journal of Japanese Society of Nursing Research* (in Japanese) ,Vol. 4, pp.17-26.

Speca, M.; Carlson, L.E.; Goodey, E, et al. (2000). A randomized, wait-list controlled clinical trial: The effect of a mindfulness meditation-based stress reduction program on mood and symptoms of stress in cancer outpatients. Psychomatic Medicine 62:613-622

Shirasawa, S.; Ishida, T.; Hakoda, Y. et al. (1999). Effects of energetic arousal on memory search. *Japanese Psychonomic Science,* Vol. 17, pp. 93-99.

Kabat-Zinn, J.; Massion, A.O.; Hebert, J.R.; Rosenbaum, E. (1998). Meditation. In: Holland JF (ed) Psycho-Oncology. Oxford University Press, New York, pp 767-779

12

Rehabilitation in Cancer Survivors: Interaction Between Lifestyle and Physical Activity

Raoul Saggini[1] and Menotti Calvani[2]
[1]*Dipartimento Università G. D'Annunzio, Chieti,*
[2]*Scuola di Specializzazione in Medicina Fisica e Riabilitativa, Università G. D'Annunzio, Chieti, Italy*

1. Introduction

1.1 Physical activity, body composition and cancer

Cancer is not a new disease, there are findings of neoplasia in the mummies of ancient Egypt, there are descriptions of the Romans and the Greeks and even remains in the fossil of dinosaurs. The study of the epidemiology of cancer, however, demonstrates an increasing incidence with an alarming progression, which is also involving countries which were considered "protected" or otherwise at low risk until last century.

- The progressive industrialization has led to an increase of environmental pollution with newly synthesized toxic substances, unknown by biological systems during the evolutionary process. Technological innovation has also increased the yield in agriculture, which has resulted in an increased food availability and a profound change in eating habits both for the type and for the amount of introduced nutrients. Technological development has also radically changed lifestyle with a progressive increase in sedentariness, a reduction to the sun exposure, causing a vitamin D deficiency also in children, by altering the circadianicity of circadian rhythms which regulate, depending on sunlight, the correct functioning of our body, including cell proliferation.

In general, the standard of living has increased in many countries, it has lengthened the life expectancy and, with it has increased cancer.

The improvement of recovery rates and survival with the progressive increase in the average age, in association with a greater focus on the quality of life, has led to basic definitions for cancer rehabilitation. This aims to help both to minimize the effects induced by the disease and the treatment (surgery, chemotherapy, radiotherapy, hormone therapy) and to regain control of many aspects of life in order to become an effective means of prevention for recurrences and comorbidity (Carver, JR.; Shapiro, CL 2007).

The rehabilitative intervention, therefore, shouldn't aim only to control physical pain but also to relieve the mental, social and spiritual pain, with all the other symptoms (Mikkelsen T .2009) (Fialka-Moser, V Crevenna, R.. 2003).

Since the 80's, scientific literature has stressed the link between sedentariness and certain types of cancer (Garabrant 1984).

Physical activity is one of the modulators of the cancer risk and survival factors that awakens our attention to the possibility of implementing a strategy within our operational capabilities.

In the history of scientific analysis of data related to physical activity, the capability to monitor it has come up against many methodological difficulties which have prevented to gather uncontaminated data, due to poor sensitivity and specificity of the used methods.

In particular, seven are the highlighted weak points:

1. most of the studies used questionnaires, often in retrospective and self-administration situations , giving many problems related both to their poor reliability of self assessment, typical of overweight people (as they often are physically inactive people) and to the inconsistencies sometimes found between the body mass and the energy expenditure calculation;
2. The quantification considered the so-called occupational (work-related activities) and / or recreational activities. Monitoring involved long periods of time in which the introduced technologies in the workplace have often increased sedentary lifestyle.
3. Most of our literature hasn't revealed the composition of each person's diet both under a calorie and under a composition point of view, right now when we are focusing our attention to glycemic index of food for their capability to induce abnormal insulin elevations, an anabolic hormone but with powerful proliferative activities.
4. We can't very often have reported data on the qualitative composition of lipids or their quantitative distribution during the day: the intake of dietary fat with a "cafeteria" diet (often connected with the type of job) shows the capability to induce inflammation and to trigger a chain of pro-cancerous events.
5. We can't always find reliably identified the duration and intensity of each physical activity and not always the used algorithms are normalized for the mass of each individual.
6. The daily activities are not located in the light and dark temporal space. Furthermore we don't have any idea, even indirect, of the situation of the vitamin D connected with the sun exposure and whose lack, especially in over 60 year people, can be a risk factor for different types of neoplasia.
7. We do not always have signs of body composition, being the BMI (Body Mass Index) the parameter for measuring the individual's structure, but it does not give an idea of body fat (especially in Asian people). This is an important piece of information as body fat is a good parameter to consider the relationship between energy intake and energy expenditure in physical activity. Fat is also an active organ under an inflammatory and hormonal point of view for **carcinogenesis** processes and tumor progression, but it is also a sensitive tissue in its plasticity in physical activity.

1.2 As regards the management of physical activity after the patient's diagnosis, it should be noted that

1. the American College of Sports Medicine has recommended to everybody, healthy and tumor-bearing, to do physical activity, even if of moderate intensity, for at least 30 minutes for 5 days a week (Haskell 2007, Schmitz 2010);
2. the American Institute for Cancer Research and the Word Cancer Fund recommends to practise physical activity at least 60 minutes a day, even if of moderate intensity, or 30 minutes of intense activity (World 2007) in order to reduce cancer risk.

1.3 As regards the creation of a proper physical exercise for the individual it should be noted that

the relationship between the mass of our body and the height has always been a guide for trainers to do their job. Older clinicians spoke about constitutional types, such as brachytype to mean short people in stature or those who appeared long-limbed, basically thin and tall. Today the relationship between weight in kilograms and height in squared meters, called BMI (Body Mass Index), has become a useful indicator of easy calculation to define the population in terms of normal-weight (BMI between 19 and 25), underweight (BMI <19), overweight (BMI between 25 and 30) or obese (between 30 to 35) or super-obese (> 35). The BMI correlates with the amount of fat, with the production of inflammatory proteins, with blood pressure, with the risk of many disabling diseases or life-threatening conditions such as diabetes, dementia, arthritis, depression, cardiovascular diseases and, with increasing evidence, cancer. The World Health Organization estimates that worldwide there are at least 1.6 billion overweight people (WHO 2006). Obese people exceed 400 millions whose incidence in Western countries has now reached and in some cases exceed 20% of the entire population (CDC 2006).

- The link between the weight gain and the incidence of cancer has been linked to biochemical factors that characterize the increase of fat mass like the increase of insulin, of IGF (Insulin Like Growth Factor), of Adipokine, Steroids, but also hypoxia linked to obesity and the entering into circulation of stromal fat cells (IARC 2002, World Cancer Research 2007, Renehan 2006, 2008, 2009).
- Today there are a lot evidences of a strong correlation between obesity and cancer, with specificity for each sex, with the involvement of a growing type of cancer in different populations.
- The obesity is linked to 20% of all cancer deaths in women and 14% in men (Calle 2003)
- It is evident that in case of obesity, exercise becomes an important moment to fight what described above.
- Tumors associated with increased BMI are cancer of breast in post-menopausal women, of prostate, of kidney, of esophagus, of endometrium, and it was determined that there is an increased risk for each increment of 5 Kg/m^2 at the BMI (Roberts 2010)
- There is a direct correlation between BMI and plasma insulin levels (McKeown-Eyssen 1994, Giovannucci 1995)
- High levels of insulin are associated with insulin resistance and low plasma levels of Insulin like Growth Factor Binding Protein 1 and 2 (IGFBP1/2), proteins which bind IGF-1 (Insulin-like Growth Factor 1) which in turn has an activity to promote cell proliferation. The reduction of IGFBP1 and IGFBP2 increases the levels of free IGF-1.
- Many epidemiological studies have shown that high plasma levels of insulin before eating, C peptide (an insulin secretion indicator of the pancreas), are related to risk of endometrial, pancreatic, colorectal, postmenopausal breast cancer (Goodwin 2002, Pisani 2008; Wolpin 2009)
- Obese individuals usually have high plasma levels of IGF-1 (Frystyk 2004), and high plasma levels of IGF-1 have been linked to high risk for cancer of the colon and the rectum, the prostate and the premenopausal breast (Renehan 2004) and, with less evidence, in the postmenopausal phase (Renehan, 2006). The IGF-1 elevation in adipose tissue results in an increase of aromatase, an enzyme involved in the conversion of androgen hormones into estradiol hormone at high mitogenic activity on the epithelium of the mammary gland (Travis 2003).

1.4 Breast cancer and the management of physical exercise

Breast cancer is the most common female cancer in many countries.

1.4.1 As regards risk factors for breast cancer it should be noted that

these have been identified in the:

- Excess weight
- Excess body fat
- High insulin on an empty stomach
- Insulin resistance
- Increased plasma levels, Insulin Like Growth Factor
- Increased plasma levels of hormones at estrogen and androgen activity

All the listed factors above are involved in the proliferative in vitro and in vivo cancer processes (Stephenson, 2003; Del Giudice 1998; Bruning 1995; Sachdev 2001; IARC 2002).
In literature there are few data about the effects of physical activity on women related to the parameters listed above (Schmitz 2005)

- There is evidence that obesity is a risk factor for breast cancer (Stephenson 2003, World Cancer Research Fund 2007)
- The high caloric intake in relation to the energy needs has been indicated as a possible cause of increased risk of breast cancer, but studies have given conflicting results. A positive relationship was described by 7 out of 15 case control studies (Franceschi 1996; Iscovitch 2004; Katsouyanni 1994, Levi 1993; Toniolo 1989; vant'Veer 1990, Yu 1990), 2 out of 10 prospective studies (Gaard 1995; Barrett -Connor 1993), with a relative risk between 1.3 and 3.5. Instead, no relationship was found by other authors (Malin 2005; Graham 1991.1992; Holmberg 1994, Ingram 1991; Katsoiyanni 1988, Miller 1978, Rohan 1995, Yuan 1995, Holmes 1999, Howe 1991, Jones 1999; Kushi Velie 1992 2000; van der Brandt 1993) and an author found an inverse relationship (Knekt 1990).
- In a latest prospective study, 38.660 women aged from 55 to 74 years were monitored in the U.S.A. between 1993-2003. In that period of time, 764 new cases of breast cancer were diagnosed. The use of questionnaires allowed us to quantify the contribution of energy, the amount of physical activity, the weight, the height and the BMI of the population. The relative risk (RR) of breast cancer for patients with the highest quartile of caloric intake compared with women with the lowest quartile was equal to 1.25 BMI > 30Kg/m2 compared with BMI < 22.5 kg/m2 and led to a risk equal to 1.35. Women with intense physical activity > 4 hours weekly reduced their RR to 0.78% compared to less active ones. Patients with the highest energy intake, with a higher BMI, doing less physical activity than the others, have a RR of 2.10 (Chang, 2006).
- Obesity, at the moment of diagnosis, is an unfavorable prognostic factor both for recurrence and for survival (Chlebowsky 2002, Boyd 1981, Goodwin 2002, Kumar 2000, Newman 1986)
- The weight gain after the diagnosis is a common phenomenon (Rock 1999; Demark-Wahnefried 1997, 2001; McInnes 2001; Goodwin 1999; Asiani 1999; Harvie 2004; Freedman 2004; xxDonegan 1978; Donegan 1978; Dixon 1978; Hernandez 1983; Bonomi 1984; Foltz 1985; Heasman 1985; Hunington 1989; Chlebowski 1986, 1993, Goodwin 1988, 1998, Gordon 1990; Levine 1991; Demark-Wahnefried 1983,1997; Faber-Langendoen 1996, Cheney 1997).
- In the Health Eating and Lifestyle Study (HEAL), 514 women with breast cancer, stage 0-IIIA, were monitored for body composition by DEXA for a period of 2 years. At the

end of the first year after diagnosis, 68% showed a weight gain between 1.7 and 4.7 kg and 74% increased their fat mass between 2.1 and 3.9%. Three years after diagnosis, the patients with greater weight gain were those with the higher stage, post-menopausal, younger, with greater reductions in physical activity after diagnosis (Irwin 2005).

- The chemotherapy has an important role in weight gain. The role of Tamoxifen would seem poor, instead, more important is the effect of other drugs such as Cyclophosphamide, Metrotexate, Epirubicin, Fluorouracil (Demark-Wahnefried 1993, Goodwin 1999, Cheney 1998 Fisher 1997; Ascani 1999, Shepherd 2001, Faber-Lanhendoen 1996; Camora 1990)
- Weight gain after diagnosis is a negative prognostic factor for survival (Chlebowsky 1987; Camora 1990; Bonomi, 1985), however, it was denied by other authors (Levine 1991; Heasman 1985, Goodwin 1988, Costa 2002)
- Women with breast cancer have an increased risk for hypertension and diabetes (Aziz 2002; Ganz 1998)

1.5 Weight and physical exercise

- Excess weight and reduced physical activity are included in a proportion between one-quarter to one-third of breast cancer carriers (IARC 2002)
- Physical activity is considered a reliable factor for breast cancer risk reduction in postmenopausal women (IARK 2002, World Cancer Research Fund in 2007, Monninkhof 2007; Friedenreich 2008), regular physical activity in itself can reduce the risk up to 20% (Warburton 2007)
- Case-control studies (Vanio 2002, Bernstein 1994, Carpenter 1999, Carpenter 2003; Yang Bernstein 2005) and cohort studies (McTiernan, 2003; Patel 2003; Dallal 2007; Lahmann 2007) demonstrated that the risk of invasive cancer of the breast is reduced by a percentage varying from 15 to 50% in women who do physical activity. Furthermore, a reduction of 50% has been reported in women of childbearing age with 4 hours of physical activity per week or post-menopausal women with the habit of regular and intense physical activity (Carpenter 1999, 2003). The results were confirmed in geographically different populations. They involved Asian and African-American women (Yang) Bernstein 2005). The risk of carcinoma in situ is reduced in women with regular physical activity as well (Patel 2003)
- The California Teachers Study (CTS), a prospective study on 133.000 women, showed that both the invasive breast cancer and the carcinoma in situ show a level of risk inversely correlated with the amount of physical activity as long as women were involved at least 5 hours per week during all their fertile life.
- However, it should be noted that moderate or intense protracted physical activity for a long period of life has demonstrated protection only for the risk of invasive cancer, compared with positive neoplasia for estrogen receptors, but not for invasive cancers which are negative for these receptors (Dallal 2007)
- The EPIC (European Prospective Investigation into Cancer and Nutrition) showed that women with higher recreational or occupational physical activity have a lower risk than those with the lowest quartile of physical activities, both in pre and post menopause. In an absolute sense neither recreational nor occupational activity show a relation with the risk. (Lahmann 2007).
- With regard to breast cancer in postmenopausal women in a meta-analysis of 19 cohort studies and 29 case-control studies showed an inverse relationship between risk and

amount of physical activity (Monninkhof 2007). The evidence is weaker for premenopausal women in which a risk reduction of 6% per weekly additional hour of physical activity, but only in half of the studies considered of the "highest quality".

- In particular, women with breast cancer, who exercise more than 9 MET per week, show a reduction in recurrence between 40 and 67% (McTiernan, 2008; Ibrahim 2010, Irwin 2007) compared with sedentary individuals.

1.6 The management of physical exercise in case of prostate cancer

- There are a lot of studies in literature which suggest a low risk reduction. (Vanio 2002). Instead, physical activity reduces the risk of the prostatic adenoma (Platz 1998)
- There is, however, some evidence that, in the groups, the most active men show a reduced risk of 10-30%, compared with the less active ones, and that the benefit is much more evident when high-intensity physical activity has started early in life (Friedenreich 2002)
- In a case control study of patients with grade 2 or more of prostate cancer, physical activity, which they had started in adolescence and which they had continued at high intensity for the rest of life, showed no substantial risk reduction (Friedenreich 2004)
- Cohort studies didn't demonstrate significant risk reduction, but they reduced the incidence of more severe forms or the ones with a fatal outcome (Friedereich 2004, Giovannucci 2005, Patel 2005)
- The prostate cancer survivors have a reduced mortality of 61% if they do high-intensity physical activity for at least 3 hours per week (Kenfield 2011)

1.7 Cancer of the colon-rectum and the management of physical exercise during cancer disease

Colon cancer is one of the forms of neoplasia with increasing incidence, with a prevalence in some countries, reaching 10% of the population suffering from cancer (Jemal 2010, Bhatia 2008).

The improvement of diagnostics and treatments has led to a substantial improvement in survival at 5 years that has passed through the most severe not localized forms (Altekruse 2010), from 51% in 1975 to 69.5% in 2006.

Survivors are at risk of developing a second cancer of the colon or of other organs, mainly breast, prostate, skin and lungs (Green 2002, Andre 2009, Birgisson 2005).

Most of the survivors of colon cancer are at risk of developing other diseases, mainly cardiovascular, pulmonary and psychiatric (Phipps, 2008, Jansen 2010; Yabroff 2004, Trentham-Dietz, 2003; Brown 1993; Denlinger 2011).

Often the survivors suffer from the consequences of therapies such as ostomy, neuropathies, chemotherapy, asthenia and depression. These may represent important limitations to the use of physical exercise as a therapeutic tool (Phipps 2008, Rauch 2004, Schneider 2007).

Physical activity has been proposed as a therapeutic but non- pharmacological tool to improve the quality of life and prognosis of patients suffering from colorectal cancer as well as a primary prevention means.

- The National Comprehensive Cancer Network recommends, during and at the end of anticancer treatment, a program of lasting and resistance physical activity to reduce asthenia.
- The American Cancer Society wishes a physical activity program to improve the quality of life, preventing recurrences or the incidence of concomitant diseases (Brown 2003)

- The American College of Sports Medicine, through a consensus, hopes for neoplastic patients a moderate-intensity physical activity of at least 150 minutes per week or 75 minutes per week of intense activity, combined with two/three weekly stretching sessions for the most important muscle groups (Schmitz 2010).

Studies on the role of physical activity in reducing the colon cancer risk are those which oncologists recognize as the most convincing (Vainio 2002). Literature provides numerous prospective studies (Lee 1995; Gerhardsson 1988, Martinez 1997, Wu 1987; Thun 1992; Dancing 1990-Barbash, Albanian 1989, Severson 1989; Lynge 1988, Paffembarger 1987, Giovannucci 1995), and retrospective (Fraser 1983 , Longnecker 1995, Wittemore 1990, Kuna 199 °, Markowitz 1992, Peters 1989, Brownson 1989, Kato 1990, Fredriksson 1989). A meta-analysis of 19 cohort studies showed a reduction in the incidence of cancer in 22% of males and in 29% of women with physical activity (Samad 2005).
Another meta-analysis of 52 observational studies showed that physical activity reduces the development of colon cancer (Wolin 2009).
However:

- data are more convincing in men than in women (Cheblowski 2004);
- the use of hormone replacement therapy alone tends to reduce the risk of cancer and this gives serious problems of interpretation when the examined women were older ;
- the combination of moderate physical activity all life long with high-intensity recreational physical activity has for women little impact on cancer risk (Mai 2007);
- women, who did physical activity in the fertile age at least 4 hours a week, have a 25% lower risk than those whose activities did not exceed 30 minutes per week (Mai 2007)
- post-menopausal women, who didn't do any hormone treatment, have a 46% risk reduction, if they did physical activity for at least 4 hours a week ;
- women with hormone therapy do not have further risk reductions with the regular practice of physical activity ;
- physical activity doesn't give any risk reduction of the rectum cancer.

In a study of 680 patients with colon cancer, who belong to a population of 51.500 subjects, recruited by the Health Professional Follow-up Study, the survivors in the period 1986-2004 were monitored every 2 years with a specific questionnaire for assessing physical activity in MET, the results showed that subjects with an energy expenditure higher than 18 MET per week had a 50% risk reduction of recurrence. An activity over
27 MET per week, compared with patients with MET <3, showed a reduction in mortality risk equal to 0.47. Free from cancer patients were 82.2% with activity <3 MET, 87.4%, those between 3 and 27 MET, 92.1% those with > 27 MET in 5 years. Free of cancer patients were, for 3 MET levels, were respectively 79.4%, 81.2%, 88.3% in 10 years. Mortality in patients with activities <27 MET had a death rate of 50% lower than the sedentary ones; this result was not related to age, disease stage, BMI, tumor location and physical activity before the diagnosis. (Meyerhardt 2009).

- From an observational prospective cohort study, the Nurses' Health Study, conducted among 121.700 subjects in the period 1986-2002, 573 women with a diagnosis of colon cancer, stage I-III, were enrolled. All participants were monitored with a questionnaire and a scale which was able to measure the activity in MET hours/week. If no response was given, they did a research aimed at establishing the evolution of the illness or the death. The level of physical activity before the diagnosis had no effect on the mortality rate.The physical activity after diagnosis reduced, in subjects with <18 MET hours /

week energy expenditure, the index of mortality risk to 0.39 compared with women with <3 MET activity. Mortality in 5 years gave the following percentages: 14.1% for patients with <3 MET activity, 14.4% for those whose activity was between 3 and 17.9 MET hours per week, 62% for the > 18 MET group. Those women who increased their physical activity compared with the pre diagnosis period reduced by 50% their risk of mortality.

- Physical activity, before the diagnosis, indirectly correlates with the reduced incidence of recurrence (Haydon 2006).
- The amount of physical activity, before the diagnosis, does not affect mortality (Meyerhardt in 2006, 2009).
- The amount of physical activity after diagnosis reduces the risk of recurrence and mortality (Meyerhardt 2006a, 2006 b).

1.8 As regards risk factors for colon cancer it should be noted that

- many studies have shown a relationship between BMI and risk of colorectal cancer (Potter, 1993, Manson 1995, Murphy 1998).
- Fat has an important role, especially in its topographic distribution (Giovannucci 1995).
- High levels of visceral adiposity are related to high levels of insulin on an empty stomach (kissenbach 1982; Bjorntorp 1990; Krotkiewsky 1983).
- The Health Professionals Follow-up Cohort Study conducted on a population of 31.400 men, highlighted that waist-thigh circumference ratio, which is a surrogate of the visceral fat measure, correlated with the risk of colon cancer in the rectum; individuals with the highest quartile showed a 3.4 RR, compared with the ones who had the lowest quartile, (Giovannucci 1995).
- The insulin and the Insulin Like Growth Factor 1 (IGF-1) have a mitogenic activity and induce cell proliferation of colon mucosa cells, in vivo and in vitro (Giovannucci 1995, Singh 1993, Tran 1996).
- Patients with type 2 diabetes have a high incidence of colon adenomas (Hu 1999, Will 1998, Nishi 2001).
- High levels of plasma insulin have been linked to higher risk of colon cancer (McKeown-Eyssen 1994, Shoen 1999, Yamada 1998).
- The observational Cardiovascular Health Study showed the onset of the colorectal cancer in 102 subjects. It was carried out in 5.849 subjects, who were monitored for 3 years. The relative risk was twice for those who belonged to the quartile with the highest glucose on an empty stomach (also insulin on an empty stomach should be tested), compared with the ones with the lowest quartile of blood glucose levels. High levels of plasma glucose and insulin, after the glucose tolerance test were related to a colorectal cancer risk of 2.4. (Shoen 1999).
- High plasma levels of C-peptide in patients with colorectal cancer are related to an unfavorable prognosis for survival (Wolpin 2009).
- High IGF-1 levels in non-cancer subjects have been associated with high risk of colorectal cancer in two important, prospective studies, the Nurses Health Study and the Physicians Health Study. This association was not confirmed by the European prospective study, EPIC (European Prospective Investigation into Cancer) (Giovannucci 2000; McPollack 1999, Rinaldi 2010)
- Two meta-analyses did not confirm the relationship between risk and pre-disease IGF-1 levels (Rinaldi, 2010; Renehan 2004).

- The IGF-1 levels during the disease are not related to the prognosis of the survivors (Haydon 2006).
- The IGFBP-3 (Insulin like Growth Factor Binding Protein-3) levels, a protein whose deficiency increases the percentage of circulating free IGF-1, correlate inversely with mortality. In subjects with higher IGFBP-3 levels, the mortality risk was reduced by 50%.

2. Our point of view with regard to an ideal physical activity in oncological patients to survive

The development of exercise in cancer rehabilitation context has as its primary goal the promotion of a better quality of life, especially in terms of individual perception.
The rehabilitation outcome has to be measured in terms of an individual perception of well-being, and it is also expressed in a collective form, involving all the interested subjects to this topic in its definition.
The outcome, in general, has to do with the return to society of people who experienced the disease, as it happens for other important but not lethal diseases.
After having expressed, in the international review, what is believed to induce positive effects in the body system which survived cancer, through the use of physical exercise, we find useful to propose a rehabilitative treatment which is not limited to recommend regular metabolic activity but aims to recover the remaining capacity of the subject, through a specific approach to the patient and the pathology but, at the same time, it aims to increase his/her residual performance with progressive metabolic load by METs .
Therefore, we divided our therapeutic intervention in 3 phases:
Phase 1 Recovery of Residual Capacity.
Phase 2 Recovery sensory-motor and functional capacity.
Phase 3 Recovery of the quality of Life.

2.1 Phase 1: Recovery of residual capacity

The rehabilitation strategy is aimed at:

1. recovering joint mobility and elasticity of muscle tissue, according to the existing damage and to the diseases;
2. increasing the uninjured muscle tone;
3. rebalancing the muscle synergies of the body system, by reprogramming the body static and dynamic scheme.

Our rehabilitation method uses instrumental and not instrumental techniques.
The aim of the therapy is to:

- induce the gradual recovery of joint mobility through passive and active exercises;
- induce a sensory stimulus for body perception in the space. This is realized by us by using tools such as PANCAFIT or similar and the postural bench system (TecnoBody, Bergamo, Italy), equipped with six independent sensors, each one positioned at the dorsal, lumbar and sacroiliac level. It allows real-time to assess the load that the patient places on each of the sensors. This feedback visual system allows the operator to assess and to work on deficient areas of the body from the proprioceptive and muscle point of view. It also allows the patient to modify, to learn and to increase his/her perception of the body in the space, inducing the acquisition of a suitable elastic posture for the two hemisomas;

- induce muscular adaptations in the recovery of muscle tone, in this regard we use a focused vibratory acoustic stimulation at high intensity (VISS, VISSMAN, Rome, Italy). Vibrations stimulate bone marrow function and the upper motor centers in order to obtain a better performance of controls, responsible for muscle recruitment; they activate the aerobic metabolism; they have an analgesic effect; they increase local circulation and bone density; they cause an increase in contractile capacity and elasticity of the skeletal muscle tissue;
- recover muscle synergies and elasticity of muscle tissue.

Rehabilitation protocol

2 sessions per week for at least 2 months with a metabolic cost of 18-21 METs.

Physical Therapies:

focused high intensity vibratory stimulation (VISS, VISSMAN, Rome, Italy).
Position: supine in the absence of muscle contraction; frequency: 300Hz; duration: 30 min.

Motor Rehabilitation:

- passive mobilization;
- passive muscle stretching exercises;
- Postural motor training using postural bench (TecnoBody, Bergamo, Italy). Position: supine; duration: 30 min.;
- isometric force exercises.

2.2 Phase 2: Sensory-motor and functional recovery

The rehabilitation strategy aims to:
replan the balance system to ensure that the brain (CNS) can use the sensory systems which are still working;
increase the tone of postural muscles, looking for an enhancement of the lower limbs and trunk muscles.
In our rehabilitation method, we use instrumental or not instrumental techniques.

The aim of therapy is to :

- induce adaptation to the pathological condition;
- induce a sensory readaptation (e.g. placing the patient on a tilting platform demanding stabilization motor tasks in closed and open kinetic chain (I-Moove Allcare Innovations Chabeuil, France);
- support a sensory substitution (e.g. trying to strengthen the role of vestibulo-spinal control by strengthening the ability to use proprioceptive afferents in a patient with sensory and/or motor neuropathy);
- induce a tone recovery and proprioception of the muscle skeletal kinetic chains by creating an unstable environment where the patient has to relate to rebalance the relationship between the kinetic chains, enhancing inter-and paravertebral muscles and searching for a core stability increase with the I -Move system or similar;
- induce a muscle strength increase, especially in the lower limbs.

Rehabilitation protocol

3 sessions per week for at least three months with a metabolic cost of 21-24 METs.

Physical Therapy:

Focused high intensity vibratory stimulation (VISS, VISSMAN, Rome, Italy)
Position: orthostatic; frequency: 300Hz; duration: 10 min

Motor Rehabilitation:

- 20 min of aerobic cycle ergometer, 80-95 bpm.
- Passive muscle stretching exercises.
- Global proprioceptive training (I-Moove Allcare Innovations Chabeuil, France). Position: orthostatic; duration: 30 min.
- Postural motor sense training using postural bench (TecnoBody, Bergamo, Italy). Position: orthostatic; duration: 10 min.
- Isometric force exercises.

2.3 Phase 3: Recovery of quality of life

The rehabilitation strategy is aimed at strengthening of the recovered **sensorimotor** capacity to allow the patient a gradual return to society, improving his/her quality of life Increasing the muscle strength needed for walking and for the orthostatic position, developing proprioception and requiring motor tasks more and more difficult and functional in daily life. In our rehabilitation method, we use instrumental or not instrumental techniques.

The aim of therapy is to:

- induce a proprioceptive increase using instruments for monitoring the performance which is achieved by biofeedback (e.g. I-Moove allows you to balance the muscle synergies through its helical movement, taking the natural, spiral course of the muscle fascia. The special movement of the platform can be expanded and strengthened specifically for the patient by increasing and improving proprioception, mobility and strength. (I-Moove Allcare Innovations Chabeuil, France);
- increase selectively the muscle strength (e.g. isotonic and isokinetic exercises, load of 60% RM for 12 repetitions for 4 series);
- stimulate motor learning;
- create a cardio circulatory metabolic adaptation.

Rehabilitation protocol

3 sessions per week for three months with a metabolic cost of 25-29 METs.

Physical Therapy:

Focused high intensity vibratory stimulation (VISS, VISSMAN, Rome, Italy). Position: supine in the absence of muscle contraction; frequency: 300Hz; duration: 30 min.
Global vibratory stimulation (PhysioPlate FIT, Globus Italy srl, Codognè (TV), Italy). Position: orthostatic; frequency: 50Hz; duration: 10 minMotor Rehabilitation:

- 40 min of aerobic cycle ergometer, 100-110 bpm;
- active and passive stretching;
- global proprioceptive training (I-Moove Allcare Innovations Chabeuil, France). Position: orthostatic; duration: 30 min;
- coordination exercises and complex motion;
- isokinetic and / or isotonic strength exercises. Our protocol is repeated after 3 months from the end of the entire project, by repeating phase 2 and 3 with a duration of 1

month per each phase in 24 months from the end of the specific medical or surgical oncology treatment.

3. Conclusions

Cancer patients suffer from persistent emotional and social distress, because of functional deficits, all that results in a reduced quality of life (QOL). The QOL assessment should include at least four functional dimensions: physical, the emotional, the social and the cognitive function. These dimensions are positively influenced by a proper rehabilitation program which includes physical exercise. It is well known that phyisical activity is an important means to prevent and to fight the problems of inactivity and disuse, and to reduce fatigue.

The information about the role of physical activity in oncology has been increasing over the years, and now is possible to confirm that " **the physical activity decreases the risk of disease; in patients who suffer from cancer, it prolongs survival, reduces the occurrence of concomitant diseases and improves the life quality" in (U.S. Department of Health and Human Services, 2008).**

4. References

Abrahamson, P.E.; Gammon, M.D.; Lund, M.J.; Britton, J.A.; Marshall, S.W.; Flagg, E.W.; Porter, P.L.; Brinton, L.A.; Eley, J.W.; Coates, R.J.; Recreational physical activity and survival among young women with breast cancer. *Cancer. 2006*;107:1777–85.

Baer*, H.J.; Tworoger,S.; Hankinson, S.; Willett W.; Body Fatness at Young Ages and Risk of Breast Cancer Throughout Life ; *American Journal of Epidemiology* Vol. 171, No. 11

Ballard-Barbash, R.; Hunsberger, S.; Alciati, M.H.; Blair, S.N.; Goodwin, P.J.; McTiernan, A.; Wing, R.; Schatzkin, A.; Physical Activity, Weight Control, and Breast Cancer Risk and Survival: Clinical Trial Rationale and Design Considerations; *J Natl Cancer Inst* 2009;101: 630 - 643

Barnett, G.C; Shah, M.; Redman, K.; Easton, D.F.; Ponder, B.A.J.; Pharoah, P.D. P. Risk Factors for the Incidence of Breast Cancer: Do They Affect Survival From the Disease? *J Clin Oncol* 26,20,10,2008

Belle, F.; Kampman, E.; McTiernan, A. et al. Dietary Fiber, Carbohydrates, Glycemic Index, and Glycemic Load in Relation to Breast Cancer Prognosis in the HEAL Cohort; *Cancer Epidemiol Biomarkers Prev* 2011;20:890-899.

Boyes, A.; Girgis, A. Exercise and Nutrition Routine Improving Cancer Health (ENRICH): The protocol for a randomized efficacy trial of a nutrition and physical activity program for adult cancer survivors and carers. *BMC Public Health* 2011, 11:236 doi:10.1186/1471-2458-11-236

Bianchini, F.; Kaaks, R.; Vainio, H,; Weight control and physicalactivity in cancer prevention. *Obes Rev. 2002*;3:5–8.

Borugian, M.J.; Sheps, S.B.; Kim-Sing, C.; Van Patten, C.; Potter, J.D.; Dunn, B.; Gallagher, R.P.; Hislop, T.G.; Insulin, macronutrient intake, and physical activity: are potential indicators of insulin resistance associated with mortality from breast cancer? *Cancer Epidemiol Biomarkers Prev. 2004*;13:1163–72.

Campbell, K.L.; McTiernan, A.; Exercise and Biomarkers for Cancer Prevention Studies; *J. Nutr.* 137: 161S–169S, 2007.

Carver, JR.; Shapiro, CL.; Ng A, Jacobs, L.; American Society of Clinical Oncology clinical evidence review on the ongoing care of adult cancer survivors: cardiac and pulmonary late effects. *J Clin Oncol. 2007* Sep 1;25(25):3991-4008. Epub 2007 Jun 18.

Chong-Do Lee, EdD; Xuemei Sui, MD; Steven N. Blair; Combined Effects of

Cardiorespiratory Fitness,Not Smoking, and Normal Waist Girth on Morbidity and Mortality in Men *Arch Intern Med. 2009;*169(22):2096-2101

Christine, M. F.; Orenstein, M.R.; Physical Activity and Cancer Prevention: Etiologic Evidence and Biological Mechanisms 0022-3166/02 $3.00 © 2002 *American Society for Nutritional Sciences.*

Courneya, K.S. ; Segal, R.J.; Mackey, J.R.; Gelmon, K.; Reid, R.D.;

Friedenreich, C.M.; Ladha, A.B.; Proulx, C.; Vallance, J.K.H.; Lane, K.; Yasui, Y.; McKenzie, D.C. Effects of Aerobic and Resistance Exercise in Breast Cancer Patients Receiving Adjuvant Chemotherapy: A Multicenter Randomized Controlled Trial ; *J Clin Oncol* 25,28,1,2007

DerSimonian, R., Laird, N.; Meta-analysis in clinical trials. *Control Clin Trials. 1986;*7:177–88.

Dessy, LA.; Monarca, C.; Grasso, F.; Saggini, A., Buccheri, EM.; Saggini, R.; Scuderi, N.; The use of mechanical acoustic vibrations to improve abdominal contour. *Aesthetic Plast Surg*. 2008 Mar;32(2):339-45.

Egger,M.; Davey Smith, G.; Schneider, M.; Minder, C.; Bias in metaanalysis detected by a simple, graphical test. *BMJ.1997;*315:629–34.

Enger ,S.M.; Bernstein, L.; Exercise activity, body size and premenopausalbreast cancer survival. *Br J Cancer. 2004;*90: 2138–41.Sternfeld B, Weltzien E, Quesenberry CP Jr, Castillo AL, Kwan

Escalante, C.P.; MD, FACP and Manzullo, E.F.; MD, FACP.; Cancer-Related Fatigue: The Approach and Treatment *J Gen Intern Med* 24(Suppl 2):412-6-2009

Fairey, A.S.; Courneya, K.S.; Field, C.J.; Bell, G.J.; Jones, L.W.; Mackey, JR.; Effects of exercise training on fasting insulin, insulin resistance, insulin-like growth factors, and insulin-like growth factor binding proteins in postmenopausal breast cancer survivors: a randomized controlled trial. *Cancer Epidemiol Biomarkers Prev. 2003;*12:721–7.

Fialka-Moser, V.; Crevenna, R.; Korpan, M.; Quittan, M.; Cancer rehabilitation: particularly with aspects on physical impairments. *J Rehabil Med.* 2003 Jul;35(4):153-62

Fossa, S. D.; Loge, J.H.; Dahl , A. A.; Long-term survivorship after cancer: how far have we come?; *Annals of Oncology 19* (Supplement 5): v25–v29, 2008

Frisch, R.E.; Wyshak, G.; Albright, N.L.; Albright, T.E.; Schiff, I.; Jones, K.P., *Witschi, J., Shiang, E., Koff, E,, Marguglio, M. Lower prevalenceof breast cancer and cancers of the reproductive system among ormer college athletes compared to non-athletes. Br J Cancer.1985;52:885–91.*

Friedenreich, C.M.; Rohan, T.E.; A review of physical activity and breast cancer. *Epidemiology. 1995;*6:311–7.

Friedenreich CM, Cust AE. Physical activity and breast cancer risk: impact of timing, type and dose of activity and population subgroup effects. *Br J Sports Med. 2008;*42:636–47 (a)

Friedenreich, C.M.; Cust, A.E.; Physical activity and breast cancer risk: impact of

subgroup effects timing, type and dose of activity and population. *Br. J. Sports Med.* 2008;42;636-647 (b)

Giovannucci, E.; Insulin, Insulin-Like Growth Factors and Colon Cancer: A Review of the Evidence; *J. Nutr.* 131: 3109S–3120S, 2001.

Goodwin, P.J.; Boyd, N.F.; Body size and breast cancer prognosis: a critical review of the evidence. *Breast Cancer Res Treat. 1990*;16:205–14.

Harvie, MN.; Howell, A.; Thatcher, N.; Baildam, A.; Campbell, I. Energy balance in patients with advanced NSCLC, metastatic melanoma and metastatic breast cancer receiving chemotherapy - a longitudinal study; *British Journal of Cancer (2005)* 92, 673 - 680

Hoffman-Goetz, L.; Apter, D.; Demark-Wahnefried, W.; Goran, MI,; McTiernan, A.; Reichman, ME.; Possible mechanisms mediating an association between physical activity and breast cancer. *Cancer.1998*;83:621–8.

Holick, C.N.; Newcomb, P.A.; Trentham-Dietz, A.; Titus-Ernstoff, L.; Bersch, A.J., Stampfer, M.; Baron J.A.; Egan, K.M.; Willett, W.C.; Physical activity and survival after diagnosis of invasive breastcancer. *Cancer Epidemiol Biomarkers Prev. 2008*;17:379–86.

Holmes, M.D.; Chen, W.Y.; Feskanich, D.; Kroenke, C.H.; Colditz, G.A.; Physical activity and survival after breast cancer diagnosis. *JAMA. 2005*;293:2479–86. Med Oncol. (a)

Holmes, M.D.; Chen, W.Y.; Feskanich, D.; et al. Physical Activity and Survival After Breast Cancer Diagnosis *JAMA*. 2005;293(20):2479-2486 (b)

Holmes, M.; MD, DrPH Wendy Chen, Y.; MD Feskanich, D.; ScD Candyce Kroenke, H.; ScD A. Colditz, G.; MD, DrPH. Physical Activity and Survival After Breast Cancer Diagnosis ; *JAMA, May 25, 2005*—Vol 293, No. 20 2479 (c)

Hutchison NA. *Cancer rehabilitation*. Minn Med. 2010 Oct;93(10):50-2

Iodice, P.; Bellomo RG.; Gialluca, G.; Fanò, G.; Saggini, R.; Acute and cumulative effects of focused high-frequency vibrations on the endocrine system and muscle strength. *Eur J Appl Physiol*. 2011 Jun;111(6):897-904.

Irwin, M.L.; Crumley, D.; McTiernan, A.; Bernstein, L., Baumgartner, R.; Gilliland, F.D.; Kriska, A.; Ballard-Barbash, R.; Physical activity levels before and after a diagnosis of breast carcinoma: the health, eating, activity, and lifestyle (heal) study. *Cancer. 2003*;97:1746–57

Irwin, M.L.; Smith, A,W.; McTiernan, A.; Ballard-Barbash, R.; Cronin, K.; Gilliland, F.D.; Baumgartner, R.N.; Baumgartner, K.B.; Bernstein, L.; Influence of pre- and postdiagnosis physical activity on mortality in breast cancer survivors: the health, eating, activity, and lifestyle study. *J Clin Oncol. 2008*;26:3958–64.

Irwin, M.L.; Physical activity interventions for cancer survivors; *Br. J. Sports Med.* 2009;43;32-38;

James, E.L.; Stacey, F.; Chapman, K.; Lubans, D.R.; Asprey, G.; Sundquist, K.;

Jernstrom, H.; Barrett-Connor, E.; Obesity, weight change, fasting insulin, proinsulin, c-peptide, and insulin-like growth factor-1levels in women with and without breast cancer: the rancho bernardo study. *J Womens Health Gend Based Med. 1999*;8:1265–72.

Kaaks, R.; Nutrition, hormones, and breast cancer: is insulin the missing link? *Cancer Causes Control. 1996*;7:605–25.

Karvinen, K.H.;. Courneya, K.S.; North, S.; et al. Associations between Exercise and Quality of Life in Bladder Cancer Survivors: A Population-Based Study; *Cancer Epidemiol Biomarkers Prev* 2007;16:984-990.

Knols, R.; Aaronson, N. K.; Uebelhart, D.; Fransen, J.; Aufdemkampe, G.; Physical Exercise in Cancer Patients During and After Medical Treatment: A Systematic Review of Randomized and Controlled Clinical Trials. *Journal of Clinical oncology vol 23,16,2005*

Laky,B.; Janda, M.; Cleghorn, G.; Obermair A.; Comparison of different nutritional assessments and bodycomposition measurements in detecting malnutrition among gynecologic cancer patients1-3. *Am J Clin Nutr 2008;*87:1678–85.

LaPorte, R.E.; Montoye, H.J.; Caspersen, C.J.; Assessment of physical activity in epidemiologic research: problems and prospects. *Public Health Rep. 1985;*100:131–46. Med Oncol

LaStayo, P.C.; Larsen, S.; Smith, S.; Dibble, L.; Marcus, R.; The Feasibility And Efficacy Of Eccentric Exercise With Older Cancer Survivors: A Preliminary Study ; *J Geriatr Phys Ther. 2010* ; 33(3): 135–140

Lau, J.; Ioannidis, J.P.; Schmid, C.H., Quantitative synthesis in systematic reviews. *Ann Intern Med. 1997;*127:820–6.

Lee, IM.; Physical activity in women: how much is good enough? *JAMA. 2003;*290:1377–9.

Ligibel, J.A.; Campbell, N.; Partridge, A.; Chen, W.Y.; Salinardi, T.; Chen, H.; Adloff, K.; Keshaviah, A.; Winer, E.P. Impact of a Mixed Strength and Endurance ExerciseIntervention on Insulin Levels in Breast Cancer Survivors; *J Clin Oncol 26,.6, 2008* (a)

Ligibel, J.A.; Campbell, N.; Partridge, A.; Chen, W.Y.; Salinardi, T.; Chen, H.;Adloff, K.; Keshaviah, A.; Winer E.P. Impact of a Mixed Strength and Endurance Exercise Intervention on Insulin Levels in Breast Cancer Survivors; *J Clin Oncol* 26,6,20,2008 (b)

Lyman, G.H.; Kuderer, N.M.; The strengths and limitations of metaanalysesbased on aggregate data. *BMC Med Res Methodol.2005;*5:14.

Mathur N.; Pedersen B.K.; Exercise as a Mean to Control Low-Grade Systemic Inflammation ; *Mediators of Inflammation* Volume 2008, Article ID 109502, 6 pages doi:10.1155/2008/109502

McNeely, M.L.; Campbell, K.L.; Rowe, B.H.; Klassen, T.P.; Mackey, J.R.; Courneya K.S. Effects of exercise on breast cancer patients and survivors: a systematic review and meta-analysis; *CMAJ* • July 4, 2006 • 175(1) | 34

McTiernan, A.; Rajan, K.B.; Tworoger, S.; Irwin, M.; Bernstein, L.; Baumgartner, R.; Gilliland, F.; Stanczyk, F.; Yasui, Y.; Ballard-Barbash R. Adiposity and Sex Hormones in Postmenopausal Breast Cancer Survivors ; *Journal of Clinical Oncology,* Vol 21, No 10 (May 15), 2003: pp 1961-1966

McTiernan, A.; Tworoger, S.S.; Ulrich, C.M.; Yasui, Y.; Irwin, M.L.; Rajan, K.B.; Sorensen, B.; Rudolph, R.E.; Bowen, D.; Stanczyk, F.Z.; otter JD, Schwartz, R,S.; Effect of exercise on serum estrogens inpostmenopausal women:a 12-month randomized clinical trial. *Cancer Res. 2004;*64:2923–8.

McTiernan, A.; Irwin, M.; VonGruenigenWeight, V.;Physical Activity, Diet, and Prognosis in Breast and Gynecologic Cancers.*J Clin Oncol 28.© 2010 (a)*

McTiernan, A.; Irwin, M.; VonGruenigen, V.; Weight, Physical Activity, Diet, and Prognosis in Breast and Gynecologic Cancers; *J Clin Oncol* 28,26,10,2010 (b)

Meyerhardt, J.A.; Giovannucci, E.L.; Holmes, M.D.; Chan, A.T.; Chan, J. A.; Colditz, G. A., Fuchs, C.S.; Physical Activity and Survival After Colorectal Cancer Diagnosis; *J Clin Oncol* 24,22,1,2006 (a)

Meyerhardt, J.A.; Heseltine, D.; Niedzwiecki, D.; Hollis, D.; Saltz, L.B. Robert; Mayer, J.; Thomas, J.; Nelson, H.; Whittom,, R.; Hantel, A.; Schilsky, R. L.; Fuchs, C.S. Impact of Physical Activity on Cancer Recurrence and Survival in Patients With Stage III Colon Cancer: Findings From CALGB 89803; *J Clin Oncol 24,22,, 2006* (b)

Meyerhardt, J. A.; Niedzwiecki, D.; Hollis, D.; Saltz, L. B;. Mayer, R. J.; Nelson,H.; Whittom, R.; Hantel, A.; Thomas, J.; Fuchs, S.C,; Impact of Body Mass Index and Weight Change After Treatment on Cancer Recurrence and Survival in Patients With Stage III Colon Cancer: Findings From Cancer and Leukemia Group B 89803. *Journal of Clinical oncology vol 28,25,2008*

Meyerhardt, J. A.; MD, MPH; Giovannucci, E. L.; MD, ScD; Ogino, S.; MD, PhD; Kirkner; G. J.;Chan, A. T. ; MD, MPH; Willett, W.; MD, DrPH; Fuchs, C. S.; MD, MPH Physical Activity and Male Colorectal Cancer Survival. *Arch Intern Med. 2009;169(22):2102-2108*

Mikkelsen, T.; Sondergaard, J.; Sokolowski, I.; Jensen, A.; Olesen, F.; *Cancer survivors' rehabilitation needs in a primary health care context*. Fam Pract. 2009 Jun;26(3):221-30. Epub 2009 Mar 5.

Monninkhof, E.M., Elias, S.G.; Vlems, F.A.;, van der Tweel, I.; Schuit, A.J.; Voskuil, D.W.; van Leeuwen, F.E.; Physical activity and breastcancer: a systematic review. *Epidemiology. 2007;*18:137–57.

Mustian, K.M. Ph.D., M.P.H., A.C.S.M, F.S.B.M., Sprod, L.K. Ph.D.; Palesh, O.G.; Ph.D.; Luke, M.P.H. ; Peppone, J. Ph.D.; Janelsins, M.C. Ph.D.; Mohile, S.G.; M.D., Carroll, J. M.D.; Exercise for the Management of Side Effects and Quality of Life among Cancer Survivors. *Curr Sports Med Rep. 2009* ; 8(6): 325–330.

Neilson, H. K.; Friedenreich, C.M.; Brockton, N.T.; Millikan R.C. Physical Activity and Postmenopausal Breast Cancer: Proposed Biologic Mechanisms and Areas for Future Research; *Cancer Epidemiol Biomarkers Prev 2009;*18(1). (a)

Neilson, H.; Friedenreich, C.; Brockton, N.T.; et al. Physical Activity and Postmenopausal Breast Cancer:Proposed Biologic Mechanisms and Areas for Future Research *Cancer Epidemiol Biomarkers Prev* 2009;18:11-27. (b)

Noble, M.; Caryl, R.; Kraemer L.; Sharratt, M.; UW WELL-FIT: the impact of supervised exercise programs on physical capacity and quality of life in individuals receiving treatment for cancer; *Support Care Cancer* DOI 10.1007/s00520-011 1175-z

Parmar , M.K.; Torri, V.; Stewart, L., Extracting summary statistics to perform meta-analyses of the published literature for survival endpoints. *Stat Med. 1998;*17:2815–34.

Pierce, J.P.; Stefanick, M.L.; Flatt, S.W.; Natarajan, L.; Sternfeld, B., Madlensky, L.; Al-Delaimy, W.K., Thomson, C.A.; Kealey, S.; Hajek, R.; Parker, B.A.; Newman, V.A.; Caan, B.; Rock, C.L.; Greater survival after breast cancer in physically active women with high vegetable- fruit intake regardless of obesity. *J Clin Oncol.2007;* 25:2345–51.

Pietrangelo, T.; Mancinelli, R.; Toniolo, L.; Cancellara, L.; Paoli, A.; Puglielli, C.; Iodice, P.; Doria, C.; Bosco, G.; D'Amelio, L.; di Tano, G.; Fulle, S.; Saggini, R.; Fanò, G.; Reggiani, C.; Effects of local vibrations on skeletal muscle trophism in elderly people: mechanical, cellular, and molecular events. *Int J Mol Med.* 2009 Oct;24(4):503-12.

Protani, M.; Coory, M.; Martin, J.H. Effect of obesity on survival of women with breast cancer: systematic review and meta-analysis; *Breast Cancer Res Treat* (210) 123:627–635

Robinson-Cohen, C.; MS; Katz, R.; Phil, D.; Mozaffarian, D.; MD, DrPH; Dalrymple, L.S.; MD, MPH; Ian de Boer, MD, MS; Sarnak, M.; MD, MS; Mike Shlipak, MD, MPH;David Siscovick, MD, MPH; Bryan Kestenbaum, MD, MS Physical Activity and Rapid Decline in Kidney Function Among Older Adults *Arch Intern Med. 2009;169(22):2116-2123*

Saggini, R.; Scuderi, N.; Bellomo, R.G.; Dessy, R.A.; Cancelli, F.; Iodice, P.; (2006) Selective development of muscular force in the rehabilitative context. *Eur Med Phys 2006*;42(suppl.1 to No.3) pag. 69-75

Sandhu, M.S.; Dunger, D. B.; Giovannucci, E.L.; Insulin, Insulin-Like Growth Factor-I (IGF-I), IGF Binding Proteins, Their Biologic Interactions, and Colorectal Cancer; *Journal of the National Cancer Institute*, Vol. 94, No. 13, July 3, 2002

Schmitz, K. H. 1; Holtzman J. 3,4,; Courneya K.S. 5; Masse, L.C. 6; CA Controlled Physical Activity Trials in Cancer Survivors: A Systematic Review and Meta-analysis. *Cancer J Clin 2003*;53;268-291

Schmitz, K. H.; Holtzman, J.; Courneya, K.S.; Ma^sse, L.C.; Duval, S.; Kane, R.; Controlled Physical Activity Trials in Cancer Survivors: A Systematic Review and Meta-analysis. *Cancer Epidemiol Biomarkers Prev* 2005;14:1588-1595.

Segal, R.; Evans, W.; Johnson, D.; Smith, J.; Colletta, S.; Gayton, J.; Woodard, S.; Wells, G.; Reid, R.;Structured Exercise Improves Physical Functioning in Women With Stages I and II Breast Cancer: Results of a Randomized Controlled Trial; *J Clin Oncol* 19:657-665. 2001

Slattery, M.L.; Caan, B.J.; Physical activity and risk of recurrenceand mortality in breast cancer survivors: findings from the lace study. *Cancer Epidemiol Biomarkers Prev. 2009*;18:87–95.

Stacey, A.; Kenfield,, Meir J;. Stampfer Giovannucci, E.; Chan, J.M.; Physical Activity and Survival After Prostate Cancer Diagnosis in the Health Professionals Follow-Up Study. *J Clin Oncol 28. © 2011*

Stoll, B.A.; Diet and exercise regimens to improve breast carcinoma prognosis. *Cancer. 1996*;78:2465–70.

Thune, I.; Furberg, A.S.; Physical activity and cancer risk: dose responseand cancer, all sites and site-specific. *Med Sci Sports Exerc. 2001*;33:S530–50. discussion S609-510.

Torjesen, P.A.; Birkeland, K.I.; Anderssen, S.A.; Hjermann, I.; Holme, I.; Urdal, P.; Lifestyle changes may reverse development of the insulin resistance syndrome. The oslo diet and exercise study: a randomized trial. *Diabetes Care. 1997*;20:26–31.

Trinh, L. 1; Plotnikoff R. C. 1,2,5; Rhodes R.E. 4; Scott North 3, and Courneya K. S.; Associations Between Physical Activity and Quality of Life in a Population-Based Sample of Kidney Cancer Survivors, *Cancer Epidemiol Biomarkers Prev;* 2011;20:859-868 (a)

Trinh, L.; Plotnikoff, R.C.; Rhodes, R.E. et al. Associations Between Physical Activity and Quality of Life in a Population-Based Sample of Kidney Cancer Survivors ; *Cancer Epidemiol Biomarkers Prev* 2011;20:859-868.(b)

Trinh, L.; Plotnikoff, R.C.; Rhodes, R. E.; et al. In a Population-Based Sample of Kidney Cancer Survivors Associations Between Physical Activity and Quality of Life *Cancer Epidemiol Biomarkers Prev* 2011;20:859-868. (c)

Vainio, H.; Kaaks, R.; Bianchini, F.; Weight control and physical activity in cancer prevention: international evaluation of the evidence. *Eur J Cancer Prev. 2002;* 11(Suppl 2):S94–100..

Wilson, D.B. ;Porter, J.S.; Parker, G.; Kilpatrick, J.; Anthropometric changes using a walking intervention in African American breast cancer survivors: a pilot study. *Prev Chronic Dis. 2005;*2:A16.

13

Fertility Preservation for Pre-Pubertal Girls and Young Female Cancer Patients

R. Gerritse[1,2], L. Bastings[1,3], C.C.M. Beerendonk[1], J.R. Westphal[1], D.D.M. Braat[1] and R. Peek[1,4]
[1]*Radboud University Nijmegen Medical Centre, Department Obstetrics and Gynaecology Nijmegen,*
[2]*Koningin Beatrix Ziekenhuis Winterswijk, The Netherlands,*
[3]*Jeroen Bosch Hospital 's Hertogenbosch, The Netherlands*

1. Introduction

New protocols in the early diagnosis and treatment of cancer have led to major improvements in the long-term survival of patients. However, aggressive chemotherapy or radiotherapy of the pelvic region, often lead to infertility, due to the damage of the follicles and/or oocytes that are present in the ovaries. In women the probability of sterilization due to cancer therapy varies with age, the type of treatment, and the follicular reserve in the ovary. Safeguarding their reproductive potential is a very important issue for women that have not yet started or completed their family, and even more so in pre-pubertal girls. Several options, some of which are still in the experimental phase, can now be offered to these women to (partially) preserve their fertility.

In this review, we will, after briefly describing the anatomy and physiology of an ovary, discuss the detrimental effects of chemotherapy and radiation on ovarian function. Subsequently, the various options that are currently available or are still in an experimental phase, for preserving fertility in women and pre-pubertal girls, will be discussed. These options (with the exception of option (i)), deal with cryopreserving either oocytes, embryos or ovarian tissue until the patient has been cured.

i. Minimizing the effects of radiation of the inner pelvic region by transposing the ovaries from the radiation area.
ii. Standard IVF procedures can be offered to women who are awaiting chemotherapy and radiotherapy for neoplastic disease. This procedure results in the generation of embryos that can be transferred after recovery of the disease. This option has its limitations, since it not only requires the presence of a male partner, but also delays cancer treatment during ovarian stimulation. In addition, the number of embryos that can be produced is restricted, and the chance of achieving a pregnancy after transfer of a cryo-preserved embryo is only 8-30%. Furthermore, the presence of estrogen-sensitive tumors is a contra-indication for this type of treatment, as high estradiol levels are induced during a normal IVF procedure, although alternative stimulation protocols with aromatase-inhibitors are nowadays available for these specific patients. Most importantly, this

treatment is not an option for pre-pubertal girls, or for post-pubertal girls who are not yet involved in a stable relationship.

iii. Aspiration of oocytes, followed by cryopreservation and IVF (if necessary preceded by *in vitro* maturation). This option has already been applied to a number of patients. Although the same drawbacks that apply to standard IVF are applicable, this procedure is mainly aimed at the treatment of post-pubertal girls/young women without a stable relationship. Only limited scientific data are currently available to substantiate its efficacy and long-term safety.

iv. As an alternative, cryopreservation of small ovarian cortex strips containing primordial follicles can be offered. After the patient has been cured, these cortex strips can subsequently be retransplanted either heterotopically or orthotopically. This procedure has been successfully used to re-establish female fertility in humans in a limited number of cases. A major problem with these avascular implants however is their relative short life expectancy and follicular loss due to long term ischemic injury directly after reimplantation.

v. Cryopreservation and subsequent reimplantation of intact ovaries may be a valuable addition to the existing array of options, especially for pre-pubertal girls and post-pubertal girls/women without a stable relationship. An important safety issue of this procedure is obviously the chance of reintroduction of malignant cells that may be present in the cryopreserved intact ovary. For this reason, patients with solid types of tumor and diffuse types of cancer such as leukemia that have a high chance of metastasizing to the ovaries, will have to be excluded from this kind of therapy. The cryobiological and surgical aspects of the preservation and retransplantation of an organ *in toto*, is technically clearly more challenging than the cryopreservation and transfer of isolated cells or tissue strips. The advantages of this approach are obvious; immediate revascularization of the transplanted ovary ensures that less ischemic damage is inflicted to the ovarian tissue post-thawing, and that more follicles will survive. In addition menses, normal long term reproductive functions, and normal hormonal status will be restored.

Finally, we will go into the safety of the procedure. Inevitably the autotransplantation of cortical strips or intact ovaries carries the risk of reintroducing malignant cells from the graft into the recipient.

The increase in knowledge of the biology and treatment of cancer has been accompanied by an increase in the efficacy of cancer therapies. Long term survival rates for many cancer types have therefore increased accordingly (Gatta et al., 2009). Consequently, the quality of life of cancer survivors is becoming an important issue.

The possibility to have genetically concordant progeny is for many people an event that is essential for an unrestricted quality of life as an adult (Schover, 2009). The loss of fertility that may result from cancer therapy, is therefore an additional complication on top of an already difficult period spent on conquering a devastating disease.

With this in mind, it is of the utmost importance to explore the possibilities for fertility preservation in patients that are to be treated with a gonado-toxic therapy. For post-pubertal boys and men, this can be achieved relatively easy via the cryopreservation of their semen prior to start of the therapy. For pre-pubertal boys this is not an option, as semen production is initiated during puberty. Also for this group of patients options for fertility preservation are being developed.

In this paper we confine ourselves to fertility preservation for female patients. We discuss the causes of anti-cancer therapy-related infertility, and review the current options for fertility preservation. We illustrate this matter with two case reports from our own clinical practice. In addition we discuss some as yet experimental procedures, that may in the future be offered to patients requiring fertility preservation.

2. Ovaries, oocytes and female reproduction

The human ovary is spherical structure with a mean volume of 7 cm^3 (range 2-15 cm^3; Munn et al., 1986). The inner ovarian mass, the medulla, consists mainly of stromal cells and contains the larger blood vessels. The outer layer of the ovary consists of the cortical tissue, spanning 2-3 mm. This tissue is rich in extra-cellular matrix proteins and poor in capillaries , and contains the vast majority of the follicles containing oocytes that comprise the ovarian reserve. The most important role of the follicle is to protect the oocyte, and support its development. Follicles are comprised of layer(s) of theca cells and granulosa cells. Different stages of follicles can be distinguished, ranging from primordial follicles to primary follicles, and via secondary finally to tertiary (antral) follicles.

In contrast to males in whom spermatogenesis is a continuous process resulting in the uninterrupted generation of fresh spermatozoa, in women a fixed number of oocytes is formed during embryogenesis from 1000-2000 germ cells. These germ cells are present in the human embryo at 30 days after conception. After 9-10 weeks, these cells transform to oogonia (Baker, 1972), that degenerate for the greater part between 10 and 20 weeks of gestation. After 5 months of gestation, the first meiotic division is initiated in the remaining oogonia, resulting in the differentiation to primary oocytes. At this stage the meiotic division process is arrested, and the oocytes enter a stage of dormancy (Wandji, 1996). At birth only 300.000 to 400.000 oocytes remain in the ovaries. From birth, the number of oocytes gradually decreases, and at the beginning of puberty around 200.000 oocytes remain. Under the influence of pituitary gonadotropic hormones (Gougeon, 1996; Oktay, 1997), each month a cohort of primary oocytes is recruited, and resumes development. Usually only one primary oocyt completes the first meiotic division. This secondary oocyt again enters a stage of dormancy, and is ovulated. The second dormant stage is only lifted after fertilization by a sperm cell. Around the age of 50 years, the total oocyte reserve is almost depleted and the woman enters menopause. In addition to age, several factors may affect the follicular reserve, leading to an early exhaustion and to premature ovarian insufficiency (POI). These factors include fertility-threatening therapies that are discussed in more detail in the next section.

3. Effects of radio- and chemotherapy on female fertility

3.1 Chemotherapy

Cytotoxic therapy may affect all components of the follicle, including granulosa cells, theca cells, and of course the oocyt itself (Sobrinho et al., 1971; Blumenfeld et al., 1999). In addition, interactions between these cell types that are required for oocyt development may be disturbed, resulting in the demise of the oocyt. Damage may become manifest by reduced ovarian weight, stromal fibrosis and in a reduction in the number of oocytes and ovarian follicles (Warne et al., 1973; Meirow et al., 1999; Oktem & Oktay, 2007).

The effect of chemotherapy on fertility is dependent on the type of the cytotoxic agent, the dose, and the duration of the therapy. Alkylating agents such as cyclophosphamide, Lphenyalanine mustard, and chlorambucil permanently damage ovarian tissue by interacting with DNA (Meirow et al., 1999; Manger et al., 2006; Oktem & Oktay, 2007). Analysis of a group of 138 young females receiving the alkylating agent busulfan as a preparative regimen for indicated that 83% of these women showed signs of fertility impairment, demonstrating the potentially very severe effects of this type of compounds (Borgmann-Staudt et al., 2011). Mertens et al. (1998) showed an even higher percentage of 99% in gonadal dysfunction for women receiving allogeneic haematopoietic stem cell transplantation. The cumulative dose of the cytotoxic drug being administered is an important factor in determining the level of ovarian insufficiency (Goldhirsch et al., 1990). Permanent ovarian insufficiency was more often induced when high dosages of drugs were administered during a short period of time, compared to low doses given over a longer time (Koyama et al., 1977).

In addition the age of the patient is pivotal in determining the amount of damage that is inflicted to the ovary. Older women, with an already decreased number of primordial follicles, have a higher risk of developing acute complete POI, compared with young women who still possess numerous primordial follicles (Schilsky et al., 1981; Sanders et al., 1996; Tauchmanova et al., 2002). Prepubertal girls seem less vulnerable to cytotoxic drugs than adults (Chiarelli et al., 1990). This may be explained by the fact that several chemotherapeutical drugs affect DNA replication and/or RNA and protein synthesis, and are therefore targeted at metabolically active cells. In prepubertal ovaries all follicles are in a dormant, metabolically quiescent state, and therefore less prone to chemotherapy induced damage. In contrast, in adult ovaries a number of follicles will be in an active state, and therefore more prone to chemotherapy induced damage. Nicosia et al. (1985) actually showed in ovarian autopsy material derived from patients having received chemotherapy, that the number of growing follicles was reduced, whereas the number of primordial follicles remained the same.

3.2 Radiotherapy

Similar to the effects of chemotherapeutical agents on DNA integrity, ionizing radiation, amongst other effects, also interferes with DNA function. As a consequence, also radiotherapy may negatively affect the ovarian reserve. Analogous to chemotherapy, the (cumulative) dose and the fractionation schedule determine the degree of damage to the ovary (Gosden et al., 1997). The human oocyte is exceptionally sensitive to radiation (Howell & Shalet, 1998) and the estimate of the LD50 (the lethal dose need to kill half the total number of oocytes) seems to be less than 2 Gy (Wallace et al., 2003). Also for radiation therapy, the age of the patient is an important factor in determining the level of damage. A dose of 4 Gy leads to sterility in 30% of young women, and in 100% of women over 40.

Not surprisingly, the combination of radiotherapy with chemotherapy increases the risk of POI (Williams et al., 1999; Wallace et al., 2005; Chemaitilly et al., 2006). Abdominal radiotherapy in combination with alkylating agents increased the risk of POI 27-fold (Byrne et al., 1992). By the age of 31, 42% of patients treated with this combination therapy, was postmenopausal, compared with 5% of women in the normal population.

3.3 Effects on pregnancy and health of newborns

In addition to their effects on oocytes and follicles, chemotherapy and radiotherapy may also influence uterine function. Radiation may lead to impaired uterine growth in premenarchal girls and failure of uterine development during pregnancy, leading to miscarriages, premature births and intrauterine growth retardation (Ogilvy-Stuart et al., 1997; Critchley, 1999; Critchley et al., 1992; 2002; Wallace et al., 2005). Comparable results were described by Salooja et al. (2001), who showed that in women that had received total body irradiation prior to autologous or allogeneic stem cell transplantation, are at high risk for maternal and fetal complications. These problems are probably a consequence of uterine vascular damage and reduced elasticity of the uterine musculature.

4. Current options for fertility preservation

4.1 Ovarian transposition

An way to prevent damage to the ovaries caused by ionizing radiation therapy applied to the pelvic region, is to surgically move the ovary temporarily to a location outside the field of radiation (Hadar et al., 1994; Howard, 1997). This procedure, referred to as oophoropexy, can be performed laparoscopically. Potential ovarian insufficiency following transposition may occur if the ovaries are not entirely moved outside the field of radiation, or when they spontaneously migrate back to their original position. Ovarian failure can also occur when the ovarian vascular pedicle has been compromised by the surgical procedure (Feeney et al., 1995). Oophoropexy is a safe and effective procedure, allowing preservation of ovarian function in 80% of cases (Bisharah & Tulandi, 2003).

4.2 Vitrification of oocytes

Cryopreservation of mature or immature oocytes is an obvious approach to preserve fertility. As no fertilization of the oocytes is yet required, this is option is especially suitable for women without a partner. The collection of mature oocytes requires stimulation with follicle stimulating hormone (FSH). This procedure, that may have to be repeated to obtain a sufficient number of oocytes, takes at least two weeks, and is therefore only suitable for women for whom it is safe to postpone their cancer treatment. The use of high doses of FSH makes this option unsuited for women with oestradiol-sensitive breast tumors, as high levels of oestradiol are induced by the FSH treatment (Sonmezer & Oktay, 2006) This caveat may be circumvented by the simultaneous use of aromatase inhibitors /anti oestrogens such as letrozole or tamoxifen (Oktay et al., 2005b; Sonmezer & Oktay, 2006). Alternatively, immature oocytes can be collected without prior stimulation. This procedure may also be used for young (prepubertal girls). Evidently, these immature oocytes must be matured in vitro (IVM) before they can be fertilised (Gosden, 2005).

After collection of the oocytes, they have to be cryopreserved in liquid nitrogen for long term storage. The formation of ice crystals during the freezing process may severely damage the oocyte, rendering it useless for further use. This is especially the case for mature oocytes, as they possess a fragile and sensitive meiotic spindle. Immature oocytes are in this respect less sensitive. Cryodamage can be prevented by freezing the oocytes in the presence of cryoprotective agents via specific protocols, either by slow freezing, or via vitrification (Cao et al., 2009; Chian et al., 2009; Kuwayama et al., 2005). During the latter procedure, that appears to result in more oocytes surviving the process undamaged, the oocytes are frozen extremely rapidly (> 12.000 °C/minute), in the presence of high concentrations of cryoprotectant, resulting in the prevention of ice crystal formation.

A consequence of the cryopreservation procedure (either slow freezing or vitrification) is hardening of the zona pellucida. Therefore, cryopreserved oocytes can only be fertilized via intracytoplasmatic sperm injection (ICSI). As the pregnancy rate per cryopreserved oocyte is approximately 3% (Kuwayama et al., 2005; Cobo et al., 2007; Homburg et al., 2009), a large number of oocytes, equivalent to several stimulation cycles and/or oocyte retrieval procedures, are required to achieve a reasonable chance of progeny. The exact number of children conceived with cryopreserved oocytes is unknown, but it is estimated to be over 500 worldwide. Postnatal parameters such as birth weight and incidence of congenital anomalies, were comparable with the reference population, indicating the safety of this procedure (Borini et al., 2007; Chian et al., 2008).

4.3 Cryopreservation of embryos

For women with a partner, the generation and cryopreservation of embryos is a suitable option. Obviously, this option will generally require ovarian stimulation, and is therefore subject to the same limitations as mentioned previously for the collection and cryopreservation of mature oocytes - the cancer treatment has to be postponed to allow for one or more ovarian stimulation(s), and extreme caution has to be taken when stimulating women with hormone sensitive tumors. The factor time may be circumvented by skipping the stimulation with FSH and collect immature oocytes instead. Evidently, in that case IVM has to be performed prior to fertilisation of the oocytes. Employing tamoxifen or letrozole based stimulation regimes may be used in the case of hormone sensitive tumors (see previous paragraph) (Oktay et al., 2005a, 2005b; Sonmezer & Oktay, 2006). Oktay et al. (2005b) has shown that in cancer patients who had been stimulated with this compound, recurrence rates were not elevated compared to cancer patients who had not been receiving any ovarian stimulation. Although we should keep in time that the follow up period was confined to only a limited number of years.

Theoretically, in women with hormone sensitive tumors oocytes can also be collected in a spontaneous (non-stimulated) cycle. However, the very limited number of oocytes that can be collected this way (one or two per cycle) makes this a very inefficient option and is therefore not advisable (Brown et al., 1996).

Embryo cryopreservation is an established and efficient technique, with reported implantation rates per thawed embryo between 8 and 30% (Frederick et al., 1995; Selick et al., 1995; Wang et al., 2001; Son et al., 2002; Senn et al., 2006), that has resulted in the birth of tens of thousands of children worldwide. In the future, new cryopreservation techniques such as vitrification may further improve the efficiency of this technique (Kuwayame et al., 2005).

4.3.1 Case report A: Emergency IVF in a patient with breast cancer

Mrs. X was diagnosed 3 years ago with breast cancer. She then underwent a lumpectomy of the right breast, and received radiotherapy. Shortly thereafter a unilateral recurrence was found, and a mastectomy with lymph node dissection was performed. Pathologic examination revealed an invasive ductal carcinoma, positive for estrogen and progesterone receptors. No tumor cells were found in the lymph nodes, and no other indications for metastatic disease were found. Additional chemotherapy courses were planned.

At this stage the patient, now 35 years of age, and her partner visited the Centre for Reproductive Medicine of our hospital, and expressed their interest in fertility preservation. After establishing that the current reproductive status of herself as well as of her partner showed no abnormalities, the possibilities for fertility preservation were discussed. Although oocyte vitrification and ovarian tissue banking were in theory viable options, the couple was counseled to proceed with an emergency IVF-

ICSI attempt, followed by cryopreservation of the embryos, as this would probably give the highest chance of progeny within the time limit set by the oncologist.
The ovarian stimulation protocol was started one month after the mastectomy. Regarding the hormone receptor positive status of the tumor, a regimen combining FSH and letrozol was selected in order to avoid the high oestradiol levels associated with ovarian hyperstimulation. The treatment eventually resulted in the retrieval of 13 oocytes, 12 of which could be inseminated via ICSI. Of the 7 resulting embryos, 3 were eligible for cryopreservation. The efficacy of the letrozol treatment was demonstrated by the finding that during the stimulation with FSH, oestradiol levels did not rise beyond 1000 pmol/L.
The patient than completed 5 cycles of chemotherapy. In addition, she received adjuvant hormonal therapy. Menses had stopped and the patient suffered from hot flushes. Two years later at age 37, the patient wanted to achieve pregnancy. After discontinuation of medication, the hot flushes diminished and menses did resume. Five months later the patient conceived spontaneously, but unfortunately the pregnancy ended in an abortion. As further spontaneous conceptions did not occur, two cycles of fresh IVF were performed. Although the second cycle resulted in a pregnancy, this again ended in an abortion. The patient is now being prepared to receive the embryos that were cryopreserved prior to the start of her chemotherapy.

4.4 Cryopreservation of ovarian cortical tissue strips

As mentioned previously, each fertility preservation option is aimed at a specific group of patients. When the patient is prepubertal, when there is no partner is available for the generation of embryos, or when the cancer treatment cannot be postponed in order to perform ovarian stimulation, cryopreservation of ovarian tissue strips may be an alternative approach. Silber et al. (2005) showed previously that transplantation of fresh (non cryopreserved) ovarian cortex strips between identical twin sisters was actually feasible. The development of efficient freezing and thawing protocols for cortex strips has rendered this technique applicable for fertility preservation purposes and has recently led to the thirteenth live birth (Donnez et al., 2011).
Although still experimental, this option is nowadays being performed on an increasing scale. Cortical fragments can be obtained laparoscopically, and slow frozen using DMSO as a cryoprotectant. Care should be taken to minimize the thickness of the cortical strips to 1 mm, to facilitate diffusion of the cryoprotectant into the tissue. In addition, thin fragments will suffer less from ischemic damage, which is a serious problem after retransplantation. A significant proportion (60-95%) of (growing) follicles that survive the freezing and thawing process, is actually lost due to warm posttransplantation ischemia (Baird et al., 1999; Nisolle et al., 2000; Candy et al., 2000; Aubard et al., 1999, Aubard, 2003; Liu et al., 2002). Cortical strips can be autotransplanted heterotopically (for instance subcutaneous in the forearm), or orthotopically. Thus far, only orthotopic transplantation has led to the birth of a number of healthy offspring (Donnez et al.,2004; Meirow et al.,2005, 2007; Demeestere et al., 2006; 2007; 2010; Andersen et al.,2008; Schmidt et al., 2011; Ernst et al., 2010).
Cryopreservation of ovarian cortical strips is applicable for a wide range of different patients. Conception may require artificial reproductive techniques like IVF or ICSI, but may occur spontaneously as well. An additional advantage of this technique is resumption of the regular hormonal processes, leading to the reversal of the postmenopausal status that many patients experience after their cancer therapy. Follicular development and restoration of ovarian function usually occur 4-5 months after a transplantation procedure (Donnez et al., 2006a; 2008), as more than 120 days are required to initiate follicular growth and

approximately 85 days to the reach final maturation stage from a pre-antral follicle (Gougeon, 1985, Oktem & Oktay, 2008). Unfortunately, the survival time of a single autotransplanted number of strips is usually limited to a few months, with exceptions of survival up to approximately 3 years (Kim et al., 2009; Meirow et al., 2007; Silber et al., 2008a), requiring another surgical intervention to transplant a new set of cortex strips.

4.4.1 Case report B: Ovarian tissue cryopreservation in a patient with Hodgkin's lymphoma

Mrs. Y was diagnosed with Hodgkin's lymphoma at the age of twenty. As she was to start with six cycles of chemotherapy the next month, she visited our fertility Centre to discuss the options for fertility preservation.

Although the patient was at the time in a steady relationship, she regarded herself to young to start emergency IVF, as this would confront both herself and her partner with the definitive choice of having children together in the future. Ovarian hyper stimulation followed by cryopreservation of the retrieved oocytes was not considered an optimal option, as the time to the start of her chemotherapy was relatively short, allowing for only one cycle of hyperstimulation. As a consequence, only a limited number of oocytes would be obtained.

Eventually the choice was made for cryopreservation of ovarian cortical strips. At that time we could not offer her this procedure ourselves so we referred her to another centre. Biopsies of both ovaries were taken via a laparoscopic procedure, and 13 strips were cryopreserved. She then started with the chemotherapy. Since then, she has had two relapses, that were treated with chemotherapy, radiotherapy, and stem cell transplantation.

At the age of 27, the patient and her partner visited our Centre as she wished to conceive. She had now been in complete remission for 3 years. Hormonal examination showed that she was postmenopausal, indicating that both spontaneous conception as well as IVF treatments were no options to achieve pregnancy. The couple was referred back to the clinic where her ovarian tissue was cryopreserved, and is now considering autotransplantation of the ovarian cortical strips.

5. Future options for fertility preservation

Several alternative procedures are being evaluated to expand the current array of fertility preservation options. These include the isolation and cryopreservation of follicles from ovarian tissue that is harvested laparoscopically (Bedaiwy & Falcone, 2007; Feigin et al., 2007). However, isolation of follicles by either mechanical or enzymatic means is difficult, especially from human ovaries (Dolmans et al., 2006). In addition, this approach requires different cryopreservation techniques then for oocytes and embryos, and sophisticated *in vitro* maturation protocols to obtain oocytes that can be fertilized *in vitro* by IVF or ICSI.

A more promising future option may comprise the cryopreservation of an intact ovary, including its vascular pedicle. The vascular pedicle can be used to reconnect the thawed ovary to the circulation, thereby preventing the devastating effects of warm ischemia that is known to deplete the follicles in ovarian tissue transplanted without vascular anastomosis (Newton et al., 1996; Nisolle et al., 2000; Candy et al., 1997; Aubard et al., 1999; Baird et al., 1999; Aubard, 2003; Liu et al., 2008). However, the successful cryopreservation of an intact organ represents an immense technical challenge. Pioneering work by Parrot (1960) on murine ovaries provided proof of principle. Later reports showed that also in other mammalian species this proved to be a viable approach. Freezing and autologous grafting of whole ovaries has now been performed in rabbits (Chen et al., 2005), pigs (Imhof et al.,

2004), and sheep (Bedaiwy et al., 2003; Arav et al., 2005; Imhof et al., 2006), yielding promising results. In rats (Wang et al., 2002) and sheep (Imhof et al., 2006), this procedure has actually resulted in live offspring. In humans, transplantation of fresh (non-cryopreserved) intact ovaries has also been performed successfully. Ovarian autotransplantation in the upper arm was performed before pelvic irradiation (Leporrier 1987, Hilders et al., 2004). Over a period of 16 years, the ovary remained functional (Leporrier et al., 2002). A first full-term pregnancy was obtained using orthotopic fresh whole ovary transplantation between identical twin sisters (Silber et al., 2008b).

Cryopreservation of an intact human ovary with its vascular pedicle has been described previously (Martinez-Madrid et al., 2004, 2007; Bedaiwy et al., 2006). These authors showed that perfusion of the ovary with cryoprotectants led to a certain degree of protection from cryodamage. The subsequent autotransplantation of frozen and thawed human ovaries, however, has thus far not been performed. Major obstacle in this respect is the much larger volume of human ovaries compared to murine and ovine ovaries (Gerritse et al., 2008). This larger volumes hampers the sufficient diffusion of cryoprotectant into the tissue (Donnez et al., 2006b). In addition, the freezing kinetics in a bulky organ are bound to be completely different from those in a small volume organ (Pegg, 2005). Finally, all components of the organ, including the vascular pedicle, the inner vasculature, the stromal tissue and of course the follicles, should be verifiably protected before retransplantation to human subjects can be even considered. This requires the development of biologically relevant assays that are able to quantify cryodamage in a reliable fashion. Understandably, efforts have focused mainly on the survival of the follicles within the intact cryopreserved ovary. This has been done by conventional histology (Bedaiwy et al., 2003, Arav et al., 2005 Courbiere et al., 2005, 2006; Martinez-Madrid et al., 2004; Imhof et al., 2006; Baudot 2007), immunohistochemistry (Arav et al., 2005; Bedaiwy et al., 2006), determining the frequency of apoptosis (Bedaiwy et al., 2003, 2006; Martinez-Madrid et al., 2007), using survival/viability/proliferation assays (Bedaiwy et al., 2003, 2006; Martinez-Madrid et al., 2004, Arav et al., 2005, Courbiere et al., 2005, 2006; Imhof et al., 2004; Baudot et al., 2007, Onions et al., 2008), transmission electron microscopy (Martinez-Madrid et al., 2007) and estradiol assays (Huang et al., 2008; Isachenko et al., 2007; Gerritse et al., 2010). These studies have produced relevant information on the prevention of cryodamage in follicles, but have largely left out the main component of the ovary, namely the stromal cell compartment that constitutes over 95% of the ovarian mass. An additional reason to focus also on survival of stromal cells is the observation that these cells are vital for optimal follicular development (McLaughlin and McIver, 2009). Finally, the metabolically active stromal cells have been described to be more sensitive to cryodamage than the quiescent primordial oocytes (Kim *et al.*, 2004). These observations emphasize the need for a cryopreservation protocol that not only efficiently preserves the follicles/oocytes, but the stromal cell compartment as well.

We therefore decided to develop an assay that is capable of quantifying the basal metabolism of the bulk of the tissue as a measure of cryodamage. For this purpose we measured the uptake of glucose and the release of lacate by cultured ovarian tissue fragments. We used bovine ovaries as a model system, as they are comparable to human ovaries with respect to size, monthly cycle, and number of follicles that mature per cycle (Gerritse et al., 2008). In this model system we were able to test different cryopreservation protocols. Our results show that both immersion of the bovine ovary in cryoprotectant, combined with perfusing it for a prolonged period of time, resulted in a nearly complete protection of the ovarian metabolism. This procedure did not affect the endothelium of the vascular pedicle and the inner vasculature (Gerritse et al., submitted). We plan to xenotransplant optimally cryopreserved bovine ovaries into immune deficient rats, in order to test the ability of the follicles to develop *in vivo* and produce mature oocytes.

6. Safety aspects of ovarian tissue autotransplantation

A major point of concern when autotransplanting ovarian tissue to cured cancer patients, is the possibility that (metastasized) tumor cells are present in the ovarian graft and are reintroduced to the patient (Shaw et al., 1996). Thus far a limited number of patients has received an autransplantation, and up to now no relapses have been reported. It should be noted, however, that most patients receiving an autotransplantation suffered from early stage cancer when their tissue was harvested. In addition, the follow up period after the transplantation has been relatively short. As a consequence, the experience with this matter is only limited, and retransplantation of the malignancy can never be ruled out completely. Shaw et al. (1996) actually showed that lymphoma could be transmitted via cryopreserved ovarian tissue in a mouse model. The physician therefore has the responsibility to counsel the patient comprehensively on the risk of malignant cells being present in the ovarian tissue, and the possible consequences after autotransplantation. Two different approaches can be used to draft an advice.First, one can extrapolate on statistical data describing the frequency with which a certain tumor in a certain stage will metastasize to the ovary. For a number of solid tumor types, ovarian metastases have been described for advanced stages but not for early stage tumors (Rosendahl et al., 2011). These include Hodgkin's disease (Khan et al., 1986), renal cell carcinoma (Insabato et al., 2003) and breast cancer (Horvath et al., 1977). It should be noted, however, that systematically collected data are missing for most tumor types, giving only a limited idea of the risk of tumor dissemination to the ovary. In contrast to solid tumors, diffuse malignancies such as leukemia are likely to be present in all blood-filled organs, including the ovary. Therefore, patients suffering from these kind of diseases should probably be excluded from using (cryopreserved) ovarian tissue as a means for fertility preservation. The second, and probably preferable, option, is to tailor a patient specific approach, i.e. analyzing (part of) the tissue that is to be autotransplanted in the future for the presence of (residual) disease. In an ideal situation, sensitive and specific tests would be available for the detection of each tumor type in a tissue. Techniques that have been used to asses the presence of malignant cells in ovarian tissue include conventional histology (Azem et al., 2010; Donnez et al., 2011), immunohistochemistry (Rosendahl et al., 2011), PCR amplification of tumor specific RNA/DNA (Rosendahl et al., 2010), and xenotransplantation of ovarian tissue fragments to immune deficient mice (Dolmans et al., 2010). In real life, however, these approaches encounter several obstacles. Histology is relatively non-sensitive as individual tumor cells can be missed, and usually only a limited number of sections is analyzed. Whereas immunohistochemistry is generally more sensitive than histology, it requires specific tumor cell markers that are not available for most type of cancers. While PCR in itself is a very sensitive technique, the ratio between the few malignant cells that are potentially present in the graft and the large number of normal ovarian cells impairs the reliability and sensitivity of this test. PCR results that indicate the presence of residual tumor cells are therefore mostly qualitative and not quantitative. Furthermore, PCR detects only the presence of relatively short stretches of specific RNA/DNA sequences and not viable cells. Xenotransplantation experiments may provide biologically relevant information, but are expensive and cumbersome and probablyl not routinely applicable. Apart from these practical issues, positive tests results raise some more questions. First, we do not know when a positive signal becomes biologically significant,. i.e. predictive of relapse after transplantation. Examples of this notion are a positive PCR signal that may be derived from a number of deceased cells and may therefore not be of clinical relevance. We currently we do not know exactly how many malignant cells are required for reintroduction of the tumor. In animal models as few as 200 lymphoblasts were sufficient to introduce leukemia (Hou et al., 2007), but the same may not apply to the human situation. Next, the ovarian tissue fragment that is being analyzed for residual disease, is evidently no longer available for transplantation. The outcome of the analysis will therefore not necessarily be applicable to the cortical fragments that are actually transplanted. The importance of this notion was substantiated by the finding that malignant cell DNA was found in an ovarian cortex fragment by PCR analysis, whereas the adjacent cortex fragment from the same ovary was found to be PCR-negative (Rosendahl, 2010). Finally, the autotransplantation of small volume cortex fragments is much less likely to reintroduce the malignancy then the autotransplantation of an intact ovary.

7. Concluding remarks

The last decade has seen the development of a number of options for fertility preservation for cancer patients. All the options that are currently available have their own specific indications and contraindications. The choice for the appropriate option will be a shared decision of both the patient and her physician, requiring a careful evaluation and counseling. Increasing the awareness of physicians to address the issue of fertility preservation before starting gonadotoxic therapy should be an integral part of medical education.

Current research, including intact ovary cryopreservation, may lead to several exciting new options for fertility preservation. It should be noted that this option is not intended to replace the current possibilities, but will rather have its own specific patient population that may benefit most from this procedure. The obvious risk of intact ovary autotransplantation is reintroduction of the malignancy. Evidently, more research into the development of valid and biologically relevant tumor detection methods in ovarian tissue, as well as in the prevalence of ovarian metastases in cancer patients with different types of primary tumors, is urgently needed.

8. Acknowledgements

The authors would like to thank the Kika Foundation and Stichting Pink Ribbon for their financial support. MSD/N.V. Organon is acknowledged for providing an unconditional grant.

9. References

Andersen, C.; Rosendahl, M.; Byskow, A.; Loft, A.; Ottosen, C.; Dueholm, M.; Schmidt, K.; Andersen A. & Ernst, E. (2008). Two successful pregnancies following autotransplantation of frozen/thawed ovarian tissue. *Hum. Reprod.* 23: 2266-2272.

Arav, A.; Reve,l A.; Nathan, Y.; Bor, A.; Gacitua, H.; Yavin, S.; Gavish, Z.; Uri, M. & Elami, A. (2005). Oocyte recovery, embryo development and ovarian function after cryopreservation and transplantation of whole sheep ovary. *Hum. Reprod.* 20:3554-9

Aubard, Y.; Piver, P.; Cognie, Y.; Fermeaux, V.;, Poulin, N. and Driancourt, M. (1999). Orthotopic and heterotopic autografts of frozen-thawed ovarian cortex in sheep. *Human. Reprod.* 14:2149-2154.

Aubard, Y.(2003). Ovarian tissue xenografting. *Eur. J. Obstet. Gynecol. Reprod. Biol.*108:14-18.

Azem, F.; Hasson, J.; Ben-Yosef, D.; Kossoy, N.; Cohen, T.; Almog, B.; Amit, A.; Lessing, J. & Lifschitz-Mercer, B. 2010. Histologic evaluation of fresh human ovarian tissue before cryopreservation. *Int. J. Gynecol. Pathol.* 29(1):19-23.

Baird, D.; Webb, R.; Campbell, B.; Harkness, L. & Gosden, R. (1999). Long-term ovarian function in sheep after ovariectomy and transplantation of autografts stored at -196°C. *Endocrinology* 140:462-471.

Baker, T. Oogenesis and ovarian development. In "Reproductive Biology" (Eds, Balin H and Glasser S) 1972; p.398. Excerpta Medica, Amsterdam.

Baudot, A.; Courbiere, B.; Odagescu, V.; Salle, B.; Mazoyer, C.; Massardier, J. & Lornage, J. (2007). Towards whole sheep ovary cryopreservation. *Cryobiology* 55(3): 236-248.

Bedaiwy, M. & Falcone, T. (2007). Harvesting and autotransplantation of vascularized ovarian grafts: approaches and techniques. *Reprod. Biomed. Online* 14(3):360-371.

Bedaiwy, M.; Hussein, M.; Biscotti, C. & Falcone, T. (2006). Cryopreservation of intact human ovary with its vascular pedicle. *Hum. Reprod.* 21(12):3258-3269.

Bedaiwy, M.; Jeremias, E.; Gurunluoglu, R.; Hussein, M.; Siemianow, M.; Biscotti, C. & Falcone, T. (2003). Restoration of ovarian function after autotransplantation of intact frozen-thawed sheep ovaries with microvascular anastomosis. *Fertil. Steril.*79(3):594-602.

Bisharah, M. & Tulandi, T. (2003). Laparoscopic preservation of ovarian function: an underused procedure. *Am. J. Obstet. Gynecol.*188(2):367-370.

Blumenfeld, Z.; Avivi, I.; Ritter, M. & Rowe, J.(1999). Preservation of fertility and ovarian function and minimizing chemotherapy-induced gonado-toxicity in young women. *J. Soc. Gynecol. Investig.* 6:229-239.

Borgmann-Staudt, A.; Rendtorff, R.; Reinmuth, S.; Hohmann, C.; Keil, T.; Schuster, F.; Holter, W.; Ehlert, K.; Keslova, P.; Lawitschka, A.; Jarisch, A. & Strauss, G. (2011).Fertility after allogeneic haematopoietic stem cell transplantation in childhood and adolescence. *Bone Marrow Transplantation* 11:1-6.

Borini, A.; Cattoli, M.; Mazzone, M.; Trevisi, M.; Nalcon, M.; & Iadarola, I. (2007). Survey of 105 babies born after slow- cooling oocyte cryopreservation. *Fertil. Steril.* 88:suppl 1:13-14.

Brown, J.; Modell, E.; Obasaju, M. & Ying, Y. (1996). Natural cycle in-vitro fertilization with embryo cryopreservation prior to chemotherapy for carcinoma of the breast. *Hum. Reprod.*11:197-199.

Byrne, J.; Fears, T.; Gail, M.; Pee, D.; Connelly, R.; Austin, D.; Holmes, G.; Holmes, F.; Latourette, H.; Meigs, J.; Strong, L.; Myers, M. & Mulvihill, J. (1992). Early menopause in long-term survivors of cancer during adolescence. *Am. J. Obstet. Gynecol* .166:788-793.

Candy, C.; Wood, M. & Whittingham, D. (2000). Restoration of a normal reproductive lifespan after grafting of cryopreserved mouse ovaries. *Hum. Reprod.*15:1300-1304.

Candy, C.; Wood, M. & Whittingham, D. (1997). Effect of cryoprotectants on the survival of follicles in frozen mouse ovaries. *J. Reprod. Fertil.*110(1):11-19.

Cao, Y.; Xing, Q.; Li, L.; Cong, L.; Zhang, Z.; Wei, Z. & Zhou, P.(2009). Comparison of survival and embryonic development in human oocytes cryopreserved by slow-freezing and vitrification. *Fertil. Steril.* 92(4):1306-1311..

Chian, R.; Huang, J. & Tan, S. (2008). Obstetric and perinatal outcome in 200 infants conceived from vitrified oocytes. *Reprod. Biomed. Online* 16:608-610.
Chian, R.; Huang, J.; Gilbert, L.; Son, W.; Holzer, H.; Cui, S.; Buckett, W.; Tulandi, T. &Tan, S. (2009). Obstetric outcomes following vitrification of in vitro and in vivo matured oocytes. *Fertil. Steril* .91(6):2391-2398.
Chemaitilly, W.; Mertens, A.; Mitby, P.; Whitton, J.; Stovall, M.; Yasui, Y.; Robison, L. & Sklar, C. (2006). Acute ovarian failure in the childhood cancer survivor study. *J. Clin. Endocrinol. Metab.* 91 (5):1723-1728.
Chen, C.; Chen, S.; Chang, F.; Wu, G.; Liu, J. & Yu, C. (2005). Autologous heterotopic transplantation of intact rabbit ovary after cryopreservation. *Hum. Reprod.* 20:1149-1150.
Chiarelli, A.; Marrett, L. & Darlington, G. (1999). Early menopause and infertility in females after treatment for childhood cancer diagnosed in 1964-1988 in Ontario, Canada. *Am. j. Epidemiol.* 150:245-254.
Cobo, A.; Kuwayama, M.; Perez, S.; Ruiz, A.; Pellicer, A. & Remohi, J. (2007). Comparison of concomitant outcome achieved with fresh and cryopreserved donor oocytes vitrified by the Cryotop method. *Fertil. Steril.* 89:1657- 1664.
Courbiere, B.; Massardier, J.; Salle, B.; Mazoyer, C.; Guerin, J. & Lornage, J. (2005). Follicular viability and histological assessment after cryopreservation of whole sheep ovaries with vascular pedicle by vitrification. *Fertil. Steril.* 84 Suppl 2:1065-1071.
Courbiere, B.; Odagescu, V.; Baudot, A.; Massardier, J.; Mazoyer, C.; Salle, B. & Lornage, J. (2006). Cryopreservation of the ovary by vitrification as an alternative to slow-cooling protocols. *Fertil. Steril.* 86(4 Suppl):1243-1251.
Critchley, H.; Bath, L. & Wallace, W. (2002). Radiation damage to the uterus. Review of the effects of treatment of childhood cancer. *Hum. Fertil.* 5:61-66.
Critchley, H.; Wallace, W.; Shalet, S.; Mamtora, H.; Higginson, J. & Anderson, D. (1992). Abdominal irradiation in childhood: the potential for pregnancy. *Br. J. Obstet. Gynaecol.*99(5):392-394.
Critchley, H. (1999). Factors of importance for implantation and problems after treatment for childhood cancer. *Med. Pediatr. Oncol.* 33(1):9-14.
Demeestere, I.; Simon, P.; Buxant, F.; Robin, V.; Fernandz, S.; Centner, J.; Delbaere, A. & Englert, Y. (2006). Ovarian function and spontaneous pregnancy after combined heterotopic and orthotopic cryopreserved ovarian tissue transplantation in a patient previously treated with bone marrow transplantation: case report. *Hum. Reprod.* 21:2010-2014.
Demeestere, I.; Simon, P.; Moffa, F.; Delbaere, A. & Englert, Y. (2010). Birth of a second healthy girl more than 3 years after cryopreserved ovarian graft. *Hum. Reprod.* 25(6):1590-1591.
Demeestere, I.; Simon, P.; Emiliani, S.; Delbaere, A. & Englert, Y. (2007). Fertility preservation: successful transplantation of cryopreserved ovarian tissue in a young patient previously treated for Hodgkin's disease. *Oncologist* 12(12):1437-1442.
Dolmans, M.; Michaux, N.; Camboni, A.; Martinez-Madrid, B.; Van Langendonckt, A.; Nottola, S. & Donnez, J. (2006). Evaluation of Liberase, a purified enzyme blend, for the isolation of human primordial and primary ovarian follicles. *Hum. Reprod.* 21(2):413-420.
Dolmans, M.; Marinescu, C.; Saussoy, P.; Van Langendonckt, A.; Amorim, C. & Donnez, J. (2010). Reimplantation of cryopreserved ovarian tissue from patients with acute lymphoblastic leukemia is potentially unsafe. *Blood* 116(16):2908-2914.

Donnez, J.; Dolmans, M.; Demylle, D.; Jadoul, P.; Pirard, C.; Squifflet, J.; Martinez-Madrid, B. & Van Langendonckt, A. (2004). Livebirth after orthotopic transplantation of cryopreserved ovarian tissue. *Lancet* 364:1405-1410.

Donnez, J.; Dolmans, M.; Demylle, D.; Jadoul, P.; Pirard, C.; Squifflet, J.; Martinez Madrid, B. & Van Langendonckt, A. (2006a). Restoration of ovarian of ovarian function after orthotopic (intraovarian and periovarian) transplantation of cryopreserved ovarian tissue in a woman treated by bone marrow transplantation for sickle cell anaemia: case report. *Hum. Reprod.* 21:183-188.

Donnez, J.; Martinez-Madrid, B.; Jadoul, P.; Van Langendonckt, A.; Demylle, D. & Dolmans, M. (2006b). Ovarian tissue cryopreservation and transplantation: a review. *Hum. Reprod. Update* 12(5):519-35.

Donnez, J.; Squifflet, J.; Van Eyck, A.; Demylle, D.; Jadoul, P.; Van Langendonck, A. & Dolmans, M. (2008). Restoration of ovarian function in orthotopically transplantated cryopreserved ovarian tissue: a pilot experience. *Reprod. Biomed. Online*;16:694-704.

Donnez, J.; Squifflet, J.; Jadoul, P.; Demylle, D.; Cheron, A.; Van Langendonckt, A. & Dolmans, M. (2011). Pregnancy and live birth after autotransplantation of frozen-thawed ovarian tissue in a patient with metastatic disease undergoing chemotherapy and hematopoietic stem cell transplantation. *Fertil. Steril.* 95(5):1787.e1-4.

Ernst, E.; Bergholdt, S.; Jørgensen, J. & Andersen, C. (2010). The first woman to give birth to two children following transplantation of frozen/thawed ovarian tissue. *Hum. Reprod.* 25(5):1280-1281.

Feeney, D.; Moore, D.; Look, K.; Stehman, F. & Sutton, G. (1995). The fate of the ovaries after radical hysterectomy and ovarian transposition. *Gynecol. Oncol.* 56:3-7.

Feigin, E.; Abir, R.; Fisch, B.; Kravarusic, D.; Steinberg, R.; Nitke, S.; Avrahami, G.; Ben-Haroush, A. & Freud, E. (2007). Laparoscopic ovarian tissue preservation in young patients at risk for ovarian failure as a result of chemotherapy/irradiation for primary malignancy. *J. Pediatr. Surg.* 42(5):862-864.

Frederick, J.; Ord, T.; Kettel, L.; Stone, S.; Balmaceda, J. & Arsch, R. (1995). Successful pregnancy outcome after cryopreservation of all fresh embryos with subsequent transfer into an unstimulated cycle. *Fertil. Steril.* 64:987- 990.

Gatta, G.; Zigon, G.; Capocaccia, R.; Coebergh, J.; Desandes, E.; Kaatsch, P.; Pastore, G.; Peris-Bonet, R. & Stiller, C. EUROCARE Working Group. (2009). Survival of European children and young adults with cancer diagnosed 1995-2002. *Eur. J. Cancer* 45:992-1005.

Gerritse, R.; Beerendonk, C.; Tijink, M.; Heetkamp, A.; Kremer, J.; Braat, D. & Westphal, J. (2008). Optimal perfusion of an intact ovary as a prerequisite for successful ovarian cryopreservation. *Hum. Reprod.*23(2):329-335.

Gerritse, R.; Peek, R.; Sweep, F.; Thomas, C.; Braat, D.; Kremer, J.; Westphal, J. & Beerendonk, C. (2010). In vitro 17ß- oestradiol release as a marker for follicular survival in cryopreserved intact bovine ovaries. *Cryo Letters* 31(4):318-328.

Gerritse, R.; Beerendonk, C.; Westphal, J.; Bastings, L.; Braat, D. & Peek, R. Glucose/lactate metabolism of cryopreserved intact ovaries as a novel quantitative marker to assess tissue cryodamage. Submitted for publication.

Goldhirsch, A.; Gelber, R. & Castiglione, M. (1990). The magnitude of endocrine effects of adjuvant chemotherapy for premenopausal breast cancer patients. The International Breast Cancer Study Group. *Ann. Oncol.*1:183-188.

Gosden, R.; Wade, J.; Fraser, H.; Sandow, J. & Faddy, M. (1997). Impact of congenital or experimental hypogonadotrophism on the radiation sensitivity of the mouse ovary. *Hum. Reprod.*12:2483-2488.

Gosden, R. (2005). Prospects for oocyte banking and in vitro maturation. *J. Natl. Cancer Inst. Monogr.* 34:60-63.

Gougeon, A. (1985). Origin and growth of the preovulatory follicle(s) in spontaneous and stimulated cycles. In: Testart J, Friedman R (Eds.). Human In Vivo Fertilization: Insemination Symposium, 24. Amsterdam:Elsevier.

Gougeon A. (1996). Regulation of ovarian follicular development in primates: facts and hypotheses. *Endocr. Rev.*17:121- 155.

Hadar, H.; Loven, D.; Herskovitz, P.; Bairey, O.; Yagoda, A. & Levavi, H. (1994). An evaluation of lateral and medial transposition of the ovaries out of radiation fields. *Cancer* 74:774-779.

Hilders, C.; Baranski, A.; Peters, L.; Ramkhelawan, A. & Trimbos, J. (2004). Successful human ovarian autotransplantation to the upper arm. *Cancer* 101(12):2771-2778.

Homburg, R.; van der Veen, F. & Silber, S. (2009). Oocyte vitrification- women's emancipation set in Stone. *Fertil. Steril.*91:1319-1320.

Horvath, T. & Schindler, A. (1977). Ovarian metastases in breast carcinoma. Fortschr. Med. 10;95(6):358-60.

Hou, M.; Andersson, M.; Eksborg, S.; Söder, O. & Jahnukainen, K. (2007). Xenotransplantation of testicular tissue into nude mice can be used for detecting leukemic cell contamination. *Hum. Reprod.* 22(7):1899-1906.

Howard, F. (1997). Laparoscopic lateral ovarian transposition before radiation treatment of Hodgkin disease. *J. Am. Assoc. Gynecol .Laparosc.* 4:601-604.

Howell, S. & Shalet, S. (1998). Gonadal damage from chemotherapy and radiotherapy. *Endocrinol. Metab. Clin. North Am.* 27:927-943.

Huang, L.; Mo, Y.; Wang, W.; Li, Y.; Zhang, Q. & Yang, D. (2008). Cryopreservation of human ovarian tissue by solid- surface vitrification. *Eur. J. Obstet. Gynecol. Reprod. Biol.* 139(2):193-198.

Imhof, M.; Hofstetter, G.; Bergmeister, H.; Rudas, M.; Kain, R.; Lipovac, M. &, Huber, J. (2004). Cryopreservation of a whole ovary as a strategy for restoring ovarian function. *J. Assist. Reprod. Genet.* 21(12):459-465.

Imhof, M.; Bergmeister, H.; Lipovac, M.; Rudas, M.; Hofstetter, G. & Huber, J. (2006). Orthotopic microvascular re- anastomosis of whole cryopreserved ovine ovaries resulting in pregnancy and life birth. *Fertil. Steril.* 85:1208- 1215.

Insabato, L.; De Rosa, G.; Franco, R.; D'Onofrio, V. & Di Vizio, D. (2003). Ovarian metastasis from renal cell carcinoma: a report of three cases. *Int. J. Surg. Pathol.* 11(4):309-12.

Isachenko, V.; Isachenko, E.; Reinsberg, J.; Montag, M.; van der Ven, K.; Dorn, C.; Roesing, B. & van der Ven, H. (2007). Cryopreservation of human ovarian tissue: comparison of rapid and conventional freezing. *Cryobiology* 55:261- 268.

Khan, M.; Dahill, S. & Stewart, K. (1986). Primary Hodgkin's disease of the ovary. Case report. *Br. J. Obstet. Gynaecol.*93(12):1300-1301.

Kim, S.; Yang, H.; Kang, H.; Lee, H.H.; Lee, H.C.; Ko, D. & Gosden, R. (2004). Quantitative assessment of ischemic tissue damage in ovarian cortical tissue with or without antioxidant (ascorbic acid) treatment. *Fertil. Steril.* 82(3):679- 685.

Kim, S.; Lee, W.; Chung, M.; Lee, H.C.; Lee H.H. & Hill, D. (2009). Long-term ovarian function and fertility after heterotopic autotransplantation of cryobanked human ovarian tissue: 8-year experience in cancer patients. *Fertil Steril.*91(6):2349-2354.

Koyama, H.; Wada, T.; Nishizawa, Y.; Iwanaga, T. & Aoki, Y. (1977). Cyclophosphamide-induced ovarian failure and its therapeutic significance in patients with breast cancer. *Cancer* 39:1403-1409.

Kuwayama, M.; Vajta, G.; Kato, O. & Leibo, S. (2005). Highly efficient vitrification method for cryopreservation of human oocytes. *Reprod. Biomed. Online*11:300-308.

Leporrier, M.; Von Theobald, P.; Roffe, J. & Muller, G. (1987). A new technique to protect ovarian function before pelvic irradiation. Heterotopic ovarian autotransplantation. *Cancer* 60:2201-2204.

Liu, J.; Van der Elst, J.; Van der Broecke, R. & Dhont, M. (2002). Early massive follicle loss and apoptosis in heterotopically grafted newborn mouse ovaries. *Hum. Reprod.*17:605-611.

Liu, L.; Wood, G.; Morikawa, L.; Ayearst, R.; Fleming, C. & McKerlie, C. (2008). Restoration of fertility by orthotopic transplantation of frozen adult mouse ovaries. *Hum. Reprod.* 23(1):122-128.

Manger, K.; Wildt, L.; Kalden, J. & Manger, B. Prevention of gonadal toxicity and preservation of gonadal function and fertility in young women with systemic lupus erythematosus treated by cyclophosphamide: the PREGO-Study. *Autoimmun. Rev.* 5(4): 269-272.

Martinez-Madrid, B.; Dolmans, M.; Van Langendonckt, A.; Defrère, S. & Donnez, J. (2004). Freeze-thawing intact human ovary with its vascular pedicle with a passive cooling device. *Fertil. Steril.* 82(5):1390-1394

Martinez-Madrid, B.; Camboni, A.; Dolmans, M.; Notolla, S.; Van Langendonckt, A. & Donnez, J. (2007). Apoptosis and ultrastructural assessment after cryopreservation of whole human ovaries with their vascular pedicle. *Fertil. Steril.* 87:1153-1165.

McLaughlin, E. & McIver, S. (2009). Awakening the oocyte: controlling primordial follicle development. *Reproduction* 137(1): 1-11.

Meirow, D.; Lewis, H.; Nugent, D. & Epstein, N. (1999). Subclinical depletion of primordial follicular reserve in mice treated with cyclophosphamide: clinical importance and proposed accurate investigative tool. *Hum. Reprod.* 14:1903-1907.

Meirow, D.; Levron, J.; Eldar-Geva, T.; Hardan, I.; Fridman, E.; Zalel, Y.; Schiff, E. & Dor, J. (2005). Pregnancy after transplantation of cryopreserved ovarian tissue in a patient with ovarian failure after chemotherapy. *N. Engl. J. Med.* 353(3):318-321.

Meirow, D.; Levron, J.; Eldar-Geva, T.; Hardan, I.; Fridman, E.; Yemini, Z. & Dor, J. (2007). Monitoring the ovaries after autotransplantation of cryopreserved ovaries tissue: endocrine studies, in vitro fertilization cycles, and live birth. *Fert. Steril.* 87:418.e7-417.e15.

Mertens, A.; Ramsay, N.; Kouris, S. & Neglia, J. (1998). Patterns of gonadal dysfunction following bone marrow transplantation.*Bone Marrow Transplant.* 22(4):345-50.

Munn, C.; Kiser, L.; Wetzner, S. & Baer, J. (1986). Ovary volume in young and premenopausal adults: US determination. Work in progress. *Radiology* 159(3):731-732.

Newton, H.; Aubard, Y.; Rutherford, A.; Sharma, V. & Gosden, R. (1996). Low temperature storage and grafting of human ovarian tissue. *Hum. Reprod.* 11(7):1487-1491.

Nicosia, S.; Matus-Ridley, M. & Meadows, A. (1985). Gonadal effects of cancer therapy in girls. *Cancer* 55:2364-2372.

Nisolle, M.; Godin, P.; Casanas-Roux, F.; Qu, J.; Motta, P. & Donnez, J. (2000). Histological and ultrastructural evaluation of fresh and frozen-thawed human ovarian xenografts in nude mice. *Fertil. Steril.*74:122-129.

Ogilvy-Stuart, A.; Stirling, H.; Kelnar, C.; Savage, M.; Dunger, D.; Buckler, J. & Shalet, S. (1997). Treatment of radiation- induced growth hormone deficiency with growth hormone-releasing hormone. *Clin. Endocrinol.* 46(5):571-578.

Oktay, K.; Briggs, D. & Gosden, R. (1997). Ontogeny of follicle-stimulating hormone receptor gene expression in isolated human ovarian follicles. *J. Clin. Endocrinol. Metab.*82:3748-3751.

Oktay, K. (2005a). Further evidence on the safety and success of ovarian stimulation with letrozole and tamoxifen in breast cancer patients undergoing in vitro fertilization to cryopreserve their embryos for fertility preservation. *J. Clin. Oncol.* 23:3858-3859.

Oktay, K.; Buyuk, E.; Libertella, N.; Akar, M. & Rosenwaks, Z. (2005b). Fertility preservation in breast cancer patients: a prospective controlled comparison of ovarian stimulation with tamoxifen and letrozole for embryo cryopreservation. *J. Clin. Oncol.* 23:4347-4353.

Oktem, O. & Oktay, K. (2007). A novel ovarian xenografting model to characterize the impact of chemotherapy agents on human primordial follicle reserve. *Cancer Res.*67(21):10159-10162.

Oktem, O. & Oktay, K. (2008). The ovary: anatomy and function throughout human life. *Ann. N. Y. Acad. Sci.* 1127:1-9.

Onions, V.; Mitchell, M.; Campbell, B. & Webb, R. (2008). Ovarian tissue viability following whole ovine ovary cryopreservation: assessing the effects of sphingosine-1-phosphate inclusion. *Hum. Reprod.* 23(3):606-618.

Parrott, D. (1960). The fertility of mice with orthotopic ovarian grafts derived from frozen tissue. *J. Reprod.* 1:230-241.

Pegg, D. (2005). The role of vitrification techniques of cryopreservation in reproductive medicine. *Hum. Fertil.* 8, 231-239.

Rosendahl, M.; Andersen, M.; Ralfkiær, E.; Kjeldsen, L.; Andersen, M.K. & Andersen C. (2010). Evidence of residual disease in cryopreserved ovarian cortex from female patients with leukemia. *Fertil. Steril.* 94(6):2186-2190.

Rosendahl, M.; Timmermans Wielenga, V.; Nedergaard, L.; Kristensen, S.; Ernst, E.; Rasmussen, P.; Anderson, M.; Schmidt, K. & Andersen, C. (2011). Cryopreservation of ovarian tissue for fertility preservation: no evidence of malignant cell contamination in ovarian tissue from patients with breast cancer. *Fertil Steril.* 95(6):2158-2161.

Salooja, N.; Szydlo, R.; Socie, G.; Rio, B.; Chatterjee, R.; Ljungman, P.; Van Lint, M.; Powles, R.; Jackson, G.; Hinterberger- Fischer, M.; Kolb, H. & Apperley, J. (2001). Late Effects Working Party of the European Group for Blood and Marrow Transplantation Pregnancy outcomes after peripheral blood or bone marrow transplantation: a retrospective survey. *Lancet* 28;358(9278):271-276.

Sanders, J.; Hawley, J.; Levy, W.; Gooley, T.; Buckner, C.; Deeg, H.; Doney, K.; Storb, R.; Sullivan, K. & Witherspoon, R. (1996). Pregnancies following high-dose Cyclophosphamide with or without high-dose Busulfan or total body irradiation and bone marrow transplantation. *Blood* 87:3045-3052.

Schilsky, R.; Sherins, R.; Hubbard, S.; Wesley, M.; Young, R. & DeVita, V. (1981). Long-term follow up of ovarian function in women treated with MOPP chemotherapy for Hodgkin's disease. *Am. J. Med.*71:552-556.

Schmidt, K.; Rosendahl, M.; Ernst, E.; Loft, A.; Andersen, A.; Dueholm, M.; Ottosen, C. & Andersen, C. (2011). Autotransplantation of cryopreserved ovarian tissue in 12 women with chemotherapy-induced premature ovarian failure: the Danish experience. *Fertil. Steril.* 2011 95(2):695-701.

Schover, L. (2009). Patient attitudes toward fertility preservation. *Pediatr. Blood Cancer.* 53(2):281-284.

Selick, C.; Hofmann, G.; Albao, C.; Horowitz, G.; Copperman, A.; Garrisi, G. & Navot, D. (1995). Embryo quality and pregnancy potential of fresh compared with frozen embryos: is freezing detrimental to high quality embryos? *Hum. Reprod.*10:392-395.

Senn, A.; Urner, F.; Chanson, A.; Primi, M.; Wirthner, D. & Germond, M. (2006). Morphological scoring of human pronuclear zygotes for prediction of pregnancy outcome. *Hum. Reprod.* 234-239.

Shaw, J.; Bowles, J.; Koopman, P.; Wood, E. & Trounson, A. (1996). Fresh and cryopreserved ovarian tissue samples from donors with lymphoma transmit the cancer to graft recipients. *Hum. Reprod.*11(8):1668-1673.

Silber, S.; Lenahan, K.; Levine, D.; Pineda, J.; Gorman, K.; Friez, M.; Crawford, E. & Gosden, R. (2005). Ovarian transplantation between monozygotic twins discordant for premature ovarian failure. *N. Engl. J. Med.* 7;353(1):58-63.

Silber, S.; DeRosa, M.; Pineda, J.; Lenahan, K.; Grenia, D.; Gorman, K. & Gosden, R. (2008a). A series of monozygotic twins discordant for ovarian failure: ovary transplantation (cortical versus microvascular) and cryopreservation. *Hum. Reprod.* 23(7):1531-1537.

Silber, S.; Grudzinskas, G. & Gosden, R. (2008b). Successful pregnancy after microsurgical transplantation of an intact ovary. *N. Engl. J. Med.* 11;359(24):2617-2618.

Sobrinho, L.; Levine, R. & DeConti, R. (1971). Amenorrhea in patients with Hodgkin's disease treated with antineoplastic agents. *Am. J. Obstet. Gynecol.*109:135-139.

Son, W.; Yoon, S.; Lee, S. & Lim, J. (2002). Pregnancy outcome following transfer of human blastocysts vitrified on electron microscopy grids after induced collapse of the blastocoele. *Human. Reprod.*18:137-139.

Sonmezer, M. & Oktay, K. (2006). Fertility preservation in young women undergoing breast cancer therapy. *Oncologist* 11(5):422-434.

Tauchmanova, L.; Selleri, C.; De Rosa, G.; Pagano, L.; Orio, F.; Lombardi, G.; Rotoli, B. & Colao, A. (2002). High prevalence of endocrine dysfunction in long-term survivors after allogenic bone marrow transplantation for hematologic diseases. *Cancer* 95:1076-1084.

Wallace, W.; Thomson, A. & Kelsey, T. (2003). The radiosensitivity of the human oocyte. *Hum. Reprod.*18:117-121.

Wallace, W.; Anderson, R. & Irvine, D. (2005). Fertility preservation for young patients with cancer: who is at risk and what can be offered? *Lancet Oncol.* ;6(4):209-218.

Wandji, S.; Srsen, V.; Voss, A. & Fortune, J. (1996). Initiation in vitro of growth of bovine primordial follicles. *Biol. Reprod.* 55(5):942-948.

Wang, J.; Yap, Y. & Mathews, C. (2001). Frozen-thawed embryo transfer: influence of clinical factors on implantation rate and risk of multiple conception. *Hum. Reprod.* 16:2316-2319.

Wang, X.; Chen, H.; Yin, H.; Kim, S.; Lin Tan, S. & Gosden, R. (2002). Fertility after intact ovary transplantation. Nature 24;415(6870):385.

Warne, G.; Fairley, K.; Hobbs, J. & Martin, F. (1973). Cyclophosphamide- induced ovarian failure. N. Engl. J. Med.289:1159-1162.

14

Human Ovarian Tissue Cryopreservation as Fertility Reserve

Elena Albani[1], Graziella Bracone[1], Sonia Di Biccari[3],
Domenico Vitobello[2], Nicola Fattizzi[2] and Paolo Emanuele Levi-Setti[1]
[1]U.O. di Ginecologia e Medicina della Riproduzione
[2]U.O. di Ginecologia
[3]Laboratorio di Medicina Quantitativa - Direzione Scientifica
Istituto Clinico Humanitas IRCCS – Cancer Center-Rozzano (MI)
Italy

1. Introduction

Oocytes designed for reproductive function in women are the largest cell in the human body. They are surrounded by granulosa cells to form the follicles that in various stages of development are present in the ovarian cortex (Fig. 1).

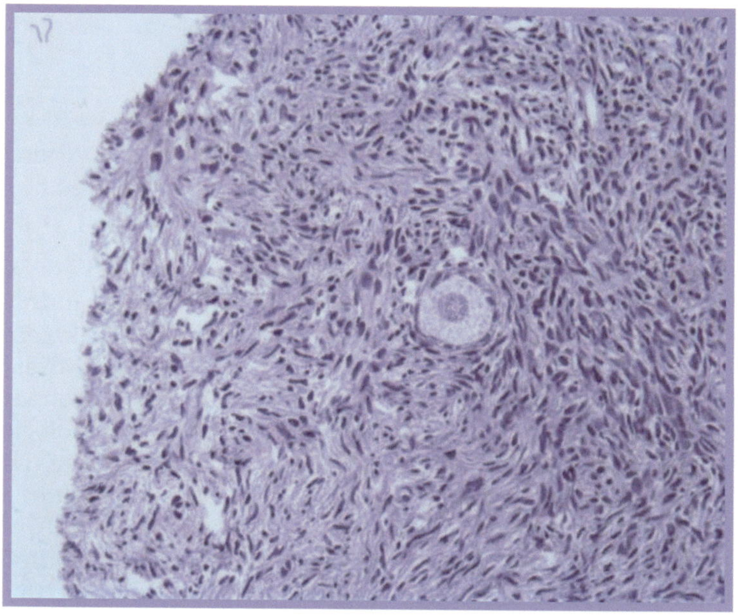

Fig. 1. Primary follicle in frozen/thawed human ovarian cortex (20X magnification)

The ovary of a healthy woman contains a finite number of follicles that decreases over time. The peak number is reached in the fifth month of gestation with approximately 7 million follicles. This number reduces progressively due to atresia, so at birth there are only 1-2

million follicles that, at puberty, become 300.000. Approximately, 400 of these follicles become mature oocytes and ovulate during the fertile life of the female.
At the age of 37, there is usually an acceleration of follicular loss, which is correlated with an increase in follicle-stimulating hormone (FSH) level.
Last year Wallace reported with a mathematical model combined with histological evidence, the establishment and decline of non-growing follicles (NGFs) in the human ovary. Wallace shows for the first time that the rate of NGF recruitment increases from birth to age 14 years and then declines with age until menopause (Fig. 2) (Wallace & Kelsey, 2010).

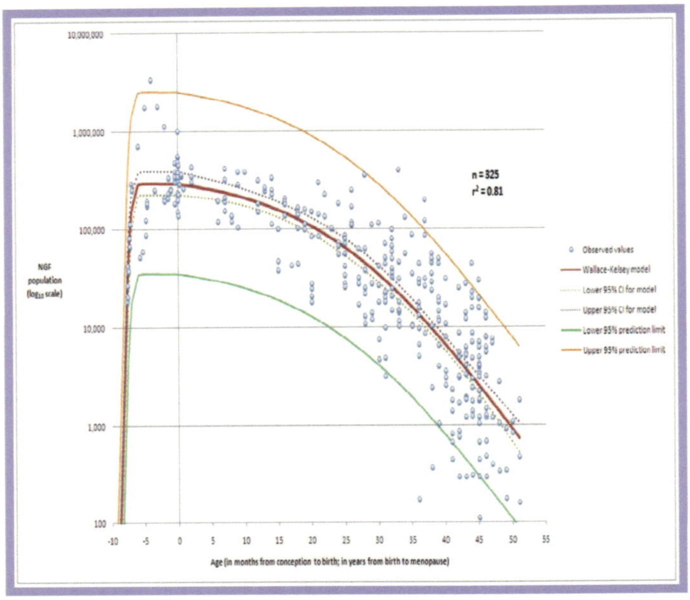

Fig. 2. The best histological model for the establishment of the NGF population after conception and the subsequent decline until menopause (Kindly provided by Professor Wallace).

However, the central dogma of ovarian biology has been questioned by new discoveries. Johnson in 2004 reported that germline stem cells (GSCs) are present in the mouse ovary, and could become new follicles (Johnson et al., 2004). It seems that female germline stem cell reside in an extragonadal location, the bone marrow, and reach the ovary through the circulatory system (Johnson et al., 2005; Lee et al., 2007). De Felici reported that germline stem cells exist in adult mouse ovaries but are quiescent under physiological conditions, contributing to the oocyte reserve only in response to ovotoxic damage (De Felici, 2010). Recently, Bukovsky showed the production of new eggs in cultures derived from premenopausal and postmenopausal human ovaries (Bukovsky et al., 2009).
Despite these exciting new prospects to indicate that oocytes are continuously formed in the female adult, at the present it is known that the pool of follicles is limited, so in case of toxic ovarian events that may affect the ovary, opportune measures should be considered to preserve the fertility of young women. According to the law in different countries regulating assisted reproductive technologies, approaches to fertility preservation include embryo, oocyte cryopreservation, or ovarian tissue banking followed by ovarian tissue transplant or in in-vitro culture.

However, cryopreservation of ovarian tissue may be the only acceptable method to preserve fertility for prepubertal girls, for women who cannot delay the start of cancer treatment for ovarian stimulation, and probably for women with hormone-sensitive malignancies. All these situations make ovarian tissue freezing the only option for female fertility preservation.

Therefore, an entire ovary or part of it, is removed laparoscopically, frozen and stored in liquid nitrogen at -196°C. After complete recovery of the patient, the tissue can be used to restore gametogenic and/or steroidogenic function.

Potential indications for ovarian tissue cryopreservation are patients diagnosed with malignant (extra-pelvic diseases: bone cancer, thyroid cancer, kidney cancer, breast cancer, melanoma, neuroblastoma; pelvic diseases: non-gynecological malignancy, gynaecological malignancy; systemic diseases: Hodkin's disease, non-Hodgkin's lymphoma, leukaemia, melanoblastoma) or benign diseases (recurrent ovarian cysts, etc), or with non malignant autoimmune diseases (systemic lupus erythematosus, rheumatoid arthritis, autoimmune thrombocytopenia or other haematological diseases). These patients are being treated successfully with chemotherapy and/or radiotherapy or repeated surgery, greatly improved in recent years, but all these therapies can be toxic to the ovary. So, it is important to focus attention on the quality of life, including fertility preservation, as well as on survival of these young women.

2. Effect of radiotherapy, chemotherapy, or other toxic drugs on female reproduction

The risk of ovarian failure after anticancer treatments is assessed in relation to patient's age, treatment protocol and type of cancer as reported by Meirow (Meirow and Nugent, 2001).

High-dose ionizing radiation is used to treat many types of cancer and hematologic malignancies. Ovarian transposition is not possible in case of total irradiation as is required for bone marrow transplantation (Meirow et al., 2010). The estimated dose at which half of the follicles are lost in humans (LD_{50}) is 4 Gy (Wallace et al., 1989), but is age-dependent. Lashbaugh reported that the toxic ovarian dose, which leads to permanent loss of fertility is higher in young women (20 Gy) than older (6 Gy) (Lushbaugh & Casarett, 1976).

Chemoterapic agents can be grouped into five classes of drugs based on their mode of action (alkylating agents, aneuploidy inducers, topoisomerase II inhibitors, antimetabolites and radiomimetics) as summarized by Meirow. It was found that alkylating agents imposed the highest risk in causing ovarian failure with an odd ratio (OR) of 3,98, followed by cisplatin with an OR of 1.77 (Meirow and Nugent, 2001).

Schmidt, reported that the ovaries of healthy young girls contain a higher number of follicles than ovaries from older women, meaning young girls are more resistant to chemotherapy. Even if chemotherapeutic agents differ in their ovarian toxicity (Schmidt et al., 2010), they are often used in combination, so their adverse effects are increased and cannot always be easily evaluated.

In 2007, Oktem and Oktay, published an interesting paper on ovarian damage from chemotherapy. They present the first quantitative evidence in humans, by histological evaluation, that alkylating agents can significantly reduce ovarian reserve, and may affect stromal cell function (Oktem & Oktay, 2007). Meirow also reported that injury from chemotherapy is in stromal cells as well as in follicles and blood vessels (Meirow, 2010).

3. Ovarian tissue cryopreservation

To preserve ovarian tissue for a lengthy period of time, it should be stored in liquid nitrogen at a temperature of -196°C. However, ovarian tissue cryopreservation is complex and requires preservation of multiple cell types, thus the ability to successfully cryopreserve would be a powerful clinical tool in an assisted reproductive laboratory.

As reported by Bakhach in 2009, is easy to imagine the cell damage when temperatures fall from +37°C to -196°C. There is a loss of about 95% of intracellular water, an increase of electrolyte concentrations in both intra and extracellular media, and ice formation in the intracellular spaces that deform cells and destroy intracellular structures (Bakhach, 2009).

Hovatta in 2005 published an interesting work on the different methods of ovarian tissue freezing which emphasizes the importance of trying to preserve most of the cellular tissue components, including even the small proportion of ovarian medulla which contain blood vessels and nerves so important for ovarian tissue function recovery after reimplantation (Hovatta, 2005). Recently, Donnez reported that revascularization of grafts depends also on the preservation of vessels in grafted tissue, and not only on neoangiogenesis from the host (Donnez et al., 2011-b).

It should be stressed that the protocol of ovarian tissue freezing is still not standardized. So, there are several freezing procedures that range from slow freezing/rapid thawing, vitrification or ultrarapid-freezing. Freezing protocols differ also depending on the cryoprotectants used, dehydration/rehydration time and temperature, different protein support, and on the containers used for storage such us cryovials, strips or other tubes.

Approaches to human ovarian tissue cryopreservation are currently characterised by the use of slow freezing/rapid thawing methods using dimethylsulphoxide (DMSO) or propanediol (PROH) as a cryoprotectant. The slow freezing requires the use of a machine that slowly decreases the temperature, so the freezing programme so takes a few hours. This procedure has the disadvantage that it can lead to the formation of ice crystals, affecting correct tissue preservation. This disadvantage is avoided by using the protocol of vitrification, where high concentrations of cryopotectants are used, which increased ovarian toxicity too. Ultra-rapid freezing should be a method somewhere between the previous two using the advantages given by vitrification with a lower concentration of cryoprotectant to act on increasing the cooling rate.

In 2003 Shaw published an interesting paper on the terminology associated with equilibrium cooling procedures or 'slow cooling' and non-equilibrium protocols such as 'vitrification', 'rapid cooling' and 'ultrarapid cooling' that is helpful in clarifying the terms often used inappropriately (Shaw & Jones, 2003).

The positive results achieved by oocyte vitrification, has been discussed in recent years, but at the present time this procedure applied to ovarian tissue has given conflicting results.

Isachenko has worked extensively on the ovarian tissue vitrification. Her paper of 2007 showed a better preservation of ovarian tissue by slow freezing in which the quality of follicles was higher compared to the rapid freezing (Isachenko et al., 2007; Isachenko et al., 2009).

In 2007 Li demonstrated that the vitrification method for cryopreservation of human ovarian tissue is effective and simple (Li et al., 2007). Kagawa in 2009 found no difference in oocyte viability between fresh and vitrified human ovarian cortical tissue (kagawa, 2009). In another paper ovarian stroma was shown to be significantly better preserved by vitrification compared to slow freezing (Keros et al., 2009).

However, data on cryopreservation of human ovarian tissues by vitrification are still modest and controversial. This may be due to the fact that the same cryopreservation procedure is often used, such as slow freezing or vitrification, but different freezing protocol (types of cryoprotectant, concentration used and time of diffusion, etc.), this creates significant bias that must be considered.

In addition vitrification presupposes direct contact with liquid nitrogen, which is a potential source of microbial contamination, as reported by Isachenko (Isachenko et al., 2009).

In conclusion, an ideal ovarian cryopreservation method has not yet been established.

4. How to use

After 4 or 5 years when the patient is considered oncologically cured, the ovarian tissue stored in liquid nitrogen can be used. There are several ways to use tissue after thawing, such us reimplantation in various anatomic sites in the same patient or in a host animal or in vitro culture to grow primordial follicles present in large number (Fig. 3).

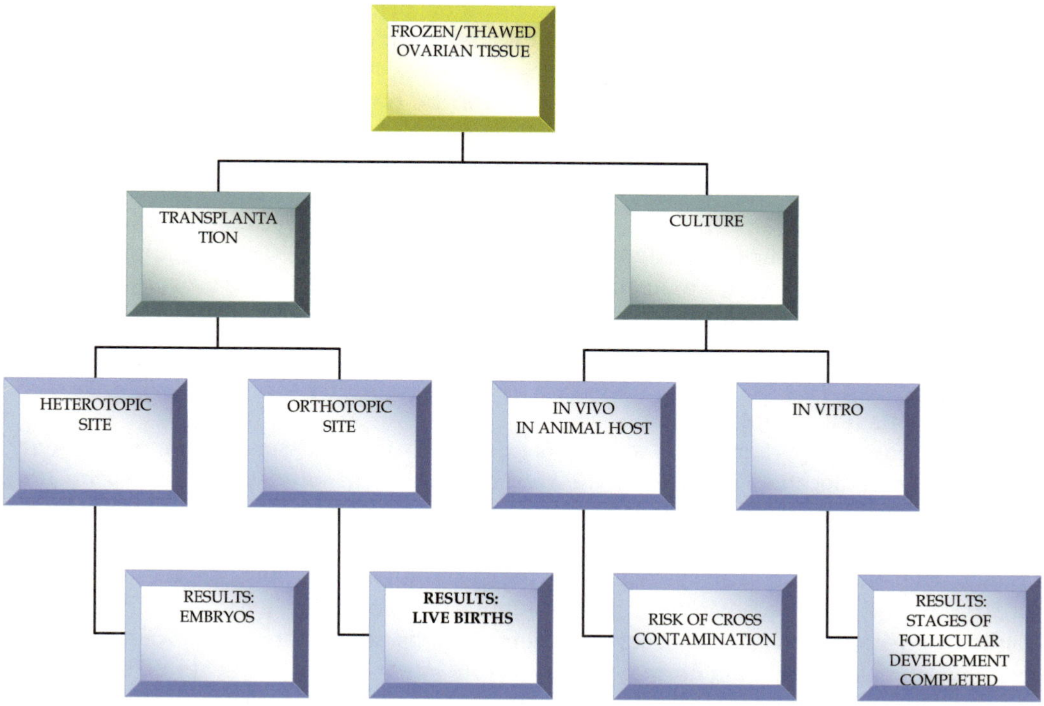

Fig. 3. Techniques using human cryopreserved ovarian tissue.

4.1 Ovarian tissue culture

When dealing with tumours that can metastasize to the ovary, ovarian tissue reimplantation should be avoided due to the risk of retransmitting cancer cells. In these cases the only option is to develop other methods in which the primordial follicles are matured in vitro within ovarian tissue pieces. Only in mice was the full maturation of primordial follicles with livebirths achieved (Eppig et al., 1996), this is difficult to replicate in large animals and humans.

In 2008 Picton published an interesting review on in vitro growth and maturation of follicles, which showed a number of different culture systems. It showed that culture of thin cortical strips has many advantages such as avoiding the damage caused by mechanical or enzymatic recovery of follicle present in the cortex, and provides a complex support system that resembles the ovary in vivo as the follicles also remain in contact with the surrounding stromal cells. This contact is very important at least until development of secondary follicles, when the follicles from the surrounding stroma should be left to facilitate further development. Thus, a multi-step strategy for the complete in vitro growth and maturation of follicles is promoted (Picton et al., 2008).

Recently another interesting review was published by Fabbri which summarizes the most relevant literature of the last ten years on in vitro cultures of ovarian cortical pieces. The conclusion was that the current optimal method for growing and maturing human follicles remains whole tissue culture. The authors underline the difficult of graduating nutrient concentration and especially what is best to add to the culture media and when (Fabbri et al., 2009).

In conclusion the culture of ovarian cortex strips is under development and currently not applicable to the human species, owing to the long period necessary for the follicle to complete development, almost six months compared to the couple of weeks in mice.

However, as suggested by Picton before these strategies can be utilised therapeutically, extensive testing is required to confirm the epigenetic health and genetic normality of in vitro growth derived oocytes (Picton et al., 2008).

We must not forget that oocytes are matured in vitro, after full development of follicles in vitro for a period exceeding 90 days, with the addition of nutrients that are not exactly what you get in their natural anatomic site, both as concentration and as timing of administration. So, even if complete follicle development in vitro is far from being clinically applicable, this does not mean that patients with malignancies that metastasize to the ovary should be excluded from the eventuality of cryopreserved tissue. We cannot know whether the study of in vitro cultures will make progress in a few years time.

4.2 Ovarian tissue reimplantation

The main option of this strategy is to transplant cortical ovarian tissue into the pelvic cavity, into its original location (orthotopic site) or in a different site, such as forearm, arm, abdominal wall, etc. (heterotopic site) when anticancer treatment is completed and the patient is disease-free.

Human transplantation history begins in the heterotopic site, such as the arm or the forearm. First studies on heterotopic reimplantation of an organ date back to 1975 and were applied to parathyroid gland. Several authors demonstrated that parathyroid autografts secret hormone and maintain normal serum calcium in the host (Wells et al., 1975; Hickey & Samaan, 1975). Oktay was the first to begin reimplanting of heterotopic tissue in the forearm, paving the way to human reimplantation history. In 2004 Oktay published a paper on the first embryo development after heterotopic transplantation of cryopreserved ovarian tissue (Oktay et el., 2004).

Successful orthotopic transplantation of ewe cryopreserved ovarian tissue was first performed by Gosden in 1994 (Gosden et al., 1994). The orthotopic transplantation is the site most suitable compared to the heterotopic site, because it is the natural environment, with comfortable temperatures and pressures for proper follicular development.

After several animal studies, ten years later, the first live human birth after frozen-thawed ovarian cortex orthotopic reimplantation was achieved by the Belgian group led by Donnez

(Donnez et al., 2004), followed recently by other live births (Donnez et al., 2011-a; Donnez et al., 2011-b; Meirow & Levron, 2005; Meirow et al., 2007; Demeestere et al., 2007; Demeestere et al., 2009; Anderson et al., 2008; Ernst et al., 2010; Silber et al., 2010; Piver et al., 2009; Sanchez-Serrano et al., 2010; Revel et al., 2011; Roux et al., 2010), as shown in table 1.
The major disadvantage of transplanting ovarian cortical strips is that revascularization of the graft needs several days, according to the species. So, revascularization occurrs within 48h after transplantation in rats and within 1 week of grafting in sheep. This leads to great loss of follicles from the grafts in transplantation due to ischemic injury, which can however be avoided by performing a whole ovarian transplantation thus providing immediate revascularization of the transplant (Onions et al., 2009; Bedaiwy & Falcone, 2004; Bedaiwy et al., 2006; Bromer & Patrizio, 2009). However, whole ovarian transplantations have a high rate of vascular complication, such as risk of thrombosis. Therefore, further work is needed before whole ovarian tissue transplantation can be considered a viable option for fertility preservation.
Exogenous factors such as antioxidants, growth factors or hormones have been tested to improve follicular survival in ovarian grafts by reducing ischaemia-reperfusion injury (Nugent et al., 1998; Torrents et al., 2003; Demeestere et al., 2009).
Until now, slow programmed ovarian tissue freezing is the only procedure that has resulted live births following orthotopic transplantation of frozen/thawed human ovarian tissue slices, but it is unknown or difficult to quantify how many women have attempted ovarian tissue reimplant.
The risk of ovarian tissue reimplantation includes transplantation of the primary tumour. However, most malignant diseases encountered during the reproductive years do not metastasize to the ovaries, except blood-borne malignancies such as leukemias, neuroblastoma and Burkitt's lymphoma. In the 1996 Shaw reported the transmission of lymphoma from a donor to a graft recipient (Shaw et al., 1996). Recently, Dolmans demonstrated, by quantitative RT-PCR, ovarian contamination by malignant cells by reimplant cryopreserved ovarian tissue in acute and chronic leukaemia patients (Dolmans et al., 2011).
So, it is highly recommended to use the best assessment to detect micro-metastases on a small portion of the harvested tissue before cryopreservation, it is also useful to freeze a less valuable part of the cortex, such as ovarian medulla.
As suggested by Von Wolff, sophisticated techniques are required to exclude first macroscopic ovarian pathology, such as ovarian metastasis, using imaging (sonography, CT scan, etc.). Then immunohistochemistry and polymerase chain reaction (PCR) to exclude single malignant cells, and identified minimal residual disease (MRD) by highly sensitive RT-PCR. Another effective method is xenotransplant small sample of ovarian tissue in a immunodeficient animal host (Von Wolff et al., 2009).

4.3 Xenotransplantation

Xenotransplantation falls between reimplantation and in vitro culture, so the follicles within the tissue are growing in vivo in an animal host (T-and B-cell-deficient SCID mice). It has been applied to assess the risk of reimplanting malignant cells after human ovarian tissue reimplantation, and to observe follicle development.
Last year Dath compared four grafting (intraperitoneal, ovarian bursa, sub-cutaneous, and intramuscular) sites for xenotransplantation of human ovarian tissue to nude mice, concluding that all four sites equally supported early follicular growth and preserved some

quiescent follicles (Dath et al., 2010). However, Sonmezer reported an asynchrony between oocytes and granulosa cell development (Sonmezer & Oktay, 2010).

FIRST AUTHOR YEAR	WHERE	DIAGNOSIS	AGE at cryo	FRESH or CRYO-PRESERVED	SLICES or WHOLE	REIMPLANTATION SIDE	OUTCOME
Donnez, 2004	Belgium	Stage IV Hodgkin's lymphoma	25	Frozen/thawed	Slices	Orthotopic: ovarian fossa peritoneum	Spontaneous pregnancy: **live birth**
Donnez, 2011-a	Belgium	Neuroectodermic tumour	17	Frozen/thawed	Slices	Orthotopic: ovary	Spontaneous pregnancy: **live birth**
Meirow, 2005, 2007	Israel	Non Hodgkin's lymphoma	28	Frozen/thawed	Slices	Orthotopic: ovary	Mild ovarian stimulation - IVF: **live birth**
Demeestere, 2007, 2010	Belgium	Stage IV Hodgkin's lymphoma	24	Frozen/thawed	Slices	Orthotopic (+ heterotopic)	Spontaneous pregnancy: **live birth in 2007** **live birth in 2009**
Andersen, 2008	Denmark	Hodgkin's lymphoma	27	Frozen/thawed	Slices	Orthotopic: ovary	Ovarian stimulation - IVF: **live birth**
Andersen, 2008; Ernst, 2010	Denmark	Ewing sarcoma	27	Frozen/thawed	Slices	Orthotopic: ovary	Mild ovarian stimulation - IVF: **1 live birth.** Spontaneous pregnancy: **1 live birth**
A- Silber, 2010 B- (Donnez, 2011 b)	USA	Stage IIIb Hodgkin's lymphoma	20	Frozen/thawed	Slices	Orthotopic	A- Ongoing pregnancies **B -live birth**
Silber, 2010	USA		24	Frozen/thawed	Slices	Orthotopic	**1 live birth + 1 live birth**
Piver, 2009	France	Microscopic polyangiitis	27	Frozen/thawed	Slices	Orthotopic	IVF: **live birth**
Sanchez-Serrano, 2010	Spain	Breast cancer	36	Frozen/thawed	Slices	Orthotopic	Ovarian stimulation, IVF: **2 live births** (twins)
Revel, 2011	Israel	Thalassemia major	19	Frozen/thawed	Slices	Orthotopic	IVF: **live birth**
Roux, 2010	France	Homozygous sicule cell anemia	20	Frozen/thawed	Slices	Orthotopic: ovary and few strips deposited in the peritoneal window	Spontaneous pregnancy: **live birth**

Table 1. Live births after frozen/thawed orthotopic transplantation of human ovarian tissue.

In conclusion, xenotransplantation should be carefully considered in its human clinical application because of the risk of cross-species retroviral infection.

5. Conclusion

As reported by Maltaris it is important to assess the 'ovarian reserve' that is the available pool of primordial follicles in the ovary and is a major determinant of female fertility potential. This information is important for a correct strategy of fertility preservation before cancer treatment. In general, ovarian reserve tests are either biochemical or biophysical (Maltaris et al., 2006), but new methods are required.

In conclusion, a common goal of life-saving methods must be to protect the fertility of young women to this aim it is important to form a closely collaborative team comprising gynaecologists, surgeons, oncologists, haematologists, biologists and psychologists. Specifically, it is important that the oncologist gives an assessment of the degree of ovarian damage in order to decide how much ovarian tissue to retrieve and store.

It is known that for each malignant disease only few protocols are commonly used, so it is possible to analyse the risk of ovarian failure. Meirow reported that the ovarian failure rate was 50% for breast cancer, 44% for non-Hodgkin's lymphoma, and 32% for Hodgkin's disease (Meirow & Nugent, 2001).

Before proceeding to cryopreserve ovarian tissue, it is important to identify a series of tests for morphological analyses (such as staining with hematoxylin and eosin for observation by an optical microscope, or a more thorough evaluation of cell components by electron microscopy), for functional analyses (such as immunohistochemistry), or for viability analyses (such as trypan blue); in order to assess the degree of overall tissue preservation with the procedure adopted in the laboratory.

In addition, it is also important to put an age limit to the preservation of ovarian tissue. The patient can use it only after cancer remission, therefore not before few years, so the cryopreservation of ovarian tissue of a patient older than 38 years old may be a useless procedure but could give psychological support to women. In any case, patients should be properly informed about the real possibility of recovering fertility and be able to get pregnant.

In conclusion, we agree with Donnez that ovarian tissue cryopreservation should be offered before anticancer treatments in all cases where there is a high risk of premature ovarian failure and where emergency in vitro fertilization is not possible (Donnez et al., 2011-c).

If the dogma of reproductive biology is that of a finite number of follicles in the ovary which, moreover, undergo atresia during reproductive life, all procedures to preserve fertility should be carried out before acting on the ovary with drugs, therapies, surgery or potentially toxic treatments. Therefore, live births after cryoprserved ovarian tissue trasnplantation opened up new chapter in the field of infertility preservation.

6. Acknowledgment

The authors thank Rosalind Roberts for reviewing the English language, and Elena Gismano (biologist) for assistance with chapter preparation.

7. References

Andersen CY, Rosendahl M, Byskov AG, Loft A, Ottosen C, et al. (2008) Two successful pregnancies following autotransplantation of frozen/thawed ovarian tissue. Hum Reprod.;23(10):2266-72.

Bakhach J. (2009) The cryopreservation of composite tissues. Pinciples and recent advancement on cryopreservation of different type of tissues. Organogenesis 5(3):119-126.

Bedaiwy MA, Falcone T. (2004) Ovarian tissue banking for cancer patients: reduction of post-transplantation ischaemic injury: intact ovary freezing and transplantation. Hum Reprod.;19(6):1242-4.

Bedaiwy MA, Hussein MR, Biscotti C, Falcone T. (2006) Cryopreservation of intact human ovary with its vascular pedicle. Hum Reprod.;21(12):3258-69.

Bromer JG, Patrizio P. (2009) Fertility preservation: the rationale for cryopreservation of the whole ovary. Semin Reprod Med.;27(6):465-71.

Bukovsky A, Caudle MR, Virant-Klun I, Gupta SK, Dominguez R, Svetlikova M, Xu F. (2009) Immune physiology and oogenesis in fetal and adult humans, ovarian infertility, and totipotency of adult ovarian stem cells. Birth Defects Res C Embryo Today.;87(1):64-89.

Dath C, Van Eyck AS, Dolmans MM, Romeu L, Delle Vigne L, et al. (2010) Xenotransplantation of human ovarian tissue to nude mice: comparison between four grafting sites. Hum Reprod.;25(7):1734-43.

De Felici M. (2010) Germ stem cells in the mammalian adult ovary: considerations by a fan of the primordial germ cells. Mol Hum Reprod.;16(9):632-6.

Demeestere I, Simon P, Emiliani S, Delbaere and Englert Y. (2007) Fertility preservation: Successful transplantation of cryopreserved ovarian tissue in a young patient previously treated for Hodgkin's disease. The Oncol.; 12:1437-1442.

Demeestere I, Simon P, Emiliani S, Delbaere A, Englert Y. (2009) Orthotopic and heterotopic ovarian tissue transplantation. Hum Reprod Update.;15(6):649-65.

Demeestere I, Simon P, Moffa F, Delbaere A, and Englert Y. (2010) Birth of a second healthy girl more than 3 years after cryopreserved ovarian graft. Letter to the Editor, Hum Reprod 1590-1591.

Dolmans MM, Marinescu C, Saussoy P, Van Langendonckt A, Amorim C and Donnez J. (2011) Reimplantation of cryopreserved ovarian tissue from patients with acute lymphoblastic leukaemia is potentially unsafe. Blood; 116(16):2908-2914.

Donnez J, Dolmans MM, Demylle D, Jadoul P, Pirard C,. (2004) Live birth after orthotopic transplantation of cryopreserved ovarian tissue. Lancet. 16-22;364(9443):1405-10.

Donnez J, Squifflet J, Jadoul P, Demylle D, Cheron AC et al,. (2011-a) Pregnancy and live birth after autotranplantation of frozen-thawed ovarian tissue in a patient with metastatic disease undergoing chemotherapy and hematopoietic stem cell transplantation. Fert Steril.; 95(5):1787.e1-1787.e4.

Donnez J, Silber S, Andersen CY, Demeestere I, Piver P, Meirow D, Pellicer A, Dolmans MM. (2011-b) Children born after autotransplantation of cryopreserved ovarian tissue. A review of 13 live births. Ann Med, 1-14.

Ernst E, bergholdt S, Jørgensen JS, Andersen CY (2010) The first woman to give birth to two children following transplantation of frozen/thawed ovarian tissue. Hum Reprod, 25(5):1280-1.

Eppig JJ, O'Brien M and Wigglesworth K.; (1996) Mammalian oocyte growth and development in vitro. Mol Reprod Dev, 44(2):260-273.

Fabbri R, Pasquinelli G, Keane D, Mozzanega B, Magnani V, et al. (2009) Culture of cryopreserved ovarian tissue: state of the art in 2008. Fertil Steril.;91(5):1619-29.

Gosden RG, Baird DT, Wade JC, Webb R. (1994) Restoration of fertility to oophorectomized sheep by ovarian autografts stored at -196 degrees C. Hum Reprod.;9(4):597-603.

Hickey RC, Samaan NA. (1975) Human parathyroid autotransplantation: proved function by radioimmunoassay of plasma parathyroid hormone. Arch Surg.;110(8):892-5.

Hovatta O. (2005) Methods for cryopreservation of human ovarian tissue. Reprod Biomed Online.;10(6):729-34

Isachenko V, Isachenko E, Reinsberg J, Montag M, van der Ven K, et al. (2007) Cryopreservation of human ovarian tissue: comparison of rapid and conventional freezing. Cryobiology. 55(3):261-8.

Isachenko V, Lapidus I, Isachenko E, Krivokharchenko A, Kreienberg R, et al. (2009) Human ovarian tissue vitrification versus conventional freezing: morphological, endocrinological, and molecular biological evaluation. Reproduction. 138(2):319-27.

Johnson J, Canning J, Kaneko T, Pru JK, Tilly JL. (2004) Germline stem cells and follicular renewal in the postnatal mammalian ovary. Nature.11;428(6979):145-50.

Johnson J, Bagley J, Skaznik-Wikiel M, Lee HJ, Adams GB, et al. (2005) Oocyte generation in adult mammalian ovaries by putative germ cells in bone marrow and peripheral blood. Cell. 29;122(2):303-15.

Kagawa N. Successful vitrification of bovine and human ovarian tissue. (2009) RBM Online, 18(4):568-577.

Keros V, Xella S, Hultenby K, Pettersson K, Sheikhi M, et al. (2009) Vitrification versus controlled-rate freezing in cryopreservation of human ovarian tissue.Hum Reprod, 24(7):1670-1683.

Lee HJ, Selesniemi K, Niikura Y, Niikura T, Klein R, et al. (2007) Bone marrow transplantation generates immature oocytes and rescues long-term fertility in a preclinical mouse model of chemotherapy-induced premature ovarian failure. J Clin Oncol. 1;25(22):3198-204.

Li YB, Zhou CQ, Yang GF, Wang Q, Dong Y. (2007) Modified vitrification method for cryopreservation of human ovarian tissues. Chin Med J (Engl). 20;120(2):110-4.

Lushbaugh CC, Casarett GW. (1976) The effects of gonadal irradiation in clinical radiation therapy: a review. Cancer; 37(2 Suppl):1111-25.

Maltaris T, Koelbl H, Seufert R, Kiesewetter F, Beckmann MW, et al. (2006) Gonadal damage and options for fertility preservation in female and male cancer survivors. Asian J Androl.;8(5):515-33.

Meirow D. and Nugent D. (2001) The effect of radiotherapy and chemotherapy on female reproduction. Hum Reprod Update, 7(6):535-543.

Meirow D and Levron J. (2005) Pregnancy after transplantation of cryopreserved ovarian tissue in a patient with ovarian failure after chemotherapy. The New Eng J Med, 353(3):318-321.

Meirow D, Levron J, Eldar-Geva T, Hardan I, Fridman E et al. (2007) Monitoring the ovaries after autotransplantation of cryopreserved ovarian tissue: endocrine studies, in vitro fertilization cycles, and live birth. Fertil Steril, 87(2):418.e7-418.e15.

Meirow D, Biederman H, Anderson RA, Wallace WH. (2010) Toxicity of chemotherapy and radiation on female reproduction. Clin Obstet Gynecol.;53(4):727-39.

Nugent D, Newton H, Gallivan L, Gosden RG. (1998) Nugent D et al. Protective effect of vitamin E on ischaemia-reperfusion injury in ovarian grafts. J Reprod Fertil.;114(2):341-6.

Oktay K, Buyuk E, Veeck L, Zaninovic N, Xu K, et al. (2004) Embryo development after heterotopic transplantation of cryopreserved ovarian tissue. Lancet. 13;363(9412):837-40.

Oktem O, Oktay K. (2007) Quantitative assessment of the impact of chemotherapy on ovarian follicle reserve and stromal function. Cancer. 15;110(10):2222-9.

Onions VJ, Webb R, McNeilly AS, Campbell BK. (2009) Ovarian endocrine profile and long-term vascular patency following heterotopic autotransplantation of cryopreserved whole ovine ovaries. Hum Reprod.;24(11):2845-55.

Picton HM, Harris SE, Muruvi W, Chambers EL. (2008) The in vitro growth and maturation of follicles. Reproduction.;136(6):703-15.

Piver P, Amiot C, Agnani G, Pech JC, Rohrlich PS et al. (2009). Two pregnancies obtained after a new technique of autotransplantation of cryopreserved ovarian tissue. Abstract of the 25th Annual Meeting of ESHRE, Amsterdam, the Netherlands, 28 June-1 July, Hum Reprod, vol. 24 suppl. 1, session 2.

Revel A, Laufer N, Meir AB, Lebovich M and Mitrani E. (2011) Micro-organ ovarian transplantation enables pregnancy: a case report. Hum Rep, March 18, pp1-7.

Roux C, Amiot C, Agnani G, Aubard Y, Rohrlich PS, et al. (2010) Live birth after ovarian tissue autograft in a patient with sickle cell disease treated by allogeneic bone marrow transplantation. Fertil Steril,. 1;93(7):2413.e15-9.

Sánchez-Serrano M, Crespo J, Mirabet V, Cobo AC, Escribá MJ, et al. (2010) Twins born after transplantation of ovarian cortical tissue and oocyte vitrification. Fertil Steril.;93(1):268.e11-3.

Schmidt KT, Larsen EC, Andersen CY, Andersen AN. (2010) Risk of ovarian failure and fertility preserving methods in girls and adolescents with a malignant disease. BJOG.;117(2):163-74.

Shaw JM, Bowles J, Koopman P, Wood EC and Trounson AO. (1996). Fresh and cryopreserved ovarian tissue samples from donors with lymphoma transmit the cancer to graft recipients. Hum Reprod.; 11(8):1668-1673.

Shaw JM, Jones GM. (2003) Terminology associated with vitrification and other cryopreservation procedures for oocytes and embryos. Hum Reprod Update.;9(6):583-605.

Silber S, Kagawa N, Kuwayama M, Gosden R. (2010) Duration of fertility after fresh and frozen ovary transplantation. Fertil Steril 94(6):2191-2196.

Sonmezer M and Oktay K. (2010) Orthotopic and heterotopic ovarian tissue transplantation. Best Pract Res Clin Obstet Gynaecol.;24(1):113-26.

Torrents E, Boiso I, Barri PN, Veiga A. (2003) Applications of ovarian tissue transplantation in experimental biology and medicine. Hum Reprod Up, 9(5):471-481.

Von Wolff M, Donnez J, Hovatta O, Keros V, Maltaris T et al. (2009) Cryopreservation and autotransplantation of human ovarian tissue prior to cytotoxic therapy – A technique in its infancy but already successful in fertility preservation. Eu J Canc 45:1545-1553.

Wallace WH, Shalet SM, Hendry JH, Morris-Jones PH, Gattamaneni HR. (1989) Ovarian failure following abdominal irradiation in childhood: the radiosensitivity of the human oocyte. Br J Radiol.;62(743):995-8.

Wallace WH, Kelsey TW. (2010) Human ovarian reserve from conception to the menopause. PLoS One. 27;5(1):e8772.

Wells SA Jr, Gunnells JC, Shelburne JD, Schneider AB, Sherwood LM. (1975) Transplantation of the parathyroid glands in man: clinical indications and results. Surgery.;78(1):34-44.

15

Lung Cancer in Elderly

Anne Dagnault and Jean Archambault
Radiation Oncology Department, CHUQ-Hôtel-Dieu de Québec, Canada

1. Introduction

Lung cancer is one of the leading causes of cancer in the population. The aging population is a reality. More and more, in oncology, we are facing challenges about management of cancer in this important population. In this chapter, we will review data on lung cancer and aging. We will explore how to evaluate this particular population to offer them the best treatment possible, bearing in mind that some adjustment may be necessary compared to younger population.

2. Definition of the elderly

2.1 Chronologic aging

The cut-off point for an adult to be considered "elder" is not well defined. According to most of the literature, age 70 years is used as a chronologic marker for definition of elderly population. This is also the age most commonly used in the clinical trials in oncology as a limit for recruitment (Balducci, 2000).

2.2 Physiologic aging

In fact, elderly should be referring to a state either than a chronological age. It is well known that with time, especially at or around 70 years of age, a number of age-related physiologic changes occur affecting the physiologic reserve of the person. Many of these changes may affect the tolerance to cancer treatment as; decreased renal and liver functions, decreased volume of distribution, immune response and intestinal absorption (Avery et al., 2009). Talking more specifically about lung function, age-related pulmonary changes include a decreased response to hypoxemia or hypercapnia, decreased elasticity of the lung tissue, increased ventilation-perfusion mismatch, and decreased forced expiratory volume (Gonzalez-Aragoneses et al., 2009).

3. The aging population

Population age is increasing in developed country. In the United States, in 2000, there were 35 million persons aged over 65 years old. This proportion is expected to continue to increase from 40 million in 2010 to 81 million in 2040 (U.S. Census Bureau). In Canada, the situation is similar. In 2036, Statistics Canada estimates the population of persons aged 70 years and older to be situated between 10 and 10.8 million.

The National institute of Aging has characterised the aging of the American Society as a "silver tsunami for which we are unprepared" (Fried & Hall, 2008).

4. Cancer as an aging problem

Is is recognized that the risk of cancer increases with age. In Canada, 43% of all new cancer cases and 61% of cancer deaths will occur among those who are at least 70 years old.
Figure 1 represents the number of new cases of cancer for Canadian males together with the corresponding age-standardized rates for 1981-2006 and estimates to the year 2010. It shows that despite the relative stability in age-standardized rates, the number of new cancer cases continue to rise steadily as the Canadian population grows and ages. The figure shows the major contribution of the population's growth and the aging population to the rising numbers of new cases from cancer.

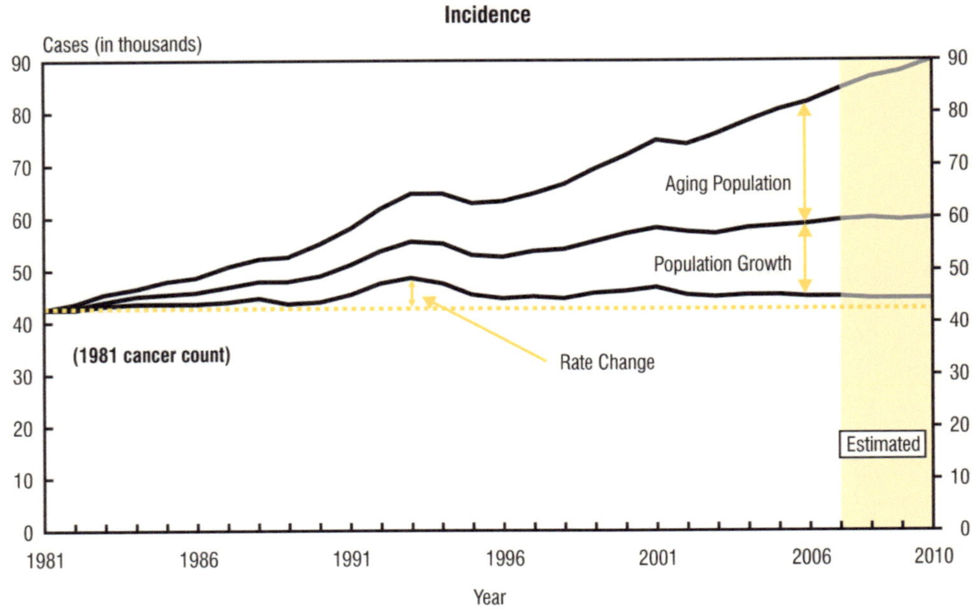

Fig. 1. Incidence of cancer for Canadian males with age-standardized rates (1981-2006) (from Canadian Cancer Statistics 2010).

The lowest line represents the total number of new cancer cases that would have occurred each year if the population size and age structure had remained in the same as it was in 1981, reflecting the impact of changing risk. The middle line represents the number of new cases that would have occurred if the age structure had remained the same as it was in 1981, reflecting the impact of changing risk and population growth. The top line, the actually occurring number of new cancer cases, represents the combined impact of changes in risk, population growth and the aging of population. This figure is similar for new cancer cases ial of adjuvant chemotherapaths rates in male and female. It indicates the importance of the impact of the aging population on the growth in the number of cancer cases that has occurred over the last 30 years (Canadian Cancer Statistics 2010).

5. Lung cancer in elderly

In Canada, both in men and women, lung cancer is the second most common cancer (13.9%) after prostate cancer in men and breast cancer in women. In 2010, it represents 24,200 new cases. More than half of all newly diagnosed cases will occur among people aged 70 years and older. More importantly, lung cancer is the leading cause of cancer death in both sex representing 20,600 deaths. Lung cancer deaths peak at age 70-79 years for both male and female in Canada.

In United States, median age for diagnosis for lung cancer was 71 years of age from 2004 to 2008 according to SEER data. 29% of cases were in persons aged between 75 and 84 and 8.3% were older than 85 years old. In the same period, the median age at death for cancer of the lung and bronchus was 72 years of age, with 30.7% between ages 75 and 84 and 9.6% in persons older than 85 years.

6. Evaluation of the elderly cancer patient

6.1 Oncologic evaluation

On the oncologic point of view, evaluation of an elderly patient should be exactly the same as for a younger one. Clinical and pathological stage of disease should be determined with the same accuracy. The complete workup for lung cancer includes at least a complete history and physical examination, a bronchoscopy, a CT scan of the chest and upper abdomen and blood tests for assessment of liver and renal function. CT scan of the head should be done if there are any suspicions of metastasis, or in advanced cases, as well as a complete bone scan. Ideally, patients must have a Pet-Scan to complete the workup. As for younger patients, biopsy of the tumour for histology is always mandatory.

When surgery or radiation therapy treatment are anticipate, pulmonary function test are essential to determine the capacity of the patient to tolerate those procedure.

Unfortunately, in the elderly population, lung cancers are less susceptible to be diagnosed at an early stage and the evaluation is more often incomplete. More than 20% of cancers in patients aged more than 85 years of age are diagnosed on a clinical or radiologic basis without pathologic confirmation (Goddwin & Osborne, 2004).

6.2 Geriatric evaluation

The geriatric assessment of a patient is also a diagnostic process. It may be done by an individual clinician, but more often, the geriatric evaluation involve a more intensive multidisplinary program. This is often referred to a comprehensive geriatric assessment (CGA). The optimal goal is to evaluate the patients' global and functional status, in order to improve treatment decisions and outcomes. His use is now recommended by the International Society of Geriatric Oncology (SIOG) for all cancer patient aged more than 70 years old. This recommendation is based on the evidence that the incidence of geriatric problems increases sharply after 70 in cancer patients (Extermann et al., 2005, as cited in Balducci et al., 1990). The CGA permits to detect unaddressed problems, improve older cancer patients functional status and possibly their survival. The SIOG was not able to recommend any specific tool or approach above others for this assessment (Extermann et al., 2005).

Whatever the approach or the tools used to complete a CGA, different aspects should be included as; functional status, comorbid medical conditions, cognitive and nutritional status, psychological state, social support and review of the medication.

6.3 Components of a comprehensive geriatric assessment

6.3.1 Functional status

Functional status represents the patient's ability to perform daily activities. The more commonly used performance status score are the Karnofsky or Eastern Cooperative Oncology Group (ECOG) scales. In older patients, these scores were showed to under-represent the degree of functional impairment (Repetto et al., 2002). For that reason, it is important to include the autonomy for Activities of Daily Living (ADL), such as feeding, grooming, transferring and toileting and for the Instrumental Activities of Daily Living (IADL) such as shopping, housekeeping, managing finances, preparing meals and taking medications in the evaluation of functional status for these patients.

A study of 566 patients with advanced non-small cell lung cancer age ≥ 70 years receiving chemotherapy explores the impact of functional status on the overall survival. Improved overall survival was associated with independence in IADLs and higher quality of life scores. Limitations in basic ADLs and the presence of comorbidity were not predictors of a decrease in overall survival (Maione et al. 2005). However, limitation in basic ADLs was previously shown to predict chemotherapy toxicity and postoperative survival and morbidity (Extermann & Huria, 2007).

6.3.2 Comorbidities

In cancer patients, comorbidity can be seen as a competitive cause of death. It is well known that with increasing age, the number or comorbid medical conditions increases. It is important to consider these comorbid conditions in life expectancy and potential treatment tolerance when balancing the risks and benefits of them. Charlson Comorbidity Index (CCI) is a way to assess the number and severity of comorbid condition (Charlson et al., 1987).

Additional issues regarding the treatment of elderly cancer patients are the presence of geriatric syndromes as; dementia, delirium, depression, falls, neglect and abuse, failure to thrive, incontinence and spontaneous bone fracture.

A review of the National Cancer Institute of Canada (NCI) Clinical Trials Group in 2008 analyzed 1,255 patients enrolled in two large, prospectively randomized trials of systemic chemotherapy for NSCLC. Patients aged 65 and older were more likely to have a CCI score of ≥ 1 (42 % versus 26%). Age did not influence overall survival, but the Charlson Comorbidy Index ≥ 1 appeared prognostic for poorer survival (Asmis et al., 2008). The impact of comorbidity was recently studied in a population of 83 untreated lung cancer patients over the age of 70. It was shown that they have a high prevalence of comorbidity but these may not cause patient's death (Gironés et al., 2011).

6.3.3 Cognitive status

Cognitive deficits are associated in the geriatric population with an increase in mortality of over 150% at 5 years. They are also associated with an increase risk of complications, depression, and functional decline.

Cognitive deficits and dementia in oncology patient is often unrecognized. However, it was demonstrated that 25-50% of older patients with cancer had abnormalities in screening cognitive exam that warranted further evaluation. Cognitive dysfunction can have significant impact in the pathway of cancer treatment; dysfunction on the ability to weigh the risks and benefits of cancer therapy, compliance with treatment, and recognition of the signs of toxicity that require medical attention (Extermann & Hurria, 2007). It was previously demonstrated than even when treated in a specialized geriatric oncology program, cognitively impaired patients had a survival of cancer one third of that of nonimpaired patients in various tumor type and stages, even if they received similar treatments (Extermann & Hurria, 2007, as cited in Callen et al. 2004). Therefore, screening for cognition should be part of the evaluation in the elderly patient afflicted with lung cancer.

6.3.4 Nutritional status

The importance of malnutrition on overall survival and morbidity is well known in the general cancer population. It is also demonstrated that aging is a factor for an increase risk of malnutrition. Other than mortality, poor nutritional status can have an impact on the quality of life, response to chemotherapy, and any other medical complications.

6.3.5 Psychological state

Many reports have shown that the incidence of psychological distress is approximately one-third of older patient with cancer. Studies of geriatric assessment show that 14% to 40% of older patients have depressive symptoms (Extermann & Hurria, 2007). A large epidemiologic studies of 24,696 older breast cancer in the SEER database (ages 67 to 90 years) revealed that a recent diagnosis of depression put them at risk for receiving less-than-definitive treatment for their cancer, and they also experienced shorter survival (Extermann & Hurria, 2007 as cited in Goddwin et al, 2004). In addition, depressive symptoms have impact on quality of life, increased utilization of healthcare resources and can affect treatment compliance.

6.3.6 Social support

Social support is a major factor that puts patients at risk for psychological distress. Even monthly telephone call was shown to reduce depression in older patients with cancer. This method was demonstrated to reduce significantly anxiety ($p<0.0001$), depression ($p=0.0004$), and overall distress ($p<0.0001$) compare to no similar support (Extermann & Hurria, 2007 as cited in Kornblith et al., 2006).

6.3.7 Review of the medication

Polypharmacy is a significant problem in the geriatric population. Many physiologic changes in the elderly may have impact on pharmacokinetic; a decrease in total body water, an increase in body fat, a decrease in renal function, decrease in hepatic mass and blood flow, and decrease in bone marrow reserve. The combination of those changes and polypharmacy is associated with an increase risk of drug interactions, adverse drug events and problem with compliance. Therefore, it is essential to regularly review the medication list to discontinue any unnecessary medications and avoid potential drug interactions.

6.4 Impact of the CGA

Many trials have studied the impact of a CGA on outcome of elderly patients with cancer. A meta-analysis of 28 controlled trials had demonstrated that CGA if linked to geriatric interventions reduced early re-hospitalisation and mortality in older patients through early identification and treatment of problems (Pallis et al. 2010, as cited in Stuck et al., 1993). In a

recent French study it was shown that comprehensive geriatric evaluation did significantly influence treatment decisions in 82% of the older cancer patients. In this 161 patients group, with a median age of 82.4 years, cancer treatment was change in 79 patients (49%), including delayed therapy in 5 patients, less intensive therapy in 18% and more intensive therapy in 28% of patients (Chaïbi et al. 2010).
It is interesting to notice that even a simplified geriatric assessment, adapted to cancer and quicker to perform than a CGA was recently demonstrated effective in patients with thoracic cancer. It is an important aid to decision-making in the management of elderly patients with bronchial cancer (Cudennec et al., 2010).

Aim	Method
Social evaluation	Place of residence: home, type of residence for an elderly, dependent patient Helpers, aids around the home
Iatrogenic risk	Number and classes of drugs
Existence of ≥3 co-morbidities significant in geriatrics	Dementia, confusion, depression, incontinence, falls, malnutrition, progressive heart failure, other cancer
Nutritional status	Loss of weight over the previous 3 months (≥5%), albuminemia levels
Cognitive functions	Mini Mental State Examination (MMSE), Clock drawing task
State of mind	Mini-Geriatric Depression Scale (mini-GDS)
Risk of fall	Timed "Get up and go" test
Sense organs	Vision and hearing
Autonomy	Instrumental Activities of Daily Living (IADL)

Table 1. Simplified Geriatric Assessment of patients with bronchial cancer (Cudennec et al., 2010).

7. Surgery

Surgery remains the mainstay of treatment for early stage NSCLC. Unfortunately, according to most published reports, elderly have a significant lower resection rates compared to younger patients and age is one of the factor influencing the decision for surgical treatment. Sigel retrospectively analyzed 27 850 patients with stage I lung cancer. The rate of lung surgery was 95% for patients less than 60 years and 79% in patients > 80 years (Sigel et al., 2009). An analysis of Riquet showed that patients older than 70 years of age represents 21.7% of patients who had surgery for lung cancer, patients of 75 years and older represents 8.8% and older than 80 years old are only 1.9% in proportion (Riquet et al., 2001).
These observations are still true, even considering the significant improvement in anesthesia, in technical procedures of lung resection and post-operative care that greatly enhanced the security of the surgery, even in a frail population. In patients with stage I and II, surgical option is still the prefer treatment option. The 5-year overall survival rates for pathological stage I range between 67% for pT1pN0 and 57% for pT2pN0 tumors. The corresponding values based on clinical stage are 61% for cT1cN0 and 37% for cT2cN0.

7.1 Evaluation and selection of patients

Patients must have a very good evaluation and adequate scrutiny is necessary to evaluate those who will really benefit from surgery. Preoperative assessment of cancer in the elderly (PACE) incorporates validated instruments including the CGA, an assessment of fatigue and performance status and an anaesthesiologist's evaluation of operative risk. It is considered to be a valuable tool in enhancing the decision process concerning the candidacy of elderly patients for surgical intervention. It also reduce inappropriate age-related inequity in access to surgical intervention (PACE, 2008).

7.2 Different types of surgery are used for the elderly. But which one is better?

Survival data from the SEER database with patient of all ages shown that survival for lung cancer stage I and II were 56 and 34% respectively (Chang et al., 2007). The most important question regarding surgical resection for lung cancer is how aggressive should it be? The choice of the type of surgery is particularly important in the elderly. Right pneumonectomy is likely to be avoided in octogenarians (Broks et al., 2007; Port et al., 2004; Van Meerbeeck et al., 2002), but low rate of pneumonectomy in different series make this difficult to assess. As an indication, the British Thoracic Society Guidelines indicates that pneumonectomy is associated with higher risk of mortality.

The sublobar pulmonary resection remains controversial in patients of any age. In a SEER analysis of 14,555 patients with stage I or II NSCLC, it was showed that benefit of a lobectomy was not evident for patients older than 71 years compared with limited resection (Meryet al., 2005). Okami did a non-randomized study to evaluate the different types of surgery in the elderly patients. A total of 764 patients, including 133 elderly and 631 younger patients had lobectomy or sublobar resection. The survival after sublobar resection was significantly lower than that after standard lobectomy in the younger group (64% vs 90.9%). Comparatively, no difference was seen in the elderly (67.6% vs 74.3%). However, locoregional recurrences were higher in patients with sublobar resection than lobectomy in young and older patients (Okami et al., 2009). A phase III study regarding this specific topic would be necessary to confirm this information.

Another study done in Pittsburg has compared lobectomy to the segmentectomy for stage I lung cancer. In a subgroup of 99 octogenarian patients, the segmentectomy was associated with an improvement of the 3-year survival ($p=0.02$) (Schuchert et al., 2009).

7.3 The impact of comorbidities on surgical outcomes

A review of 10,761 patients with lung cancer stage IA showed the age of 67 years or more as an independent factor associated with long-term survival worse after surgery. One of the major criticisms of this study is that patients were not stratified based on their functional status or their comorbidities. It is known that these two factors are associated with advanced age and are predictors of mortality in elderly patients suffering from lung cancer (Maione et al., 2005; Frasci et al., 2000; Asmis et al., 2008; Schuchert et al., 2009).

In another study of 126 patients 70 years of age or older with lung cancer, the Charlson Comorbidity Index has been performed in patients for lung surgery. A low score was a predictor of major complications after surgery (Birim et al., 2003). Some studies in patients older than 80 years of age were also conducted (Brokx et al., 2007; Okami et al., 2009; Wada et al., 1998). At the Mayo Clinic, 294 patients aged between 80 and 94 years underwent pulmonary resection and their 1-year survival was 80% and 2-year survival was 62% (Dominguez-Ventura et al., 2007).

A review of 297 articles was done by Chambers (2010) to consider the impact of lung resection on morbidity, mortality and postoperative quality of life for patients aged over 70 years. They found twelve articles to answer this question. The collective analysis of these 12 articles showed a five-year survival following surgery for early stages in those under age 70 between 69 and 77%, for those over 70 years, the five-year survival ranges from 59 to 78%. The 30-day mortality rate was 5.7% in patients younger than 70 years against 1.3 to 3.3% in those over 70 years, length of hospital stay after thoracoscopy was respectively 4.6 and 4.9 to 5.2 days. The post-operative lung functions were also equivalent between the two groups. FEV_1 decreased 13% compared to 18% in patients older than 70 years (p=0.34) comparing the functional vital capacity decrease were equivalent between both groups (9% vs 14%).
Lung function was also compared among young and elderly patients after lobectomy for early stage NSCLC. Changes in FEV_1 and functional vital capacity were not significant although postoperative complications occurred in 32% of younger patients and 48% in the elderly (Sullivan et al., 2005).

8. Adjuvant chemotherapy

The use of adjuvant chemotherapy in the elderly is increasingly popular (Wang et al., 2008). In a SEER database, 25.8% of patients aged between 66 and 69 years received adjuvant treatment compared to 19.8% for those aged 70 to 74, 13.7% for those of 75 to 79 and only 9% for patients older than 80 years old. In the LACE meta-analysis of 4,584 patients with adjuvant chemotherapy, the hazard ratio for mortality was 0.89 and favored chemotherapy, with a 5-year absolute survival benefit of 5.4%. The authors concluded that the benefit of chemotherapy is similar between the elderly and their younger counterpart (Pignon et al., 2006). Another meta-analysis of the impact of adjuvant chemotherapy done by the Non-Small Cell Lung Cancer Collaborative Group and regrouping 52 trials with 9,387 patients between 1963 and 1992 has showed the same absolute benefice on survival of 5% at 5 years. The odds ratio for survival is similar between the different groups of age (Cochrane review, 2000).
Pepe et al. at ASCO meeting in 2006 presented an age-specific evaluation of BR10 study, a phase III trial with patients with stage Ib and II NSCLC and comparing four cycles of cisplatin and vinorelbine with observation. 155 patients of the 482 enrolled in this study were aged 65 years and older. Baseline characteristics were similar between age cohorts except for the histology with more elderly patients with squamous cell cancer. In general, elderly received a lower mean dose intensity of chemotherapy. Overall survival was in favor of the younger patients, but chemotherapy led still to a benefit effect compared with standard observation in elderly. There were few patients aged over 75 and without regard to treatment, survival was still poor at 26% at 5 years (Pepe et al., 2007).
Other studies have been conducted on adjuvant chemotherapy, but the elderly subgroup was either absent, very little or without subgroup analysis as in the IALT study (Arriagada et al., 2004), Anita study (Douillard et al., 2006), Italian study Alpi (Scagliotti et al., 2003), Big Lung Trial (Waller et al., 2004) and CALGB (Strauss et al., 2004, 2006).
Because studies on this subject are retrospective, it is still difficult to conclude on the exact role of surgery in elderly patients with lung cancer. However, surgery should be considered for patients in good condition. Lobectomy is preferable to the limited resections if patients are medically fit (Alberts et al., 2007). Pneumonectomy is associated with greater morbidity and mortality and should only be performed in a highly selected group of patients. With

few conclusive results available from studies of adjuvant chemotherapy in elderly, it is difficult to conclude that it should be a standard treatment for older people. However, we can possibly extrapolate from studies done with younger patients and use it in selected patients aged less than 75 years of age.

9. Radiotherapy

It was demonstrated that nearly 25% of patients with disease stage I or II did not have surgery, most often because of significant comorbidities, patient preferences or poor lung functions (Bach et al., 1999; Spiro et al., 2002). For elderly who are not candidates for surgery, radiation therapy is possible. Unfortunately, it usually gives poor results with a 5-year survival estimated at between 6 to 14% (Razet al., 2007; Wisnivesky et al., 2005). In this section, the curative as well as palliative indication for radiation will be discussed.

Radiation therapy has been shown to improve outcomes compared to best supportive care alone (Raz et al., 2007). A subgroup analysis, in the study of Morita, assessed the impact of age in relation with survival in irradiated patients. One hundred and forty-nine patients older than 80 years with stage I lung cancer were included in this analysis. The survival was lower in older patients compared with younger. The 3- and 5-years actuarial survival was 15.4% and 7.7% in octogenarians versus respectively 38.2% and 25.2% in younger ($p=0.035$) (Morita et al., 1997). Similar results were found by Sibley (Sibley et al., 1998). However, a retrospective study from 6 studies of EORTC with 1,208 patients has shown no difference in overall survival between patients older or younger of 70 years (Pignon et al., 1998). Other retrospective studies compared treatment outcomes in younger and older patients. The North Central Cancer Treatment Group studied the impact of age (≥ 70 years versus younger) with two different schedules of radiation, either daily or twice per day, combined with concurrent chemotherapy. The 2-year survival rates were 39% in younger and 36% in the elderly and at 5-year, it was 18% versus 13% in patients ≥ 70 years ($p=0.4$). Toxicity of grade 4 or more were significantly higher in older patients (81%) than in younger ones (62%). The conclusion of this study was that toxicity is higher in elderly, but the survival is similar. Thus for fit patients this treatment can be proposed (Schild et al., 2003).

In the treatment of locally advanced NCSLC, the standard of care is radiation with chemotherapy based on cisplatin. Two major trials demonstrated a survival advantage for the use of induction chemotherapy prior to radiation therapy (Dillman et al., 1990; Sause et al., 2000). After the publication of these results, studies have been done to test the combined treatment. These studies shown that combined chemoradiotherapy is more effective compared to radiation alone (Dillman et al., 1990; Furuse et al., 1999). Elderly were in general excluded from these studies and few trials have been done about the role of combined chemoradiation in this particular population. A phase II study in 40 elderly patients with unresectable stage III or medically inoperable stage I and II lung cancer treated with concurrent carboplatin and radiation was done. For stage IIIA/IIIB patients, the median survival time was 15.1 months and 1-and 2-year actuarial survival rates were 52.6% and 20.5%, respectively. For stage I/II patients, 1- and 3-year actuarial survival rates were 90.9% and 69.3%, respectively (Atagi et al., 2000).

A phase III trial was performed by Atagi in 2005 with patients older than 70 years with stage III NSCLC. Patients were randomly assigned to either radiation therapy (dose of 60 Gy) with concurrent carboplatin or radiation therapy alone. 4 patient's death may have resulted from poor compliance in the design of the radiation fields. This trial was closed early with only 46 randomised patients.

A retrospective study of Langer (2002b) examined 104 patients older than 70 years with good performance status and minor weight loss receiving either sequential chemotherapy followed by daily radiotherapy, concomitant chemotherapy with daily radiotherapy or concomitant chemotherapy with twice daily radiation in phase III RTOG protocol 94-10. Concurrent treatment was proved to be favourable in the elderly, but toxicities were increased in this group. Median survival was 22.4 months for concurrent therapy with daily radiation, 16.4 months for concurrent chemotherapy with twice daily radiation treatment and 10.8 months for sequential treatment (p=0.069).

Patients over 70 years of prospective studies performed by CALGB were retrospectively analyzed by Rocha Lima (2002). In CALGB 9130, patients were randomised between vinblastine and cisplatin followed by radiation alone at dose of 60 Gy or neoadjuvant vinblastine and cisplatin followed by concurrent radiation with carboplatin. 22% of the patients enrolled in this study had between 70-79 years and no patients had more than 80 years of age. Age was not found to be a factor in survival or response rate, but elderly had more neutropenia and renal toxicity of grade 3 or more.

Hayakawa (2001) showed an alteration of performance index in only 5% of patients between 75-79 years and 8% in those more than 80 years when they are treated with radiation alone of 60 Gy. Another study presenting results about toxicity in 51 patients older than 65 years shows no augmentation of the toxicity in these patients in function with age, but survival was significantly correlated with performance status and importance of comorbidities (Fiorica et al., 2010).

Retrospective case series of older patients treated with curative radiation alone have demonstrated a median survival of up to 37 months for stage I-II and 8 months pour stage III (Bonfili et al., 2009; Lonardi et al., 2000; San José et al., 2006 & Tombolini et al., 2000).

It is recommended to provide elderly patients with advanced lung cancer disease in good general condition radiotherapy combined with chemotherapy. Concomitant treatment gives better results, but it is also more toxic to patients. For those that concomitant treatment is not possible, chemotherapy may be given before sequential radiotherapy. If the general condition of the patient or his comorbidities do not allow use of chemotherapy, he should receive radiation therapy alone either for curative or palliative purpose.

9.1 Radiotherapy planning

9.1.1 Treatment volume

There would be an increase of interruption of radiation treatment with the increased volume of the radiation field in patients over 80 years (Zachariah et al., 1997). For patients over 90 years, Ikeda (1999) showed that radiotherapy is better tolerated if treatment is limited to the macroscopic volume. In Pergolizzi (2002), 40 patients with stage IIIA, aged older than 75 years, were treated with involved field with median dose of 60 Gy. The overall survival was 18% at 3-years and 12% at 5 years.

9.1.2 Radiation technique

Technique of radiation could also influence the response to treatment in elderly population. Thus, Park's study evaluate whether complex radiotherapy planning with 3D techniques was associated with improvement outcomes in elderly compared with intermediate analysis with 2D planning. They found a better survival in patients treated with a more complex planning (Park et al., 2010).

In 2008, Yu conducted a multicenter prospective study in older patients with Intensity Modulated Radiotherapy (IMRT), an inverse planning technique. 80 patients had stage I and II disease and were medically inoperable or refused surgery. Patients received 66 Gy to involved field including primary tumor and clinical enlarged nodes. Objective response rate was 88.6%, with 1-, 2- and 5-year overall survival rates of 65.8%, 55.7% and 25.3% respectively and local progression-free survival was 84.8%. Toxicity was minimal. This study confirms that involved field radiation is a reasonable treatment for elderly patients.

9.2 Stereotactic radiation

Stereotactic body irradiation (SBRT) is a technique that utilizes precisely targeted radiation to tumor while minimizing radiation to adjacent normal tissue. This is accomplished by using multiple beams (typically 10 to 12) or large angle arc rotations. This technique is promising in the elderly. SBRT accurately delivers highly hypofractionated doses of radiation. High biologically effective radiation doses are generally of advantage with regard to tumor cell kill and local tumor control. SBRT is in general well tolerated and local control is similar than for patients treated with surgery.

In Zimmermann study, 68 patients were treated with a mean dose of 37.5 Gy in 3-5 fractions. The mean age was 76 years. Actuarial local tumor control at 1, 2 and 3 years was 96%, 88% and 88%. Disease-specific survival was 96%, 82% and 73% at 1, 2, and 3 year follow-up. 2 patients died by local tumor progression and a total of 8 patients died from their lung cancer disease. 55% of patients had mild acute and subacute toxicities (Zimmerman 2006). In Indiana University study, patients received in a phase I trial 66 Gy in 3 fractions for T2 tumors. The maximum tolerated dose was not reached for T1 tumors at 60 Gy in 3 fractions (McGarry et al., 2005; Timmerman et al., 2003). A RTOG multicenter study treated 59 patients with T1-T2N0 tumor with 54 Gy in 3 fractions. Three-year local control of the tumor was 98%. The three-year disease-free and overall survivals were 48% and 56% respectively (Timmerman, 2010).

In general, the results for stereotactic radiotherapy appear better than those of standard radiotherapy. Local control at 3 years vary from 86-95% (Baumann et al., 2006, 2009; Onishi et al., 2007; Xia et al., 2006; Zimmermann et al., 2006) for patients treated with SBRT while for external radiotherapy, local recurrences are more than 50% (Rowell et al., 2001 & Qiao et al., 2003) with 5-years survival around 10 to 30%.

Moreover a Palma analysis on 875 elderly patients shown that SBRT introduction was associated with an improvement of 16% in the use of radiation, and a decline in the number of untreated elderly patients (Palma et al., 2010).

9.3 Palliative radiation

The main goal of palliative radiation is to decrease the pulmonary symptoms of the patients. The number of treatment may vary according to the general functional status of the patients. According to a review of 13 randomized trials, no significant difference was observed for specific symptom control end points, but there is an improvement in survival favoured with high dose radiotherapy. For good functional status patients, it is recommended to use a palliative dose of radiation with a biological effective dose (BED) of at least 35 Gy_{10} (Fairchild et al., 2008). Another review of 12 randomized controlled studies recommends a short course (one or two fraction) of hypofractioned radiotherapy for the majority of the patients. Selected patients with good performance status should be considered for higher dose regimens as this could increase their survival (Toy et al., 2003).

9.3.1 Brachytherapy as palliation

Another way to treat lung cancer disease is using palliative brachytherapy. This treatment is effective to treat endobronchial disease. This often causes cough, hemoptysis and dyspnea. Stout compared external beam radiation therapy (EBRT) with endobronchial brachytherapy. He showed that EBRT offers a better palliation. Furthermore, there was slightly improved in survival (Stout et al., 2000). However, some patients cannot be treated with external beam radiation and brachytherapy could be offered to them. This approach seems to be more effective than other types of treatment, such as cryotherapy, cauterization or phototherapy, which only superficially destruct cancer cell (Hetzel et al., 1985; Sutedja et al., 1994; Walsh et al., 1990). High-dose rate brachytherapy is cost-effective and convenient owing to its short irradiation time and the fact that it can be provided on an outpatient basis. Endobronchial brachytherapy treats tumors up to 1-cm deep with 100% of prescribed dose and a decreasing dose can reach up to 2-cm deep.

A retrospective study with inoperable endobronchial lung cancer or metastasis had shown a significant improvement of symptoms and a good survival. 85% of patients had an improvement of the dyspnea during or shortly after the end of the treatment. Hemoptysis was stopped in all 23 patients of the study and 77% of them had an improvement of their cough. Patients had received 4 weekly fractions of 5 Gy each time. The complication rate during treatment was low (Dagnault et al., 2010).

Thus, for palliation, hypofractionated external beam radiation therapy and brachytherapy are alternatives to proper treatment for the relief of symptoms.

10. Chemotherapy

The treatment of advanced lung cancer requires chemotherapy. The standard combination is based on a combination of platinum and either vinorelbine, gemcitabine, paclitaxel or docetaxel. Few studies have yet been made to assess the best chemotherapy agents in elderly people. Many of the available data are from analysis of subgroups. The American College of Chest Physician guidelines recommends chemotherapy for stage IV NSCLC for selected patients older than 70 years. They caution that the benefits of chemotherapy in patients over 80 years of age are unknown and recommend instead a case by case assessment (Socinski et al., 2007).

The first important question is to determine if older people tolerates chemotherapy as well as younger patients and if the outcome of the treatments is the same. Some studies have been done in this direction. Nguyen (1999) compared cisplatin and gemcitabine to cisplatin alone and showed that tolerance to treatment and outcome of patients were identical for patients aged more or less than 70 years. In a subset analysis of an Eastern Cooperative Oncology Group study (ECOG 5592) patients received cisplatin and etoposide or paclitaxel. A total of 574 patients were included in this trial, which 15% were 70 or older. The response rate, the time to progression and the survival rate did not differ across groups but there was higher hematological and neuropsychiatric toxicities in the elders. There was no difference in the quality of life (Langer et al., 2002a). In the CALGB 7730 trial, 561 patients received paclitaxel compared to paclitaxel and carboplatin. The total of patients aged more than 70 years included in this trial was 27% or 155 patients. In that study, there was no formal subgroup analysis based on age, but the general data revealed no obvious difference between age groups (Lilenbaum et al., 2005). Further studies with subgroup analysis showed similar results (Belani et al., 2005; Earle et al., 2001; Hensinget al., 2003; Iberti et al., 1995; Langer et al., 2003; Rocha Lima et al., 2002). We can then conclude that the survival benefit is similar in elderly as in younger patients.

10.1 Importance of patient evaluation for chemotherapy treatment

As previously discussed, age by itself should not be a factor to decide if a patient will received or not chemotherapy treatment. That decision should be taken considering the global functional status of the patients and his comorbidities, particularly cardiovascular and pulmonary ones. Aging is associated with several physiologic changes in organ function. Those changes could alter drug pharmacokinetics and they could have an impact on cytotoxic chemotherapy toxicity and tolerability (Wildiers et al., 2003). Thus, it is always mandatory to know the serum creatinine, but also the creatinine clearance to assess renal function, particularly for chemotherapy agents whose main route of elimination is by the kidney, as platinum derivatives and methotrexate. It is also important to evaluate the bone marrow reserve as this reserve may diminish with increasing age, and the risk of neutropenia increases with age (Langer et al., 2002; Rocha Lima et al., 2002).

10.2 Single-agent chemotherapy versus best supportive care

This question was evaluated in elderly patients with advanced/metastatic NSCLC in the Italian phase III trial, Elderly Lung Cancer Vinorelbine Italian Group Study (ELVIS) (Ardizzoni et al., 2005). Patients over 70 years of age were randomly assigned to either receive vinorelbine (30 mg/m^2 on days 1 and 8) or to receive best supportive care (BSC). Even if the accrual of this study was poor, with only 161 evaluable patients, it demonstrated that there was a significant advantage of survival in the vinorelbine arm ($p=0.03$). The median survival was 21 weeks for BSC versus 28 weeks for vinorelbine. Survival rates were 41% at 6 months for control arm compared to 55% in the vinorelbine arm. At 12 months, survival was respectively 14% for BSC and 32% with vinorelbine. This study also shown that patients receiving chemotherapy had a significant benefit in disease-related quality-of-life (QoL) measures (decreased pain $p=0.02$, decreased dyspnea $p=0.05$). Toxicity was acceptable. Only 5 of 71 older patients discontinued treatment secondary to severe toxic events (3 patients had constipation grade 3, 1 patient had constipation grade 4 and 1 patient had grade 2 heart toxicity). Even if 4 patients had a grade 4 leukopenia, treatment had not been interrupted.

10.3 Type of single-agent chemotherapy

Others chemotherapy were tested to find the best one in elderly patients. A phase III trial of West Japan Thoracic Oncology Group Trial (WJTOG 9904) randomized 182 patients older than 70 years between two agents: docetaxel (60 mg/m^2 on day 1) or vinorelbine (25 mg/m^2 on days 1 and 8). Patients received 4 cycles every 21 days. Median survival was not significantly different between two arms with docetaxel group being 14.3 months compared to 9.9 months with vinorelbine ($p=0.138$). However, others outcomes were significantly in favour of docetaxel. Thus, the progression-free survival was 5.5 months versus 3.1 months ($p<0.001$) and the response rate was 22.7% compared to 9.9% ($p=0.019$). Even if no significant differences in global QoL were observed between the two groups, it is interesting to notice that patients in the docetaxel group had a significant greater improvement in overall symptom score than those in vinorelbine group. One disadvantage of docetaxel is that it induces significantly severe neutropenia more frequently. To conclude, docetaxel in monotherapy can be considered as an option of treatment in older patients (Kudoh et al., 2006). A phase 2 study performed in older patients compared gemcitabine and docetaxel and these agents had comparable efficacy and tolerability profiles (Leong et al., 2007).

In 2010, a phase II trial was published on the role of single-agent vinorelbine in patient older than 70 years with poor performance status (ECOG 2 or more). Forty-three patients received oral vinorelbine at the dose of 60 mg/m^2 on days 1 to 8 every 3 weeks. Overall response rate was 18.6%, median time to progression was 4.0 months and median overall survival was 8.0 months. This treatment was safe, without grade 3 or 4 toxicity, exception of a single non-febrile grade 3 neutropenia. Therefore, vinorelbine is safe for elderly patient, even in those with poor performance status (Camerini et al., 2010). Previously, another study with docetaxel in monotherapy, comparing weekly to 3-weekly administration, had also conclude that this treatment is effective and well tolerated in older patients, even with poor performance status (Lilenbaum et al., 2007).

An international expert panel ruled in favour of the use of single-agent chemotherapy in the elderly cancer patient. A third-generation agent is recommended for patients with any performance status and a platinum-based chemotherapy is recommended for those with performance status 0 or 1 and no contre-indications for comorbidities (Gridelli et al., 2005).

10.4 Combination versus single-agent chemotherapy

When studies revealed that single-agent chemotherapy improved survival, the search for more effective treatment continued and studies with combinations of chemotherapy have been done. Few randomized trials compared a combination of chemotherapy to a single agent. A French Intergroup study randomly assigned 451 patients of 70-89 years with performance status 0-2 that previously had untreated stage III or IV disease. Patients received a combination of carboplatin (AUC 6 on day 1) plus paclitaxel (90 mg/m^2, days 1, 8 and 15) every 4 weeks for a total of four cycles or a single agent (gemcitabine or vinorelbine, as predetermined by each institution). Gemcitabine (1,150 mg/m^2) or vinorelbine (30 mg/m^2) were given on days 1 and 8 for 5 cycles, every 3 weeks. At ASCO meeting in 2010, preliminary results were presented. For the first 313 patients, overall survival was significantly better in the combination arm with 10.4 months versus 6.2 months for single agent chemotherapy. Progression-free survival was significantly improved with combination chemotherapy (6.3 versus 3.2 months) and this difference was significant. The combined treatment was well tolerable even if neutropenia grade 3 and 4 were more frequent with the combination chemotherapy (Quoix et al., 2010).

A phase III study done by The South Italian Cooperative Oncology Group (SICOG) randomized patients between vinorelbine (30 mg/m^2 days 1 and 8 every 3 weeks), versus vinorelbine/gemcitabine (vinorelbine 30 mg/m^2 and gemcitabine 1,200 mg/m^2, days 1 and 8 every 3 weeks). In this study an interim analysis of survival with the first 60 patients was done. This analysis showed a significant survival advantage for the combination arm, with median survival of 29 weeks versus 18 weeks for the single arm. Following these results, the study was closed prematurely. The estimated 6-months and 1-year survival were 56% and 30% for the combination group and 32% and 13% in the single-agent arm ($p<0.01$). Patients receiving monotherapy treatment had more symptoms and deterioration of quality of life.

Toxicity for the combination arm resulted in grade 3-4 neutropenia and thrombocytopenia in 38% and 13% respectively, and it was more prevalent than in the vinorelbine arm (Frasci et al., 2000).

The Cancer and Leukemia Group B reported results of a phase III trial (CALGB-9730) that compared a combination of carboplatin and paclitaxel with paclitaxel in monotherapy. In this study, in which 155 patients had over 70 years, the response rate was 36% versus 21% respectively. The median survival was better in patients treated with the combination compared with monotherapy (8.0 vs 5.8 months respectively- non significant) (Lilenbaum et al., 2005).

Docetaxel and cisplatin doublet was compared with docetaxel in monotherapy in a phase III trial for elderly patient with NSCLC (Ansari et al., 2007). The planned sample size was 115 patients per arm, but the study was closed when the planned interim analysis showed that the doublet may be beneficial for patient aged 70 to 74 years.

However, results remain conflicting about the impact of a combination of chemotherapy. Multicenter Italian Lung cancer in the elderly Study (MILES) is another randomized study that involves patients aged 70 years or older. 698 patients were randomly assigned to gemcitabine alone (1,200 mg/m^2 days 1 and 8, every 3 weeks), vinorelbine alone (30 mg/m^2 on days 1 and 8, every 3 weeks) or gemcitabine (1,000 mg/m^2) plus vinorelbine (25 mg/m^2) both administrated on days 1 and 8 every 3 weeks (Gridelli et al., 2003). In this study, there was no difference between each single-agent and the combination arm for progression-free survival and overall survival. The estimated 1-year survival was 38% and 28% for patients respectively with vinorelbine and gemcitabine alone. In the combination arm, the overall survival was 30%. Median survival was 36 weeks for vinorelbine, 28 weeks for gemcitabine alone and 30 weeks for the combination. Toxicities were more frequent in the patients receiving combination chemotherapy. Thus, the combination of vinorelbine and gemcitabine was not shown to be more effective than single agent vinorelbine or gemcitabine in elderly patients with NSCLC (Gridelli et al., 2003).

A study analysed the baseline assessment of functional status, comorbidity and quality of life in elderly patients randomised in MILES trial. The presence of comorbidity was assessed with a checklist of 33 items, items 29 and 30 of the European Organisation for research and Treatment of Cancer (EORTC) core questionnaire QLQ-C30 were used for the quality of life and the Charlson scale was used to summarize cormorbidity. Better values of activities of instrumental activities of daily living (IADL) (p=0.04) and of baseline quality of life (p=0.0003) were significantly associated with better prognosis. Two others factors, either activities of daily living (ADL) and the Charlson scale score had no prognostic value (Maione et al., 2005).

An analysis from SEER data on patients with NSCLC over 65 years old evaluated the role of chemotherapy. Of over 21,000 patients evaluated, only 25.8% received first-line chemotherapy. After adjusting for comorbidities, age and performance status, patients with chemotherapy had an increased adjusted 1-year survival rate of 27% when compared to those without chemotherapy (11%) and a reduction of the adjusted risk of death, with a hazard ratio of 0.558. In this study, the use of combination of platinum agents was associated with an increase survival at 30.1% compared with single-agent at 19.4% (Davidoff et al., 2010).

A meta-analysis involving 2,867 patients of randomized controlled trial had shown superior results for efficacy and tolerability of docetaxel compared with vinorelbine or vindesine (Douillard et al., 2007; Laporte et al., 2007). The overall survival was 11% greater in patients with doxetaxel compared with vinca alkaloid-based regimen (HR 0.89). This benefit was observed when docetaxel was used with or without a platinum agent as part of the regimen. In this meta-analysis, the benefit of docetaxel was at least as much important in older patients than in younger (Laporte et al., 2007).

In conclusion, for fit elderly patients, combination chemotherapy with a platinum-based regimen can improve survival without much toxicity. For patients without a good performance status a single-agent may be proposed.

10.5 Second-line therapy

No definitive studies have been conducted in the second-line setting in older patients with NSCLC. A phase II study has shown utility of docetaxel as second-line therapy. Tibaldi's trial demonstrated an objective response rate of 21% (Tibaldi et al., 2006). A subset analysis of a phase III trial compared docetaxel with pemetrexed, in 86 patients older than 70 years. This study demonstrated an objective response rate of 6% and a median overall survival of 9.5 months in the pemetrexed group and 7.7 months in docetaxel (not statistically significant) (Weiss et al., 2006).

10.6 EGFR-thyrosin kinase inhibitors

Over the last years, many biologic and targeted therapies have been approved. Molecules which target epidermal growth factor receptor (EGFR) include erlotinib and gefitinib. Some monoclonal antibodies are also now approved for the use in lung cancer like cetuximab which targets EGFR and bevacizumab which targets the vascular endothelial growth factor (VEGF).

Thanks to their oral administration and their toxicity profile, the EGFR may be alternative treatments in chemotherapy-naïve elderly. In a phase II trial, chemotherapy-naïve patients older than 75 years with advanced NSCLC received gefitinib in monotherapy. The primary objective of this study was the objective response rate. 49 patients were eligible. The response rate was 25% with median survival of 10 months and 1-year survival of 50%. Skin disorders were the most frequent adverse side effects, in 76% of patients (Ebi et al., 2008).

A phase II trial, INVITE, compared gefitinib versus vinorelbine in chemotherapy-naïve elderly patients with advanced non-small-cell lung cancer. 97 patients were randomly assigned to gefitinib and received 250 mg/d orally and 99 patients received vinorelbine (30 mg/m^2 infusion on days 1 and 8 of a 21-day cycle). The primary endpoint was progression-free survival and the hazard ratio was 1.19 (gefitinib versus vinorelbine). Overall survival was 2.7 months for gefitinib versus 2.9 months for vinorelbine and hazard ratio was 0.98. Disease control rates were 43.3% for gefitinib and 53.5% for vinorelbine. The quality of life (QoL) was also analysed in this study. There was no statistical difference between gefitinib and vinorelbine for pulmonary symptom improvement (PSI) and QoL. The improvement of overall QoL and PSI were 24.3% and 36.6% for gefitinib and 10.9% and 31.0% for vinorelbine respectively. 54 patients had EGFR FISH-positive and the hazard ratio were 3.13 for PFS and 2.88 for OS (Crinò et al., 2008).

A phase III trial, TOPICAL, compared erlotinib versus placebo in chemotherapy-naïve patients with poor performance status who were not candidate for first line chemotherapy. Overall survival was not significantly different between both groups (Lee et al., 2010).

For elderly patients whose tumor contains an EGFR mutation, it is recommend to treat with an EGFR TK inhibitor, as erlotinib or gefitinib, rather than chemotherapy.

Regarding the use of bevacizumab, few subsets analyses were done. In ECOG 4599, patients over 70 years were randomized to carboplatin and paclitaxel, with or without the addition of bevacizumab. The overall incidence of severe or fatal (grade 3 to 5) toxicity was significantly higher (87% versus 61%) in those receiving bevacizumab and treatment-related deaths were more frequent (6.3% versus 2.6%). This trial revealed a trend toward improvement in disease response (29% versus 17 %) and progression-free survival (5.9 versus 4.9 months), without benefit in overall survival (Ramalingam et al., 2008).

11. Conclusion

Lung cancer is already a significant problem in our population. It is one of the major causes for cancer mortality in the younger population, even more in the elderly. The aging population will continue to grow and the proportion of elderly with lung cancer will increase in coming decades. Oncologist will have to develop their abilities to better evaluate them and to give them the appropriate treatment for their condition. Actually, no specific assessment tool is proved to be better than other, but we demonstrated the importance of a form of CGA and all his components in the evaluation of these persons.

Many treatment options are available and proved to be effective in the elderly. It can vary from standard treatment, as for younger patient, to more adapted treatment, in regard to the general functional status of the person and his comorbidities.

For patients with early stage disease, surgery remains the treatment of choice with or without adjuvant chemotherapy. When it is not possible, radiation therapy is an excellent alternative, well tolerated with limited side effects. In case of advanced disease, radiation combined or not to chemotherapy is the option, according to the general functional status of the patient. Palliative treatment, either radiation or chemotherapy can also be offered to the elderly patient, according to their symptoms and wishes.

A good evaluation of the patient and realistic goal for treatment remain essential in this population, but treatment decisions based solely on chronological age is no longer acceptable at this time.

12. References

Alberts, W. M. et al. (2007). Diagnosis and management of lung cancer : ACCP evidence-based clinical practice guidelines (2nd edition). *Chest*, Vol. 132. No.3 suppl, (September), pp. 1S-19S, ISSN 0012-3692.

Ansari, R. H. et al. (2007). Elderly subgroup analysis of a randomized phase 3 trial of gemcitabine (G) in combination with carboplatin (Cb) or paclitaxel (P) compared to paclitaxel plus carboplatin in advanced (stage IIIB, IV) non-small-cell lung cancer. *Proceeding of American Society of Clinical Oncology*, ISSN 0732 183X, Chicago, IL, June 2007.

Ardizzoni, A. et al. (2005). Platinum-etoposide chemotherapy in elderly patients with non-small lung cancer: results of a randomized multicenter phase II study assessing attenuated-dose or full-dose with lenograstim prophylaxis- a Forza Operativa Nazionale Italiana Carcinoma Polmonare and Gruppo Studio Tumori Polmonari Veneto (FONICAP-GSTPV) study. *Journal of Clinical Oncology*, Vol.23, No.3, (January 2005). pp. 569-75, ISSN 0732-183X.

Arriagada, R. et al. (2004). International Adjuvant Lung Cancer Trial Collaborative Group: cisplatin-based adjuvant chemotherapy in patients with completely resected non-small-cell lung cancer. *New England Journal of Medicine*, Vol.350, No.4, (January 2004), pp. 351-60, ISSN 0028-4793.

Asmis, T. R. et al. (2008). Age and comorbidity as independent prognostic factors in the treatment of non small-cell lung cancer: a review of National Cancer Institute of Canada Clinical Trials Group trials. *Journal of Clinical Oncology*, Vol. 26, No.1, (January 2009), pp. 54-59, ISSN 0732-183X.

Atagi, S. et al. (2000). Phase II trial of daily low-dose carboplatin and thoracic radiotherapy in elderly patients with locally advanced non-small cell lung cancer. *Japan Journal of Clinical Oncology*, Vol.30, No.2, (February 200), pp. 59-64, ISSN 1465-3621.

Atagi, S. et al. (2005). Standard thoracic radiotherapy with or without concurrent daily low-dose carboplatin in elderly patients with locally advanced non-small cell lung cancer: a phase III trial of the Japan Clinical Oncology Group (JCOG9812). *Japan Journal of Clinical Oncology*, Vol.35, No.4, (April, 2005), pp. 195-201, ISSN 1465-3621.

Avery, E. J., Kessinger, A. & Ganti, A. K. (2009). Therapeutic options for elderly patients with advanced non-small cell lung cancer. *Cancer Treatment Reviews*, Vol. 35, No.4, (June 2009), pp. 340-344, ISSN 0305-7372.

Bach, P.B. et al. (1999). Racial differences in the treatment of early-stage lung cancer. *New England Journal of Medicine*, Vol.341, No.14 , (October 1999), pp. 1198-1205, ISSN 0028-4793.

Balducci, L. (2000). Geriatric oncology; challenges for the new century. *European Journal of Cancer*, Vol. 36, No. 14, (Septembre 2000), pp. 1741-1754, ISSN 0959-8049.

Baumann, P. et al. (2006). Factors important for efficacy of stereotactic body radiotherapy of medically inoperable stage I lung cancer. A retrospective analysis of patients treated in the Nordic countries. *Acta Oncologica*. Vol.45, No,7, pp. 787-95, ISSN 1651-226X.

Baumann, P. et al. (2009). Outcome in a prospective phase II trial of medically inoperable stage I non-small cell lung cancer patients treated with stereotactic body radiotherapy. *Journal of Clinical Oncology*, Vol. 27, No.20, (July 2010), pp. 3290-3296, ISSN 0732-183X.

Belani C. P. & Fossela F. (2005). Elderly subgroup analysis of a randomized phase III study of docetaxel plus platinum combinations versus vinorelbine plus cisplatin for first-line treatment of advanced non-small cell lung carcinoma (TAX326). *Cancer*, Vol.104, No. 12, pp. 2766-74, (December 2005), ISSN 1097-0142.

Birim, O. et al. (2003). Lung resection for non-small cell lung cancer in patients older than 70: mortality, morbidity, and late survival compared with the general population. *The Annals of Thoracic Surgery*, Vol.76, No.6, (December 2003), pp. 1796-801, ISSN 1552-6259.

Bonfili, P. et al. (2009). Hypofractionned radical radiotherapy in elderly patients with medically inoperable stage I-II non-small-cell lung cancer. *Lung Cancer*, Vol. 67, No.1, (January 2010), pp. 81-5, ISSN 0169-5002.

Brokx, H.A. et al. (2007). Surgical treatment for octogenarians with lung cancer: results from a population-based series of 124 patients. *Journal of Thoracic Oncology*, Vol.2, No.11, (November 2007), pp. 1013-1017, ISSN 1556-0864.

Canadian Cancer Society's Steering committee: Canadian Cancer Statistics 2010. (2010) Toronto: Canadian Cancer Society, (April 2010), ISSN 0835-2976.

Camerini, A. et al. (2010). Phase II of single-agent oral vinorelbine in elderly (> or =70 years) patients with advanced non-small-cell lung cancer and poor performance status. *The Annals of Oncology*, Vol.21, No.6, (June 2010), pp. 1290-95, ISSN 1552-6259.

Chaïbi, P. et al. (2010). Influence of geriatric consultation with comprehensive geriatric assessment on final therapeutic decision in elderly cancer patients. *Critical Reviews in Oncology/Hematology*, Epub ahead of print, (December 2010), ISSN 1040-8428.

Chambers, A. et al (2010). In elderly patients with lung cancer is resection justified in terms of morbidity, mortality and residual quality of life? *Interactive CardioVascular and Thoracic Surgery*, Vo.10, No.6, (June 2010), pp. 1015-1021, ISSN 1569-9293.

Chang, M.Y. et al. (2007). Factors predicting poor survival after resection of stage IA non-small cell lung cancer. *Journal of Thoracic Cardiovascular Surgery*, Vol.134, No.4, (October 2007), pp. 850-6, ISSN 0022-5223.

Charlson, M.E. et al. (1987). A new method of classifying prognostic comorbidity in longitudinal studies: development and validation. *Journal of Chronic Disease*, Vol. 40, No.5, (1987), pp. 373-383, ISSN 0021-9681.

Cochrane Lung Cancer Group (2000). Chemotherapy for non-small cell lung cancer. Non-small Cell Lung Cancer Collaborative Group. *Cochrane Database Systematic Reviews*, 2000,Vol. 2, ISSN 1469-493X.

Cudennec, T. et al. (2010). Use of a simplified geriatric evaluation in thoracic oncology. *Lung Cancer*, (February 2010), Vol.67, No2, pp. 232-6, ISSN 0169-5002.

Crinò, L. et al. (2008). Gefitinib versus vinorelbine in chemotherapy-naïve elderly patients with advanced non-small-cell lung cancer (INVITE): a randomized phase II study. *Journal of Clinical Oncology*, Vol.26, No.26, (September 2010), pp. 4253, ISSN 0732-183X.

Dagnault, A. et al (2010). Retrospective study of 81 patients treated with brachytherapy for endobronchial primary tumor or metastasis. *Brachytherapy*, Vol.9, No.3, (July-September 2010), pp. 243-7, ISSN 1538-4721.

Davidoff, A. J. et al. (2010). Chemotherapy and survival benefit in elderly patients with advanced non-small-cell lung cancer. *Journal of Clinical Oncology*, Vol.28, No.13, (may 2010), pp. 2191-7, ISSN 0732-183X.

Dillman, R. O. et al. (1990). A randomized trial of induction chemotherapy plus high-dose radiation versus radiation alone in stage III non-small-cell lung cancer. *New England Journal of Medicine*, Vol.323, No.14, (October 1990), pp. 940-945, ISSN 0028-4793.

Dillman, R. O. et al. (1996). Improved survival I stage III non-small-cell lung cancer: seven-year follow-up of cancer and leukemia group B (CALGB) 8433 trial. *Journal of National Cancer Institute*, Vol. 88, No.17, (September 1996), pp. 1210-1215, ISSN 1052-6773.

Dominguez-Ventura, A. et al. (2007). Lung cancer in octogenarians : factors affecting long-term survival following resection. *European Journal of Cardiothoracic Surgery*, Vol.32, No2, (August 2007), pp. 370-4, ISSN 1010-7940.

Douillard, J. Y et al (2006). Adjuvant vinorelbine plus cisplatin versus observation in patients with completely resected stage IB-IIIA non-small-cell lung cancer (Adjuvant Novelbine International Trialist Association, Anita): a randomized controlled trial. *Lancet Oncology*, Vol. 7, No.9, (September 2006), pp. 719-27, ISSN 1470-2045.

Douillard, J. Y. et al (2007). Comparison of docetaxel- and vinca-alkaloid-based chemotherapy in the first-line treatment of advanced non-small-cell lung cancer: a meta-analysis of seven randomized clinical trials. *Journal of Thoracic Oncology*, Vol.2, No.10, (October 2007), pp. 939-946, ISSN 1556 0864.

Earle, C. C. et al. (2001). Effectiveness of chemotherapy for advanced lung cancer in the elderly: Instrumental variable and propensity analysis. *Journal of Clinical Oncology*, Vol.19, No.4, (February 2001), pp. 1064-70, ISSN 0732-183X.

Ebi, N. et al. (2008). A phase II trial of gefitinib monotherapy in chemotherapy-naïve patients of 75 years or older with advanced non-small cell lung cancer. *Journal of Thoracic Oncology*, Vol.3, No.10, (October 2008), pp. 1166-71, ISSN 1556-0864.

Extermann, M. et al. (2005). Use of comprehensive geriatric assessment in older cancer patients: recommendations from the task force on CGA of the International Society of Geriatric Oncology (SIOG). *Critical Reviews in Oncology/Hematology*, Vol. 55, No. 3, (September 2005), pp. 241-252, ISSN 1040-8428.

Extermann, M. & Hurria, A. (2007). Comprehensive geriatric assessment for older patients with cancer. *Journal of Clinical Oncology*, Vol. 25, No.14, (May 2007), pp. 1824-31, ISSN 0732-183X.

Fairchild, A. et al. (2008). Palliative thoracic radiotherapy for lung cancer: a systematic review. *Journal of Clinical Oncology*, Vol.26, No24, (August 2004), pp. 4001-4011 , ISSN 0732-183X.

Fiorica, F. et al. (2010). Safety and feasibility of radiotherapy treatment in elderly non-small cell lung cancer (NSCLC) patients. *Archives of Gerontology and Geriatrics*, Vol.5, No.2, (March-April 2010), pp. 185-91, ISSN 0167-4943.

Frasci, G.et al. (2000). Gemcitabine plus vinorelbine alone in elderly patients with advanced non-small-cell lung cancer. *Journal of Clinical Oncology*, Vol.18, No.13, (July 2000), pp. 2529-36, ISSN 0732-183X.

Fried, L. P. & Hall, W. J. (2008). EDITORIAL: Leading on Behalf of an Aging Society. *Journal of the American Geriatrics Society*, Vol.56, No.10, pp. 1791–95, ISSN 0002-8614.

Furuse, K. et al. (1999). Phase III study of concurrent versus sequential thoracic radiotherapy in combination with mitomycin, vindesine, and cisplatin in unresectable stage III non-small-cell lung cancer. *Journal of Clinical Oncology*. Vol. 17, No.9, (September 1999), pp. 2692-2699, ISSN 0732-183X.

Gironés, R. et al. (2011). Prognostic impact of comorbidity in elderly lung cancer patients: use and comparison of two scores. *Lung Cancer*, Vol. 72, No. 1, (April 2011), pp. 108-13, ISSN 0169-5002.

Goddwin J. S. & Osborne C. (2004). Factors affecting the diagnosis and treatment of older persons with cancer, In: *Comprehensive Geriatric Oncology*, Balducci L., Lyman, G.H., Ershler, W.B. Extermann, M., (Eds), pp. 56-64, Taylor & Francis, ISBN 1-84181-296-6, United Kingdom.

Gonzalez-Aragoneses, F. et al. (2009). Lung cancer surgery in the elderly. *Critical Reviews in Oncology/Hematology*,Vol. 71, No. 3, (September 2009), pp. 266-271, ISSN 1040-8428.

Gridelli, C. et al. (2003). Chemotherapy for elderly patients with advanced non-small-cell lung cancer: the Multicenter Italian Lung Cancer in the Elderly Study (MILES) phase III randomized trial. *Journal of National Cancer Institute,* Vol.95, No.5, (March 2003), pp. 362-72, ISSN 1052-6773.

Gridelli, C. (2005). Treatment of advanced non-small-cell lung cancer in the elderly: Results of an international expert panel. *Journal of Clinical Oncology,* Vol.23, No.13, (May 2005), pp. 3125-37, ISSN 0732-183X.

Hayakawa et al. (2001). High-dose radiation therapy for elderly patients with inoperable or unresectable non-small cell lung cancer. *Lung cancer,* vol.32, No.1, (April 2001), pp. 81-8, ISSN 0169-5002.

Hensing, T.A. et al. (2003). The impact of age on toxicity, response rate, quality of life and survival in patients with advanced, stage IIIB or IV non-small cell lung carcinoma treated with carboplatin and paclitaxel. *Cancer,* Vol. 98, No.4, (August 2003), pp. 779-88, ISSN 1097-0142.

Hetzel, M. R. et al. (1985). Laser therapy in 100 tracheobronchial tumors. *Thorax,* Vol.40, No.5, (May 1985). pp. 341-5, ISSN 0040-6376.

Iberti, W. et al. (1995). Chemotherapy in non-small cell lung cancer: A meta-analysis using updated data on individual patients from 52 randomised clinical trials. *Bristish Medical Journal,* Vol.311, No.7010, (October 1995), pp. 899-909, ISSN 0959-8138.

Ikeda, H. et al. (1999). Analysis of 57 nonagerian cancer patients treated by radical radiotherapy: a survey of eight institutions. *Japan Journal of Clinical Oncology,* Vol. 29, No.8, (August 1999), pp. 378-81, ISSN 1465-3621.

Kudoh, S. et al. (2006). Phase III study of docetaxel compared with vinorelbine in elderly patients with advanced non-small-cell lung cancer: results of the West Japan Thoracic Oncology Group Trial (WJTOG 9904). *Journal of Clinical Oncology,* Vol.24, No.22, (August 2006), pp. 3657-63, ISSN 0732-183X.

Langer, C. J. et al. (2002). Cisplatin-based therapy for elderly patients with advanced non-small-cell lung cancer: implications of Eastern Cooperative Oncology Group 5592, a randomized trial. *Journal of National Cancer Institute,* Vol.94, No. 3, (February 2002), pp.173-81, ISSN 1052-6773.

Langer, C. J. et al. (2002). Elderly patients with locally advanced non-small cell lung cancer benefit from combined modality therapy: Secondary analysis of Radiation Therapy Oncology Group (RTOG) 94-10. *Proceeding American Society of Clinical Oncology,* ISSN 0732-183X, Orlando, FL, June 2002.

Langer, C. J. et al. (2003). Age-specific subanalysis of ECOG 1594; fit elderly patients (70-80yrs) with NSCLC do as well as younger pts (<70). *Proceeding of American Society of Clinical Oncology,* ISSN 0732-183X, Chicago, IL, May 2003.

Laporte, S. et al. (2007). Meta-analysis comparing docetaxel and vinca-alkaloid in the first-line treatment of NSCLC. Comparison of results based on individual patient data, study report data, and published data. *Presented at the European Cancer Conference 14 (ECCO 14),* Barcelona, Spain, September, 2007.

Lee, S.M. et al. (2010). TOPICAL: Randomized phase III trial of erlotinib compared with placebo in chemotherapy-naïve patients with advanced non-small cell lung cancer and unsuitable for first-line chemotherapy (abstract #7504). *Proceeding American Society of Clinical Oncology,* ISSN 0732-183X, Chicago, IL, June 2010.

Leong, S.S. et al. (2007).A randomized phase II of single-agent gemcitabine, vinorelbine or docetaxel in patients with advanced non-small cell lung cancer who are poor status performance and/or are elderly. *Journal of Thoracic Oncology*, Vol.2, No. 3, (March 2007), pp. 230-6, ISSN 1556-0864.

Lilenbaum, R.C. et al (2005). Single-agent versus combination chemotherapy in advanced non-small-cell lung cancer ; the Cancer and Leukemia Group B (study 9730). *Journal of Clinical Oncology*, Vol.23, No.1, (January 2005), pp. 190-6, ISSN 0732-183X.

Lilenbaum, R. et al. (2007). A randomized phase II trial of two schedules of docetaxel in elderly or poor performance status patients with advanced non-small cell lung cancer. *Journal of Thoracic Oncology*, Vol.2, No.4, (April 2007), pp. 306-11, ISSN 1556-0864.

Lonardi, F. et al. (2000). Radiotherapy for non-small cell lung cancer in patients aged 75 and over: safety, effectiveness and possible impact on survival. *Lung Cancer*, Vol.28, No.1, (April 2000), pp. 43-50, ISSN 0169-5002.

Maione P,et al. (2005). Pretreatment quality of life and functional status assessment significantly predict survival of elderly patients with advanced non-small-cell lung cancer receiving chemotherapy: a prognostic analysis of the multicenter Italian lung cancer in the elderly study. *Journal of Clinical Oncology*, Vol. 23, No. 28, (October 2005), pp. 6865-72, ISSN 0732-183X.

McGarry, R. C. et al. (2005). Stereotactic body irradiation therapy of early-stage non-small-cell lung carcinoma: phase I study. *International Journal of Oncology, Biology, Physics*, Vol.63, No.4, (November 2005), pp. 1010-5, ISSN 0360-3016.

Mery, C. M. et al. (2005). Similar long-term survival of elderly patients with non-small cell lung cancer treated with lobectomy or wedge resection within the Surveillance, Epidemiology, and End results database. *Chest* Vol.128, No.1, (July 2005), pp. 237-245, ISSN 0012-3692.

Morita, K. et al. (1997). Radical radiotherapy for medically inoperable non-small cell lung cancer in clinical stage I: a retrospective analysis of 149 patients. *Radiotherapy and Oncology*, Vol.42, No.1, (January 1997), pp. 31-6, ISSN 0167-8140.

Nguyen, B. et al. (1999). The safety and efficacy of gemcitabine plus cisplatin in the elderly chemonaive NCSLC patients (age>=70 years) as compared to those with age <70 years. *Proceeding American Society of Clinical Oncology*, ISSN 0732-183X, Atlanta, GA, May, 1999.

Okami, J. et al. (2009) Pulmonary resection in patients aged 80 years or over with clinical stage I non-small cell lung cancer. *Journal of Thoracic Oncology*, Vol.4, No.10, (October 2009), pp. 1247-1253, ISSN 1556-0864.

Onishi, H. et al. (2007). Hypofractionned stereotactic radiotherapy (HypoFXSRT) for stage I non-small cell lung cancer: updated results of 257 patients in a Japanese multi-instutitional study. *Journal of Clinical Oncology*, Vol.2, No.7, supp.3, (July 2007), pp. S94-S100, ISSN 0732-183X.

PACE participants. (2008). Shall we operate? Preoperative assessment in elderly cancer patients (PACE) can help. A SIOG surgical task force prospective study. *Critical Reviews in Oncology/Hematology*, Vol. 65, No. 2, (February 2008), pp. 156-163, ISSN 1040-8428.

Pallis, A.G. et al. (2010). EORTC task force position paper: Approach to the older cancer patient. *European Journal of Cancer*, Vol.46, No.9, (June 2010), pp. 1502-1513, ISSN 0959-8049.

Palma, D. et al. (2010). Impact of introducing stereotactic lung radiotherapy for elderly patients with stage I non-small-cell lung cancer: A population-based time-trend analysis. *Journal of Clinical Oncology*, Vol.28, No.35, (December 2010), pp. 5153-59, ISSN 0732-183X.

Park, C.H. et al. (In press 2010). Effect of radiotherapy planning complexity on survival of elderly patients with unresected localized lung cancer. *International Journal of Radiation, Oncology, Biology, Physics*, pp. 1-6, ISSN 0360-3016.

Pepe, C. et al. (2007).: Adjuvant vinorelbine and cisplatin in elderly patients: National Cancer Institute of Canada and Intergroup Study JBR.10. *Journal of Clinical Oncology*, Vol.25, No. 12, (April 2007), pp. 1553-61, ISSN 0732-183X.

Pergolizzi, S. et al. (2002). Older people with non small cell lung cancer in clinical stage IIIA and co-morbid conditions. Is curative irradiation feasible? Final results of a prospective study. *Lung Cancer*, Vol.37, N0.2, (August 2002), pp. 201-6, ISSN 0169-5002.

Pignon, J.P. et al. (2006). Lung Adjuvant Cisplatin Evaluation (LACE): a pooled analysis of five randomized clinical trials including 4584 patients. *Proceeding of American Society of Clinical Oncology*, ISSN 0732-183X,Atlanta, GA, June 2006.

Pignon, T. et al. (1998). Age has no impact on acute and late toxicity of curative thoracic radiotherapy. *Radiotherapy and Oncology*, Vol.46, No.3, (March 1998), pp. 239-48, ISSN 0167 8140.

Port, J. et al. (2004). Pulmonary resection for lung cancer in the octogenarian. *Chest*, Vol.126, No.3, (September 2004), pp. 733-738, ISSN 0012-3692.

Qiao, X. et al. (2003). The role of radiotherapy in treatment of stage I non-small-cell lung cancer. *Lung Cancer, Vol.* 41, Vol.1, (July 2003), pp. 1-11, ISSN 0169-5002.

Quoix, E. A. et al. (2010). Weekly paclitaxel combined with monthly carboplatin versus single-agent therapy in patients age 70 to 89: IFCT-0501 randomized phase III study in advanced non-small-cell lung cancer (NSCLC) *Proceeding American Society of Clinical Oncology*, ISSN 0732-183X, Chicago, IL, June 2010.

Ramalingam, S. S. et al. (2008). Outcomes for elderly, advanced-stage non small-cell lung cancer patients treated with bevacizumab in combination with carboplatin and paclitaxel: analysis of Eastern Cooperative Oncology Group Trial 4599. *Journal of Clinical Oncology*, Vol.26, No1, (January 2008),pp. 60-5, ISSN 0732-183X.

Raz, D.J. et al. (2007). Natural history of stage I non-small cell lung cancer. *Chest*, Vol.132, Vol.1, (July 2007), pp. 193-199, ISSN 0012-3692.

Repetto, L. et al. (2002). Comprehensive geriatric assessment adds information to Eastern Cooperative Oncology Group performance status in elderly cancer patients: an Italian Group for Geriatric Oncology Study. *Journal of Clinical Oncology*, Vol. 20, No. 2, (January 2002), pp. 494-502, ISSN 0732-183X.

Riquet, M. et al. (2001). Non-small cell lung cancer: surgical trends as a function of age. *Revue des maladies respiratoires*, Vol.18, suppl.2, (May 2001), IssN 0761-8425.

Rocha Lima, C. et al. (2002). Therapy choices among older patients with lung carcinoma: an evaluation of two trials of the Cancer and Leukemia Group B. *Cancer*, Vol.94, No.1, (January 1994), pp. 181-87, ISSN 1097-0142.

Rowell, N. P. & Williams, C. J. (2001). Radical radiotherapy for stage I/II non-small-cell lung cancer in patients not sufficiently fit for or declining surgery (medically inoperable): A systematic review. *Thorax* Vol.56, No.8, (August 2001), pp. 628-638, ISSN 0040-6376.

Scagliotti, G.V. et al. (2003). Randomized study of adjuvant chemotherapy for completely resected stage I, II, or IIIA non-small-cell lung cancer. *Journal of National Cancer Institute,* Vol.95, no.19, (October 2003), pp. 1453-61, ISSN 1052-6773.

San José, S. et al. (2006). Radiation therapy alone in elderly patients with early stage non-small cell lung cancer. *Lung Cancer,* Vol.52, Vol.2, (May 2006), pp. 149-54, ISSN 0169-5002.

Sause, W. T. (1994). Combination chemotherapy and radiation therapy in lung cancer. *Seminar of Oncology,* Vol.21, No.3, suppl. 6, (June 1994) pp. 72-78, ISSN 0093-7754.

Sause, W.T. et al. (2000). Final results of phase III trial in regionally advanced unresectable non-small cell lung cancer: Radiation Therapy Oncology Group, Eastern Cooperative Oncology Group, a Southwest Oncology Group. *Chest,* Vol. 117. No.2, (February 2000), pp. 358-364, ISSN 0012-3692.

Schild, S. E. et al. (2003). North Central Cancer Treatment Group. The outcome of combined-modality therapy for stage III non-small cell lung cancer in the elderly. *Journal of Clinical Oncology.* Vol.21, No.17, (September 2003), pp. 3201-3206, ISSN 0732-183X.

Schild, S. E. et al. (2005). Results of combined therapy for limited-stage small cell lung carcinoma in the elderly. *Cancer,* Vol.103, No.11, (June 2005), pp. 2349-54, ISSN 1097-0142.

Schuchert, M. J. et al. (2009). Clinical impact of age on outcomes following anatomic lung resection for stage I non-small lung cancer. *Proceeding American Society of Clinical Oncology,* ISSN 0732-183X, Orlando, FL, June 2009.

Sigel, K. et al. (2009). Effect of age on survival of clinical stage I non-small-cell lung cancer. *Annals of surgical Oncology,* Vol.16, No.7, (July 2009), pp.1912-7, ISSN 1068-9265.

Sibley, G. S. et al. (1998). Radiotherapy alone for medically inoperable stage I non-small cell lung cancer: the Duke experience. *International Journal of Radiation, Oncology, Biology, Physics,* Vol.40, No.1, (January 1998), pp. 149-54, ISSN 0360-3016.

Socinski, M. A. et al. (2007). Treatment of non-small cell lung cancer, stage IV :ACCP evidence-based clinical practice guidelines (2nd edition). *Chest,* Vol.132, No.3 suppl., (September 2007), pp. 277S-289S, ISSN 0012-3692.

Spiro, S. G, & Porter, J. C. (2002). Lung cancer: Where are we today? Current advances in staging and nonsurgical treatment. *American Journal of Respiratory Critical Care Medicine,* Vol.166, No.9, (November 2002), pp.1166-1196, ISSN 1073-449X.

Stout, R. et al. (2000). Clinical and quality of life outcomes in the first United Kingdom randomized trial if endobronchial brachytherapy (intraluminal radiotherapy) vs. external beam radiotherapy in the palliative treatment in inoperable non small cell lung cancer. *Radiotherapy and Oncology,* Vol.56, No.3, (September 2000), pp. 323-327, ISSN 0167-8140.

Strauss, G. M. et al. (2004). Randomized clinical trial of adjuvant chemotherapy with paclitaxel and carboplatin following resection in stage IB non-small cell lung cancer (NSCLC): report of a Cancer and Leukemia Group B (CALGB) protocol 9633. *Proceeding American Society of Clinical Oncology,* ISSN 0732-183X, New Orleans, LA, June 2004.

Strauss, G. M. et al. (2006). Adjuvant chemotherapy in stage IB non-small cell lung cancer (NSCLC) : report of a Cancer and Luekemia Group B (CALGB) protocol 9633.

Proceeding American Society of Clinical Oncology, ISSN 0732-183X, Atlanta, GA, June 2006.

Sullivan, V. et al. (2005). Advanced age does not exclude lobectomy for non-small cell lung carcinoma. *Chest,* Vol.128, No.4, pp. 2671-2676, ISSN 0012-3692.

Sutedja, G. et al. (1994). Fiberoptic bronchoscopic electrosurgery under local anesthesia for rapid palliation n patients with central airway malignancies. A preliminary report. *Thorax,* Vol.49, No.12, (December 1994), pp. 1243-46, ISSN 0040 6376.

Tibaldi, C. et al. (2006). Second-line chemotherapy with a modified schedule of docetaxel in elderly patients with advanced-stage non-small-cell lung cancer. *Clinical Lung Cancer,* Vol.7, No.6, (May 2006), pp. 401-405, ISSN 1526-7304.

Timmerman, R. et al. (2003). Extracranial stereotactic radioablation: results of a phase I study in medically inoperable stage I non-small cell lung cancer, *Chest* Vol. 124, No.5, (November 2003), pp. 1946-55, ISSN 0012-3692.

Timmerman, R. et al. (2006). Excessive toxicity when treating central tumor in a phase II study of stereotactic body radiation therapy for medically inoperable early-stage lung cancer. *Journal of Clinical Oncology,* Vol.24, No.30, (October 2006), pp. 4833-4839, ISSN 0732-183X.

Timmerman, R. et al. (2010). Stereotactic body radiation therapy for inoperable early-stage lung cancer. *JAMA,* Vol.303, No.11, (March 2010), pp. 1070-6, ISSN 0098-7484.

Tombolini, V.et al. (2000). Radiotherapy alone in elderly patients with medically inoperable stage IIIA and IIIB non-small cell lung cancer. *Anticancer Research,* Vol.20, No.6C, (November-December 2000), pp. 4829-33, ISSN 0250-7005.

Toy, E. et al (2003). Palliative Thoracic radiotherapy for non-small-cell lung cancer: A systematic review. *American Journal of Clinical Oncology,* Vol. 26, No.2, (April 2003), pp. 112-123, ISSN 0277-3732.

Van Meeerbeeck, J.P.; Damhuis, R. A. & Vos de Wael, M. L. (2002). High post-operative risk after pneumonectomy in elderly patients with right-sided lung cancer cancer. *Euopean Respiratory Journal,* Vol.19, No.1, (January 2002), pp. 141-145, ISSN2042-4884.

Wada, H. et al (1998) Thirty-day operative mortality for thoracotomy in lung cancer. *Journal of Thoracic Cardiovascular Surgery,* Vol. 115, No.1, (January 1998), pp. 70-73, ISSN002-5223.

Waller, D. et al. (2004). Chemotherapy for patients with non-small cell lung cancer: the surgical setting of the Big Lung Trial. *European Journal of Cardiothoracic Surgery,* Vol.26, No.1, (July 2004), pp. 173-82, ISSN 1010-7940.

Wang, J. et al. (2008). Temporal trends and predictors of perioperative chemotherapy use in elderly patients with resected non-small cell lung cancer. *Cancer,* Vol.112, No.2, (January 2008), pp. 382-390, ISSN 0012-3692.

Walsh, D. et al. (1990). Bronchoscopic cryotherapy for advanced bronchial carcinoma. *Thorax,* Vol.45, no.7, (July 1990), pp. 509-513, ISSN 0040-6376.

Weiss, G. J. et al. (2006). Elderly patients benefit from second-line cytotoxic chemotherapy: A subset analysis of a randomized phase III trial of pemetrexed compared with docetaxel in patients with previously treated advanced non-small-cell lung cancer. *Journal of Clinical Oncology,* Vol.24, No.27, (September 2006), pp. 4405-4411, ISSN 0732-183X.

Wildiers, H. et al. (2003). Pharmacology of anticancer drugs in the elderly population. *Clinical Pharmacokinetics* Vol.42, No.14, pp. 1213-42, ISSN 0312 5963.

Wisnivesky, J.P. et al. (2005). Radiation therapy for the treatment of unresected stage I-II non-small cell lung cancer. *Chest,* Vol.128, No.3, (September 2005), pp. 1461-1467, ISSN 0012-3692.

Xia, T. et al. (2006). Promising clinical outcome of stereotactic body radiation therapy for patients with inoperable stage I/II non-small-cell lung cancer. *International Journal of Radiation, Oncology, Biology, Physics,* Vol.66, No.1, (September 2006), pp. 117-25, ISSN 0360-3016.

Yu, H.M. et al. (2008). Involved-field radiotherapy is effective for patients 70 years old or more with early stage non-small cell lung cancer. *Radiotherapy and Oncology,* Vol.87, No.1, (April 2008), pp. 29-34, ISSN 0167-8140.

Zachariah, B. et al. (1997). Radiotherapy for cancer patients aged 80 and older: a study of effectiveness and side effects. *International Journal of Radiation, Oncology, Biology, Phyics* Vol.39, No.5, (December 1997), pp. 1125-9, ISSN 0360-3016.

Zimmermann, F. B. et al. (2006). Stereotactic hypofractionned radiotherapy in stage I (T1-2 N0 M0) non-small-cell lung cancer (NSCLC). *Acta Oncologica,* Vol.45,No.7, pp. 796-801, ISSN 1651-226X.

Electronic Sources

U.S. Census Bureau. (2009) Date of access: April 21, 2011. Available from: <http://www.census.gov/popest/national/asrh/NC-EST2009-sa.html>

U.S. Census Bureau. (2008) Date of access: April 21, 2011. Available from: <http://www.census.gov/population/www/projections/summarytables.html>

Statistics Canada. Date of access: April 21, 2011. Available from: <http://www40.statcan.gc.ca/l02/cst01/demo08d-fra.htm>

Canadian Cancer Society. Date of access: April 21, 2011. Available from: <htttp://www.cancer.ca/Quebec/About%20cancer/Cancer%20statistics/Stats%20at%20a%20glance/General%20cancer%20stats.aspx?sc_lang=en>

U.S. National Institues of Health, Surveillance Epidemiology and End Results. Date of access: April 21, 2011. Available from: < http://www.seer.cancer.gov/statfacts/html/lungb.html>

16

Prediction of Postoperative Lung Function

Seung Hun Jang
*Division of Pulmonary, Allergy and Critical Care Medicine,
Hallym University Sacred Heart Hospital,
Republic of Korea*

1. Introduction

Lung cancer is the leading cause of cancer death in many counties. Despite significant improvement in chemotherapy and radiotherapy, surgery is still the cornerstone of non-small cell lung cancer treatment. The lung cancer is categorized into non-small cell lung cancer or small cell lung cancer according to the histology. The patients with stage IA-IIB non-small cell lung cancer and stage I small cell lung cancer are good candidates for lung resection which can offer the best chance for cure. In a series of 407 individuals with resectable cancer, the 346 who went to thoracotomy had a median survival of 30.9 months compared with 15.6 months in the 57 who did not go to surgery (Loewen, et al. 2007). A part of individuals with stage IIIA non-small cell stage may also be the surgical candidates if they are adequately treated with chemotherapy and/or radiotherapy before and/or after surgery. The long term goals of lung cancer surgery include cancer control improving survival and quality of life of the patients.

Smoking is the important risk factor not only for lung cancer but also for other comorbid diseases such as chronic obstructive pulmonary disease (COPD) and coronary heart disease. The patients with lung cancer and COPD have reduced ability to tolerate further losses in lung function. Because of relatively high incidence of postoperative complications, the hospital mortality, as well as disappointing long-term survival after surgical resection of lung cancer, the appropriate selection of patients for pulmonary resection is a continuing challenge. It was reported that only about 30% of individuals with lung cancer were determined to be candidates for lung resection because of the advanced stage (Damhuis & Schutte 1996). In addition, a report showed that 37% of individuals who present with anatomically resectable disease deemed not to be surgical candidates based on poor lung function alone (Baser, et al. 2006). If a patient is deemed a candidate for surgery, it must be realized that pulmonary function will be affected by the resection. The decline in lung function varies with the extent of the resection. Accordingly, it is important to be informed about the risk factors and how they affect postoperative morbidity, mortality, and long-term survival.

Pulmonary function measures such as the forced expiratory volume in one second (FEV1) and the diffusing capacity for carbon monoxide (DLco) are useful predictors of postoperative outcome (Bousamra, et al. 1996; Ferguson, et al. 1988; Markos, et al. 1989). Postoperative value of FEV1 is certainly the most widely used parameter for preoperative risk stratification. It has been shown to be an independent predictor of complications including mortality (Kearney, et al. 1994; Mitsudomi, et al. 1996; Ribas, et al. 1998). The assessment of regional lung function to predict postoperative function is integral to preoperative evaluation of pulmonary resection candidates who have impaired lung function. There are four validated ways to predict postoperative FEV1. However, all of them tend to underestimate the predicted value compared with the actual postoperative lung function. Although predicted postoperative FEV1 (ppoFEV1) somewhat exactly correlates with actual postoperative FEV1 (apoFEV1), the correlation can be affected by several clinical factors. If actual postoperative lung function quite differs from predicted value, it may be a cause of serious clinical outcome especially in the patients with marginal postoperative lung function; someone may undergo life-threatening lung resection, and someone may lose the opportunity to be cured by surgery. Therefore, we need to know clinical factors as many as possible which can affect the discrepancy between apoFEV1 and ppoFEV1. The aim of the chapter is to review the accuracy of the prediction methods for postoperative lung function, especially FEV1, and the clinical factors affecting the prediction accuracy. This will confer the ideas about the appropriate selection of patients for pulmonary resection and perioperative management for risk reduction.

2. The physiologic evaluation for the decision about operability

2.1 Lung function test

Among lung function measures, FEV1 and DLco are the most useful predictors of postoperative outcomes. Both absolute values and percent predicted normal values have been studied and proved as a predictors of postoperative complications including mortality (Licker, et al. 2006). The generally accepted lung function for minimal postoperative mortality is preoperative FEV1 > 1.5 L for a lobectomy, and > 2L for a pneumonectomy. Those who have lung function above this level can undergo surgery without further evaluation. There is little evidence that one cutoff absolute value of FEV1 should be used to permit resection of varying extent. Although the absolute value for ppoFEV1 that would allow resection has not been found, the previous studies suggested the values greater than 0.8-1 L for acceptable postoperative mortality (Boysen, et al. 1981; Wernly, et al. 1980). The values of pulmonary function expressed as percentage of normal are more convenient and useful because they are affected by individual's age, sex, height, and race. In terms of percentage of normal, ppoFEV1 less than 30% predicted would be very highly risky for perioperative death and ppoFEV1 greater than 40% has been suggested for tolerable resection up to calculated extent of resection (Beckles, et al. 2003; Colice, et al. 2007; Markos, et al. 1989). If ppoFEV1 is between 30% and 40%, the decision had better to incorporate the result of maximal oxygen consumptions (VO2max).

Cardiopulmonary exercise testing has been used as a means to access a patient's fitness for lung resection. Several studies have identified exercise capacity (VO2max) as a predictor of postoperative complications as well as of postoperative long term mortality (Bolliger, et al. 1995; Brutsche, et al. 2000). Risk for perioperative complications can generally be stratified by VO2max. Several studies demonstrated that preoperative VO2max > 20 mL/kg/min was not associated with increased risk of complications or death (Bolliger, et al. 1994; Richter Larsen, et al. 1997). Patients with VO2max of 15 to 20 mL/kg/min can undergo curative lung cancer surgery with an acceptably low mortality rate (Richter Larsen, et al. 1997; Win, et al. 2005). On the contrary, the risk of perioperative death sharply increases below the level of VO2max < 15 mL/kg/min (Bolliger, et al. 1995; Win, et al. 2005). VO2max < 10 mL/kg/min has been reported as a very high risk of postoperative death (Holden, et al. 1992; Olsen, et al. 1989).

Algorithmic approaches for the candidate selection have been developed in an effort to improve decision making (Colice, et al. 2007; Wyser, et al. 1999). Wyser et al. showed that algorithmic decision reduced the complications in half compared with the author's prior series. In summary, individuals with VO2max < 10 mL/kg/min, or < 15 mL/kg/min with both ppoFEV1 and ppoDLco < 40% predicted, are at high risk for perioperative death and complications. Both preoperative FEV1 and DLco ≥ 80% predicted normal or VO2max ≥ 20 mL/kg/min allow lobectomy or pneumonectomy without any further evaluation.

2.2 Stair climbing and walking test

If cardiopulmonary exercise test were not available, another simple exercise test could replace the test. Stair climbing has been investigated, and it was proven to correlate with FEV1 and VO2max very well (Bolton, et al. 1987; Pollock, et al. 1993). It is generally accepted that patient who can climb five flights of stairs has VO2max > 20 mL/kg/min, and conversely, patient who cannot climb one flight of stairs has VO2max < 10 mL/kg/min (Beckles, et al. 2003). The data about the shuttle walking or 6-minute walking test are limited, but they can also surrogate cardiopulmonary exercise test.

2.3 Arterial blood gas analysis

The results of arterial blood gas analysis reflect the cardiopulmonary functional status. Historically, hypercapnea (PaCO2 > 45 mmHg) has been regarded as an exclusion criterion for lung resection (Celli 1993). However, a few clinical studies suggested that hypercapnea did not increase perioperative complications (Harpole, et al. 1996; Kearney, et al. 1994). Hypercapnea is not an independent risk factor for increased perioperative complications, and the operability should be decided after further physiologic testing.

3. The methods for prediction of postoperative lung function

The surgical procedure depends on the stage of lung cancer and on the cardiopulmonary reserve of the patients. A prospective randomized trial comparing limited resection to lobectomy in patients with peripheral stage I lung cancers reported that the patients treated with limited resection had a three-fold increase in local recurrence, a 75% increase in combined local and distant recurrence, and a 50% increase in death with cancer (Ginsberg & Rubinstein 1995). Therefore, anatomic resection such as lobectomy or pneumonectomy should be done if physiologically feasible. Lung sparing anatomic resection like sleeve lobectomy is preferred over pneumonectomy, if anatomically appropriate and if margin-negative resection can be achieved. A study compared clinical outcomes of the elderly patients undergoing sleeve lobectomy or pneumonectomy due to non-small-cell lung cancer (Bolukbas, et al. 2011). The loss of FEV1 was 12.0% vs. 27.3% ($p = 0.001$), and 5 year survival rate was 59% vs. 0% favoring sleeve lobectomy although there was no statistical difference in postoperative mortality (6.5% in sleeve lobectomy vs. 10.3% in pneumonectomy). Sublobar resection, either segmentectomy (preferred) or wedge resection, is appropriate in selected patients if margin-negative resection can be achieved. The limited resection is appropriate especially for the patients with poor pulmonary reserve or other major co-morbidity that contraindicates lobectomy.

For the prediction of postoperative remnant lung function, the anatomy of the lung should be understood. The right lung consists of three lobes; upper, middle and lower lobe. The right upper lobe consists of 3 segments, the right middle lobe 2 segments, and the right lower lobe 5 segments. The left lung consists of two lobes; upper and lower lobe. The left upper lobe consists of 4 segments, the left lower lobe 4 segments. The anteromediobasal segment of the left lower lobe is the counterpart of anterobasal segment and mediobasal segment of the right lower lobe, but it has a common bronchial orifice. Although it is anatomically one segment, it contains two segments in volume. Therefore, the left lung is regarded to have 9 segments in terms of volume; 4 segments in the left upper lobe and 5 segments in the left lower lobe. Each segment is assumed to have same volume (1/19 of the lung function). The four validated methods to predict postoperative lung function are: 1) anatomic calculation, 2) split radionuclide perfusion scanning, 3) quantitative computed tomography (CT) scanning, and 4) dynamic perfusion magnetic resonance imaging (MRI). Using these techniques, the actual lung function was consistently underestimated, particularly if the starting value was lower (Giordano, et al. 1997; Zeiher, et al. 1995). The accuracy of prediction of anatomic calculation is slightly lower than the other methods, but the other methods effectively predict postoperative FEV1 with similar accuracy. Medical cost, local expertise and availability of equipments should be considered for the choice.

3.1 Anatomic calculation

Estimation of predicted postoperative lung function based on anatomical calculation is the simplest, but the accuracy is slightly lower than other methods. Predicted postoperative FEV1 can be calculated by simple subtraction of the FEV1 proportion of resected lung segments from the total preoperative FEV1 (Juhl & Frost 1975; Zeiher, et al. 1995).

$$\text{ppoFEV1} = \text{preoperative FEV1} \times [1 - (\text{number of segments to be resected}/19)]$$

For example, if a patient will undergo right upper lobectomy, the predicted postoperative FEV1 will be calculated to remain 16/19 (84.2%) of preoperative FEV1. This method is also applied to the other methods as a basic concept.

3.2 Split radionuclide perfusion scanning

In most clinical cases, the extent of pulmonary disease may be different in each side of the lung, which is leading cause of different regional lung function according to the disease status. This is a major violation of the assumption that each lung segment represents the same lung function. The general principle of the radionuclide scanning technique is same for the anatomic calculation method. The prediction of postoperative lung function can be calculated by the following two steps. The first step is determining the functional contribution of resected (right or left) lung by quantitative perfusion lung scan, and the second step is applying the principle of anatomical calculation to the resected lung. Postoperative lung function is then estimated to be the product of the preoperative function and the portion of lung function that will remain after resection as estimated by the scan.

$$\text{ppoFEV1} = \text{preoperative FEV1} \times [1 - \text{functional fraction of the resected lung} \times (\text{number of segments to be resected}/\text{total segments of that lung})]$$

The accuracy of these techniques has been questioned. A recent study using technetium scanning calculated values of imprecision from 18%-21% despite showing reasonable correlation (Giordano, et al. 1997).

3.3 Quantitative CT scanning

Quantitative computed tomography scanning has been studied as a technique to estimate postresection lung function. The basic concept is similar to radionuclide perfusion scanning method. This measures the split lung function using the CT attenuation density instead of radionuclide signal intensity. The volume of lung with attenuation between -500 and -910 Hounsfield units was used to estimate functional lung volume. The portion of the lung remaining postresection was predicted by calculating lung volume in the area to be resected as a portion of total lung volume. With this, predicted postoperative function correlated as well as the method using radionuclide quantitative perfusion imaging (Wu, et al. 2002).

3.4 Dynamic perfusion magnetic resonance imaging (MRI)

A study showed that magnetic resonance (MR) perfusion imaging had almost the same sensitivity and specificity for diagnosis of pulmonary perfusion defects as conventional perfusion scintigraphy (Berthezene, et al. 1999). The regional lung function is calculated from the subtraction images for normal lung parenchyma using image analysis software. The accuracy of MR perfusion for the prediction of ppoFEV1 was validated in a study (Iwasawa, et al. 2002). This study demonstrated that the correlation between perfusion ratios derived from MR perfusion image and radionuclide perfusion scanning was excellent ($R = 0.92$). The correlation between ppoFEV1 and actual postoperative FEV1 was similar when the two methods were compared ($R = 0.682$ in MR perfusion and $R = 0.667$ in radionuclide perfusion).

4. Clinical parameters affecting prediction accuracy of postoperative lung function

Prediction accuracy of postoperative lung function is affected not only by the calculation technique, but also the clinical factors associated with the actual postoperative lung function. The actual lung function closely relates to the physiology of lung volume reduction, reversibility of airway obstruction, pharmacotherapy, and postoperative respiratory rehabilitation.

4.1 Chronic obstructive pulmonary sisease

Pulmonary function is affected by lung resection and the decline in lung function varies with the extent of the resection. The degree of functional loss appears to be less in individuals with poor baseline lung function uniformly across the studies (Bobbio, et al. 2005; Boushy, et al. 1971; Edwards, et al. 2001). In patients with severe emphysema, surgery performed to remove the most emphysematous portion of the lung may lead to improvements in lung function (Fishman, et al. 2003). A case-matched study demonstrated that the patients with COPD had a three-fold higher rate of cardiopulmonary morbidity (28% versus 10%, $p=0.04$), but lower reduction in FEV1 (6% versus 13%, $p=0.0002$) compared with non-COPD patients after lobectomy for lung cancer (Pompili, et al. 2010). Importantly, although the postoperative quality of life in both groups was reduced, there were no significant differences in quality of life between the groups. This suggests that the patients with lung cancer and COPD may be unexpectedly tolerable with the curative lung resection if the candidates are carefully selected. This is attributed to lung volume reduction effect which takes place very early. The risk-benefit should be balanced based on the negative physiologic effects of thoracotomy versus positive effects of lung volume reduction in the surgical decision for the patients with lung cancer and COPD. As most lung cancer patients have more or less emphysematous changes, adequate volume reduction may open small airways, expand or overinflate functional alveoli, improve diaphragmatic movement and consequently increase postoperative FEV1 than the expected. This is consistent with the basic principle of volume reduction surgery for severe emphysema that postoperative lung function can be improved by resection of relatively functionless emphysematous lung.

4.2 Resected lung portion

Besides preoperative lung function, a study has suggested that the prediction accuracy of postoperative lung function could be influenced by other clinical factor such as resected lung portion (Sekine, et al. 2003). Sekine et al. reported that the presence of COPD and resection of the lower lung portion (lower lobectomy or middle-lower bilobectomy) were significantly associated with minimal deterioration of pulmonary function after lobectomy. The authors retrospectively analyzed 521 patients who had undergone lobectomy for lung cancer. The ppoFEV1 was calculated by modified anatomic calculation by multiplying a specific coefficient according to the baseline FEV1 categories. The apoFEV1 was measured at 1 month after operation. Minimal alteration of postoperative lung function, defined as apoFEV1 $\geq 1.15 \times$ ppoFEV1, was confirmed to be associated with COPD (vs. non-COPD) and resection of the lower lung portion (vs. upper lung portion) in multivariate analysis. Lung volume reduction theory can explain minimal alteration of apoFEV1 in the patients with COPD. The authors speculated that occasional anatomic repositioning after upper lobectomy, which causes narrowing of the orifice of lower or middle lobe bronchus, and different movement and elevation of diaphragm between upper lobectomy and lower lobectomy might be the potential causes the minimal alteration in the cases of resection of the lower lung portion (Nonaka, et al. 2000; Van Leuven, et al. 1999).

4.3 Number of resected lung segment and bronchodilator response

The writer of this chapter and his colleagues (Kim, et al. 2008) investigated another clinical factors affecting prediction accuracy. Some of the findings would like to be introduced in detail, because those may help for the selection of candidates for surgery and perioperative management of the patients.

A total of 82 patients with non-small-cell lung cancer undergoing pulmonary resection were retrospectively analyzed in this study. Forty eight patients underwent lobectomy, 11 patients underwent bilobectomy, and the remaining 23 patients underwent pneumonectomy. The ppoFEV1 was dually estimated by anatomical calculation and split radionuclide perfusion scanning method. The mean time interval between surgery and apoFEV1 was 24 ± 7 days. The ppoFEV1 calculated by split radionuclide perfusion scanning method was more accurate than that by anatomic calculation method (apoFEV1/ppoFEV1 = 1.00 ± 0.19 vs. 1.07 ± 0.23, $p < 0.001$). Multivariate linear regression analysis was performed to identify clinical parameters affecting the prediction accuracy with the covariates of age, gender, preoperative FEV1, time interval between surgery and the day of measuring apoFEV1, preoperative bronchodilator response (% increase in FEV1 after inhalation of short acting beta-2 agonist), resected lung portion, and the number of resected lung segments. Among these clinical factors, the number of resected lung segments and preoperative FEV1 were significant clinical factors affecting the prediction accuracy ($p = 0.026$ and 0.002, respectively). As the preoperative FEV1 became smaller and the more lung segments were

resected, apoFEV1 tended to be larger than ppoFEV1. It is noteworthy that the corresponding means of apoFEV1/ppoFEV1 for each number of resected lung segments gathered on a straight line of a constant slope. The apoFEV1 was closest to ppoFEV1 when four segments were resected. Contrary to the previous report, resected lung portion (upper or lower portion resection) was not related to the prediction accuracy ($p = 0.10$). However, more number of segments was resected in lower portion resection compared with upper portion resection (5.6 ± 1.1 vs. 3.7 ± 1.0, $p = 0.001$), which might be a confounding factor.
Lung functions of 46/82 patients were followed at 106 ± 30 days after surgery, which was reflecting plateau lung function of the patients undergoing lung resection. As expected, plateau apoFEV1 was increased by 13% compared with apoFEV1 measured at 24 days after surgery. In predicting plateau lung function, split radionuclide perfusion scanning method was also superior to anatomic calculation (plateau apoFEV1/ppoFEV1 = 1.11 ± 0.24 vs. 1.18 ± 0.30, $p < 0.001$). These data also indicate that the prediction methods are fitter for short-term postoperative value rather than long-term value. In general, postoperative lung function gradually improves with time (Brunelli, et al. 2007). However, the plateau apoFEV1 was lower than the apoFEV1 measured at 24 days in 9/46 (19%) patients. Their preoperative bronchodilator response values were higher than those of the others although it did not reach statistical significance ($11.2 \pm 8.4\%$ vs. $7.0 \pm 6.8\%$, $p = 0.11$). The study did not investigate prescription status of bronchodilator or the patients' adherence to the drugs. However, this finding suggests that adequate perioperative bronchodilator therapy is necessary for the patients with high bronchodilator response, especially for the patients with poor lung function. Bronchodilator response is a well known predictor of pulmonary function improvement after long term treatment with long acting beta-2 agonist. A study demonstrated that bronchodilator response, wheezing history positively correlated with improvement in FEV1 after three months inhalation treatment with salmeterol/fluticasone combination, conversely negative correlation with emphysema extent (Lee, et al. 2011). COPD is a complex and heterogeneous disorder of mixed chronic bronchitis and emphysema. Another study showed that three months inhalation treatment with long-acting beta-agonist and corticosteroid significantly improved the FEV1 of obstruction-dominant patients compared with the emphysema-dominant subgroup. Again, baseline bronchodilator response and DLco were the meaningful predictors associated with improvement of FEV1 after the treatment (Lee, et al. 2010). If the patients with high bronchodilator response do not receive regular bronchodilator treatment after surgery, the FEV1 should decrease and the prediction accuracy of postoperative lung function would be affected as a matter of course.
Preoperative FEV1 was significantly lower in the COPD group than in the non-COPD group ($67.1 \pm 8.3\%$ vs. $101.6 \pm 15.2\%$, $p < 0.001$). The apoFEV1 was about 14% larger than ppoFEV1 in the COPD group while apoFEV1 was very similar to ppoFEV1 in the non-COPD group (apoFEV1/ppoFEV1 = 1.1 ± 0.2 in COPD group and 1.0 ± 0.1 in non-COPD group, $p < 0.001$). These are the same results with the previous studies indicating that the prediction of postoperative lung function is more accurate in the non-COPD group than in the COPD group, and postoperative lung function of the COPD group may be less deteriorated than that of the non-COPD group.

5. Physiologic changes in the lung volume reduction surgery

Actual postoperative FEV1 is better than the predicted value in the patients with COPD, which is universally observed in many clinical studies. This phenomenon is explained by the physiology of lung volume reduction. In patients with COPD, inhaled air is trapped in the thorax as a result of decreased elastic recoil of the lung and early closure of the small airways during exhalation. This is manifested as hyperinflation of the chest, flattening of the diaphragm, increased intra-thoracic pressure, and reduced inspiratory capacity. These worsen during exercise and result in dyspnea and limitation of exercise capacity. After surgical volume reduction, there is expansion of the remaining lung in addition to reduction of the overall thoracic volume and pressure, and it is probable that some areas of relative compression have been reexpanded. Lung volume reduction surgery is associated with improvement in exercise capacity, lung function, quality of life, and dyspnea, but the changes after surgery are variable according to the individuals (Gelb, et al. 2001). The improvement of FEV1 and reduction in hyperinflation has been explained by the increase of lung parenchymal elastic recoil (Sciurba, et al. 1996). It is accompanied with subsequent repositioning of the diaphragm, recruitment of inspiratory muscles, and improvement of respiratory mechanics (Benditt, et al. 1997; Criner, et al. 1998).

Surgical treatment of emphysema had been tried with multiple wedge resections and plications technique which is no longer used (Brantigan & Mueller 1957), and then Cooper et al. reintroduced lung volume reduction surgery as a possible surgical therapy for selected patients with a heterogeneous form of emphysema (Cooper, et al. 1995). The most affected portions are excised about 20% to 35% of the volume of each lung for lung volume reduction. The surgical mortality rate ranges 4-15% and one-year mortality rates are as high as 17% (Argenziano, et al. 1996; Flaherty, et al. 2001; Gelb, et al. 2001). A large randomized controlled trial was conducted to compare lung volume reduction surgery with medical therapy for severe emphysema (Fishman, et al. 2003). The FEV1 of surgery arm was significantly better than that of medical treatment group after 6, 12, and 24 months follow-up. The rates of improvement versus deterioration of FEV1 compared with the baseline were 65% : 35% at 6 months follow-up, 56% : 44% at 12 months, and 43% : 57% at 24 months in the lung volume reduction surgery group. It is also observed in the bullectomy case series that FEV1 is initially improved after lung volume reduction surgery and then returns to the baseline lung function with time. The 90-day mortality was 7.9% (95% confidence interval, 5.9-10.3%) in surgery group, and 1.3% (95% confidence interval, 0.6-2.6%) in medical treatment group. The functional benefits of lung volume reduction surgery came at the price of increased short-term mortality. Overall mortality was similar in both treatment groups, but subgroup analysis showed that the survival benefit was observed in the patients with predominantly upper lobe emphysema and a low baseline exercise capacity. Patients with non–upper lobe emphysema and high baseline exercise capacity are poor candidates for lung volume reduction surgery, because of increased mortality and negligible functional gain.

The similar physiologic changes can be also expected in the giant bullae. If a giant bulla compresses the adjacent normal lung parenchyma and it is causing incapacitating dyspnea, it should be resected for the reexpansion of the normal lung. Bullectomy can produce immediate lung function improvement, but the benefit usually decline with time (Laros, et al. 1986; Schipper, et al. 2004). Giant bullae are frequently combined with emphysema.

6. COPD and lung cancer

COPD is characterized by chronic airflow limitation that is not fully reversible and usually progressive with time. The airflow limitation is usually associated with an abnormal inflammatory response of the lung to noxious particles or gases. COPD refers to patients with emphysema or chronic bronchitis, though these two disease entities are frequently mixed up to a varying ratio. It is accompanied with some significant extrapulmonary effects and comorbidities (Agusti 2005). COPD has been defined in several ways, and the differences in definitions and diagnosis affect the estimates of the burden of the disease. The Global Initiative for Chronic Obstructive Lung Disease (GOLD) defines the disease in stages of clinical severity based on FEV1 and FEV1/FVC (forced vital capacity) from post-bronchodilator spirometry (Rabe, et al. 2007). The statement recommends to use the fixed ratio post-bronchodilator FEV1/FVC < 0.7 for definition of airflow limitation despite a problematic issue of overdiagnosis.

COPD are at risk for lung cancer due to common risk factors like aging, smoking, reactive oxygen species (Azad, et al. 2008; Soriano, et al. 2005; Young, et al. 2009). Tobacco smoking is considered to be the leading cause both of lung cancer and COPD. Smokers have a higher prevalence of respiratory symptoms and lung function abnormalities, a greater annual decline rate in FEV1 and a greater COPD mortality rate than nonsmokers. Smoking accounts for more than 85-90% of all lung cancer related deaths (Doll & Peto 1976). Cancer cells proliferate in reactive oxygen species rich inflammatory environment which is promoting DNA damage, inactivation of apoptosis, upregulation of growth factors, cytokines, and activating growth supporting genes (Cook, et al. 2004). Reactive oxygen species and chronic inflammation are also important pathologic mechanisms of COPD. A meta-analysis demonstrated that overall relative risk of lung cancer for subjects with COPD was 2.22 (95% confidence interval, 1.66-2.97%). Besides COPD, previous history of pneumonia or tuberculosis also increased the lung cancer risk even in never-smoker population (Brenner, et al. 2011). Chronic inflammation has been proposed as a cause of cancer development.

An effective COPD management includes severity assessment, regular monitoring, risk factor elimination, pharmacotherapy, and rehabilitation. This multidimensional approach includes patient education, health advice, counseling about smoking cessation, instruction in exercise and nutrition. Almost all the same therapeutic approach and monitoring should be also applied to the patients with the patients undergoing lung resection. Pharmacotherapy is helpful to prevent and control respiratory symptoms, reduce the frequency and severity of exacerbation, and improve exercise capacity and quality of life. The existing medications for COPD do not modify the long-term decline in lung function, but regular treatment with long-acting anticholinergic bronchodilator (Tiotropium bromide), long-acting beta-2 agonists, inhaled glucocorticoid, and its combination can decrease the rate of decline of lung function (Celli, et al. 2008; Tashkin, et al. 2008). Bronchodilators acting on peripheral airways reduce air trapping, thereby reducing residual lung volume and improving respiratory symptoms and exercise capacity. Patient education is essential in COPD like any other chronic diseases. The component of education should include smoking cessation, disease information about pathophysiology and natural course, general approach to the therapy, and self management skill. The poor adherence of the patients with COPD to the inhaler medication has been pointed out (Bender, et al. 2006). However, it is essential to remind the patients of regular using inhaler medication, because adherence to inhaled medication has been shown to be significantly associated with reduced risk of death and admission to hospital due to exacerbation in COPD (Vestbo, et al. 2009).

COPD doubles the risk of postoperative pulmonary complications (Kroenke, et al. 1993). Strategies for reducing pulmonary complications are needed. Preoperatively, inhaled bronchodilators such as long-acting anticholinergics or beta-2 agonists are indicated for the patients with COPD. Adequate drug therapies can maximize the potential to tolerate lung resection, help us to offer potentially curative treatment to the patients as many as possible. Postoperatively, lung expansion maneuvers and pain control are the two most important methods for reducing the risk of pulmonary complications. Both the incentive spirometry and deep breathing exercise are proved to be effective for lung expansion and reducing pulmonary complications (Thomas & McIntosh 1994). A meta-analysis of randomized controlled trials of postoperative pain control and pulmonary complications demonstrated that epidural local anesthetics significantly reduce the risk of pneumonia and all postoperative pulmonary complications (Ballantyne, et al. 1998). Pulmonary function recovers up to 6 months after a lobectomy, and up to 3 months after a pneumonectomy (Bolliger, et al. 1996; Nezu, et al. 1998). There has been little research on long term postoperative optimized outcome in terms of lung function and quality of life. There is no direct evidence supporting an additional role of bronchodilators in the lung resection candidate beyond what would be standard use for COPD or asthma. A study showed that post-operative respiratory rehabilitation after lung resection for lung cancer was beneficial for the Borg dyspnea scale, exercise capacity represented by 6-minute walk distance, and maintenance of lung function (Cesario, et al. 2007). The inpatient rehabilitation program included supervised incremental exercise and educational sessions covering such topics as pulmonary physiopathology, pharmacology of patients' medications, dietary counseling, relaxation and stress management techniques, energy conservation principles, and breathing retraining. The individuals joining the rehabilitation program had the significantly improved exercise capacity and maintained FEV1, whereas the control group had the significantly decreased exercise capacity and decreased FEV1 compared with baseline values. Although the rehabilitation is not confined to pharmacotherapy, it should be kept in mind that multidimensional efforts to maintain exercise capacity and lung function should be required because they could be labile after lung resection.

7. Conclusion

Medical operability of lung cancer has been frequently determined based on preoperative FEV1, DLCO, and VO2max. Predicted postoperative FEV1 is still the most helpful indicator for the safe operation as it provides fundamental information about underlying lung function and disease status. As the concept of regional lung function is introduced to anatomic calculation, the prediction accuracy of postoperative lung function is improved. However, substantial gap is still present between ppoFEV1 and apoFEV1, which tends to be greater in COPD and large lung volume resection. This inaccuracy may be critical in the patients with marginal lung function after lung resection. We should consider that the the accuracy can be affected not only by the technique to measure the regional lung function, but also several clinical factors such as the presence of obstructive lung disease, resected lung portion, extent of lung volume resection, preoperative bronchodilator response, adherence to bronchodilator therapy, physical exercise, nutrition, postoperative pain control, patient education and so on.

The moderate to severe COPD should not hinder the curative resection of lung cancer which could increase the chance of cure, if the candidates of surgery would be properly selected, because the surgery could partly work as lung volume reduction, thereby minimizing the loss of pulmonary function in patients with COPD. Proper perioperative management regarding the aforementioned clinical factors is mandatory to improve lung function and reduce postoperative complication despite remarkable advances in anesthesia, surgery.

8. References

Agusti, A.G. (2005). Systemic effects of chronic obstructive pulmonary disease. *Proc Am Thorac Soc,* Vol.2, No.4, pp. 367-370; discussion 371-372

Argenziano, M., Moazami, N., Thomashow, B., Jellen P.A., Gorenstein L.A., Rose E.A., et al. (1996). Extended indications for lung volume reduction surgery in advanced emphysema. *Ann Thorac Surg,* Vol.62, No.6, pp. 1588-1597

Azad, N., Rojanasakul, Y., Vallyathan, V. (2008). Inflammation and lung cancer: roles of reactive oxygen/nitrogen species. *J Toxicol Environ Health B Crit Rev,* Vol.11, No.1, pp. 1-15

Ballantyne, J.C., Carr, D.B., deFerranti, S., Suarez, T., Lau, J., Chalmers, T.C., et al. (1998). The comparative effects of postoperative analgesic therapies on pulmonary outcome: cumulative meta-analyses of randomized, controlled trials. *Anesth Analg,* Vol.86, No.3, pp. 598-612

Baser, S., Shannon, V.R., Eapen, G.A., Jimenez, C.A., Onn, A., Keus, L., et al. (2006). Pulmonary dysfunction as a major cause of inoperability among patients with non-small-cell lung cancer. *Clin Lung Cancer,* Vol.7, No.5, pp. 344-349

Beckles, M.A., Spiro, S.G., Colice, G.L., Rudd, R.M. (2003). The physiologic evaluation of patients with lung cancer being considered for resectional surgery. *Chest,* Vol.123, No.1 Suppl, pp. 105S-114S

Bender, B.G., Pedan, A., Varasteh, L.T. (2006). Adherence and persistence with fluticasone propionate/salmeterol combination therapy. *J Allergy Clin Immunol,* Vol.118, No.4, pp. 899-904

Benditt, J.O., Wood, D.E., McCool, F.D., Lewis, S., Albert, R.K. (1997). Changes in breathing and ventilatory muscle recruitment patterns induced by lung volume reduction surgery. *Am J Respir Crit Care Med,* Vol.155, No.1, pp. 279-284

Berthezène, Y., Croisille, P., Wiart, M., Howarth, N., Houzard, C., Faure, O., et al. (1999). Prospective comparison of MR lung perfusion and lung scintigraphy. *J Magn Reson Imaging,* Vol.9, No.1, pp. 61-68

Bobbio, A., Chetta, A., Carbognani, P., Internullo, E., Verduri, A., Sansebastiano, G., et al. (2005). Changes in pulmonary function test and cardio-pulmonary exercise capacity in COPD patients after lobar pulmonary resection. *Eur J Cardiothorac Surg,* Vol.28, No.5, pp. 754-758

Bolliger, C.T., Jordan, P., Solèr, M., Stulz, P., Grädel, E., Skarvan, K., et al. (1995). Exercise capacity as a predictor of postoperative complications in lung resection candidates. *Am J Respir Crit Care Med,* Vol.151, No.5, pp. 1472-1480

Bolliger, C.T., Jordan, P., Solèr, M., Stulz, P., Tamm, M., Wyser, C., et al. (1996). Pulmonary function and exercise capacity after lung resection. *Eur Respir J,* Vol.9, No.3, pp. 415-421

Bolliger, C.T., Solèr, M., Stulz, P., Grädel, E., Müller-Brand, J., Elsasser, S., et al. (1994). Evaluation of high-risk lung resection candidates: pulmonary haemodynamics versus exercise testing. A series of five patients. *Respiration,* Vol.61, No.4, pp. 181-186

Bolliger, C.T., Wyser, C., Roser, H., Solèr, M., Perruchoud, A.P. (1995). Lung scanning and exercise testing for the prediction of postoperative performance in lung resection candidates at increased risk for complications. *Chest,* Vol.108, No.2, pp. 341-348

Bolton, J.W., Weiman, D.S., Haynes, J.L., Hornung, C.A., Olsen, G.N., Almond, C.H. (1987). Stair climbing as an indicator of pulmonary function. *Chest,* Vol.92, No.5, pp. 783-788

Bölükbas, S., Eberlein, M.H., Schirren, J. (2011). Pneumonectomy vs. Sleeve Resection for Non-Small Cell Lung Carcinoma in the Elderly: Analysis of Short-term and Long-term Results. *Thorac Cardiovasc Surg,* Vol.59, No.3, pp. 142-147

Bousamra, M. 2nd., Presberg, K.W., Chammas, J.H., Tweddell, J.S., Winton, B.L., Bielefeld, M.R., et al. (1996). Early and late morbidity in patients undergoing pulmonary resection with low diffusion capacity. *Ann Thorac Surg,* Vol.62, No.4, pp. 968-974; discussion 974-965

Boushy, S.F., Billig, D.M., North, L.B., Helgason, A.H. (1971). Clinical course related to preoperative and postoperative pulmonary function in patients with bronchogenic carcinoma. *Chest,* Vol.59, No.4, pp. 383-391

Boysen, P.G., Harris, J.O., Block, A.J., Olsen, G.N. (1981). Prospective evaluation for pneumonectomy using perfusion scanning: follow-up beyond one year. *Chest,* Vol.80, No.2, pp. 163-166

Brantigan, O.C. & Mueller, E. (1957). Surgical treatment of pulmonary emphysema. *Am Surg,* Vol.23, No.9, pp. 789-804

Brenner, D.R., McLaughlin, J.R., Hung, R.J. (2011). Previous lung diseases and lung cancer risk: a systematic review and meta-analysis. *PLoS One,* Vol.6, No.3, pp. e17479

Brunelli, A., Refai, M., Salati, M., Xiumé, F., Sabbatini, A. (2007). Predicted versus observed FEV1 and DLCO after major lung resection: a prospective evaluation at different postoperative periods. *Ann Thorac Surg,* Vol.83, No.3, pp. 1134-1139

Brutsche, M.H., Spiliopoulos, A., Bolliger, C.T., Licker, M., Frey, J.G., Tschopp, J.M. (2000). Exercise capacity and extent of resection as predictors of surgical risk in lung cancer. *Eur Respir J,* Vol.15, No.5, pp. 828-832

Celli, B.R. (1993). What is the value of preoperative pulmonary function testing? *Med Clin North Am,* Vol.77, No.2, pp. 309-325

Celli, B.R., Thomas, N.E., Anderson, J.A., Ferguson, G.T., Jenkins, C.R., Jones, P.W., et al. (2008). Effect of pharmacotherapy on rate of decline of lung function in chronic obstructive pulmonary disease: results from the TORCH study. *Am J Respir Crit Care Med,* Vol.178, No.4, pp. 332-338

Cesario, A., Ferri, L., Galetta, D., Pasqua, F., Bonassi, S., Clini, E., et al. (2007). Post-operative respiratory rehabilitation after lung resection for non-small cell lung cancer. *Lung Cancer,* Vol.57, No.2, pp. 175-180

Colice, G.L., Shafazand, S., Griffin, J.P., Keenan, R., Bolliger, C.T. (2007). Physiologic evaluation of the patient with lung cancer being considered for resectional surgery: ACCP evidenced-based clinical practice guidelines (2nd edition). *Chest,* Vol.132, No.3 Suppl, pp. 161S-177S.

Cook, J.A., Gius, D., Wink, D.A., Krishna, M.C., Russo, A., Mitchell, J.B. (2004). Oxidative stress, redox, and the tumor microenvironment. *Semin Radiat Oncol,* Vol.14, No.3, pp. 259-266

Cooper, J.D., Trulock, E.P., Triantafillou, A.N., Patterson, G.A., Pohl, M.S., Deloney, P.A., et al. (1995). Bilateral pneumectomy (volume reduction) for chronic obstructive pulmonary disease. *J Thorac Cardiovasc Surg,* Vol.109, No.1, pp. 106-116; discussion 116-109

Criner, G., Cordova, F.C., Leyenson, V., Roy, B., Travaline, J., Sudarshan, S., et al. (1998). Effect of lung volume reduction surgery on diaphragm strength. *Am J Respir Crit Care Med,* Vol.157, No.5 Pt 1, pp. 1578-1585

Damhuis, R.A. & Schutte, P.R. (1996). Resection rates and postoperative mortality in 7,899 patients with lung cancer. *Eur Respir J,* Vol.9, No.1, pp. 7-10

Doll, R. & Peto, R. (1976). Mortality in relation to smoking: 20 years' observations on male British doctors. *Br Med J,* Vol.2, No.6051, pp. 1525-1536

Edwards, J.G., Duthie, D.J., Waller, D.A. (2001). Lobar volume reduction surgery: a method of increasing the lung cancer resection rate in patients with emphysema. *Thorax,* Vol.56, No.10, pp. 791-795

Ferguson, M.K., Little, L., Rizzo, L., Popovich, K.J., Glonek, G.F., Leff, A., et al. (1988). Diffusing capacity predicts morbidity and mortality after pulmonary resection. *J Thorac Cardiovasc Surg,* Vol.96, No.6, pp. 894-900

Fishman, A., Martinez, F., Naunheim, K., Piantadosi, S., Wise, R., Ries, A., et al. (2003). A randomized trial comparing lung-volume-reduction surgery with medical therapy for severe emphysema. *N Engl J Med,* Vol.348, No.21, pp. 2059-2073

Flaherty, K.R., Kazerooni, E.A., Curtis, J.L., Iannettoni, M., Lange, L., Schork, M.A., et al. (2001). Short-term and long-term outcomes after bilateral lung volume reduction surgery : prediction by quantitative CT. *Chest,* Vol.119, No.5, pp. 1337-1346

Gelb, A.F., McKenna, R.J. Jr., Brenner, M. (2001). Expanding knowledge of lung volume reduction. *Chest,* Vol.119, No.5, pp. 1300-1302

Ginsberg, R.J. & Rubinstein, L.V. (1995). Randomized trial of lobectomy versus limited resection for T1 N0 non-small cell lung cancer. Lung Cancer Study Group. *Ann Thorac Surg,* Vol.60, No.3, pp. 615-622; discussion 622-613

Giordano, A., Calcagni, M.L., Meduri, G., Valente, S., Galli, G.. (1997). Perfusion lung scintigraphy for the prediction of postlobectomy residual pulmonary function. *Chest,* Vol.111, No.6, pp. 1542-1547

Harpole, D.H., Liptay, M.J., DeCamp, M.M. Jr., Mentzer, S.J., Swanson, S.J., Sugarbaker, D.J. (1996). Prospective analysis of pneumonectomy: risk factors for major morbidity and cardiac dysrhythmias. *Ann Thorac Surg,* Vol.61, No.3, pp. 977-982

Holden, D.A., Rice, T.W., Stelmach, K., Meeker, D.P. (1992). Exercise testing, 6-min walk, and stair climb in the evaluation of patients at high risk for pulmonary resection. *Chest,* Vol.102, No.6, pp. 1774-1779

Iwasawa, T., Saito, K., Ogawa, N., Ishiwa, N., Kurihara, H. (2002). Prediction of postoperative pulmonary function using perfusion magnetic resonance imaging of the lung. *J Magn Reson Imaging,* Vol.15, No.6, pp. 685-692

Juhl, B. & Frost, N. (1975). A comparison between measured and calculated changes in the lung function after operation for pulmonary cancer. *Acta Anaesthesiol Scand Suppl,* Vol.57, pp. 39-45

Kearney, D.J., Lee, T.H., Reilly, J.J., DeCamp, M.M., Sugarbaker, D.J. (1994). Assessment of operative risk in patients undergoing lung resection. Importance of predicted pulmonary function. *Chest,* Vol.105, No.3. pp. 753-759

Kim, J.K., Jang, S.H., Lee, J.W., Kim, D.G., Hong, K.W., Jung, K.S. (2008). Clinical parameters affecting prediction accuracy of postoperative lung function in non-small cell lung cancer. *Interact Cardiovasc Thorac Surg,* Vol.7, No.6, pp. 1019-1023

Kroenke, K., Lawrence, V.A., Theroux, J.F., Tuley, M.R., Hilsenbeck, S. (1993). Postoperative complications after thoracic and major abdominal surgery in patients with and without obstructive lung disease. *Chest,* Vol.104, No.5, pp. 1445-1451

Laros, C.D., Gelissen, H.J., Bergstein, P.G., Van den Bosch, J.M, Vanderschueren, R.G., Westermann CJ, et al. (1986). Bullectomy for giant bullae in emphysema. *J Thorac Cardiovasc Surg,*Vol. 91, No.1, pp. 63-70

Lee, J.H., Lee, Y.K., Kim, E.K,, Kim, T.H., Huh, J.W., Kim, W.J., et al. (2010). Responses to inhaled long-acting beta-agonist and corticosteroid according to COPD subtype. *Respir Med,* Vol.104, No.4, pp. 542-549

Lee, J.S., Huh, J.W., Chae, E.J., Seo, J.B., Ra, S.W., Lee, J.H., et al. (2011). Predictors of pulmonary function response to treatment with salmeterol/fluticasone in patients with chronic obstructive pulmonary disease. *J Korean Med Sci,* Vol.26, No.3, pp. 379-385

Licker, M..J, Widikker, I., Robert, J., Frey, J.G., Spiliopoulos, A., Ellenberger, C., et al. (2006). Operative mortality and respiratory complications after lung resection for cancer: impact of chronic obstructive pulmonary disease and time trends. *Ann Thorac Surg,* Vol.81, No.5, pp. 1830-1837

Loewen, G.M., Watson, D., Kohman, L., Herndon, J.E. 2nd., Shennib, H., Kernstine, K., et al. (2007). Preoperative exercise Vo2 measurement for lung resection candidates: results of Cancer and Leukemia Group B Protocol 9238. *J Thorac Oncol,* Vol.2, No.7, pp. 619-625

Markos, J., Mullan, B.P., Hillman, D.R., Musk, A.W., Antico, V.F., Lovegrove, F.T., et al. (1989). Preoperative assessment as a predictor of mortality and morbidity after lung resection. *Am Rev Respir Dis,* Vol.139, No.4, pp. 902-910

Mitsudomi, T., Mizoue, T., Yoshimatsu, T., Oyama, T., Nakanishi, R., Okabayashi, K., et al. (1996). Postoperative complications after pneumonectomy for treatment of lung cancer: multivariate analysis. *J Surg Oncol,* Vol.61, No.3, pp. 218-222

Nezu, K., Kushibe, K., Tojo, T., Takahama, M., Kitamura, S. (1998). Recovery and limitation of exercise capacity after lung resection for lung cancer. *Chest,* Vol.113, No.6, pp. 1511-1516

Nonaka, M., Kadokura, M., Yamamoto, S., Kataoka, D., Iyano, K., Kushihashi, T., et al. (2000). Analysis of the anatomic changes in the thoracic cage after a lung resection using magnetic resonance imaging. *Surg Today,* Vol.30, No.10, pp. 879-885

Olsen, G.N., Weiman, D.S., Bolton, J.W., Gass, G.D., McLain, W.C., Schoonover, G.A., et al. (1989). Submaximal invasive exercise testing and quantitative lung scanning in the evaluation for tolerance of lung resection. *Chest,* Vol.95, No.2, pp. 267-273

Pollock, M., Roa, J., Benditt, J., Celli, B. (1993). Estimation of ventilatory reserve by stair climbing. A study in patients with chronic airflow obstruction. *Chest,* Vol.104, No.5, pp. 1378-1383

Pompili, C., Brunelli, A., Refai, M., Xiumè, F., Sabbatini, A. (2010). Does chronic obstructive pulmonary disease affect postoperative quality of life in patients undergoing lobectomy for lung cancer? A case-matched study. *Eur J Cardiothorac Surg,* Vol.37, No.3, pp. 525-530

Rabe, K.F., Hurd, S., Anzueto, A., Barnes, P.J., Buist, S.A., Calverley, P., et al. (2007). Global strategy for the diagnosis, management, and prevention of chronic obstructive pulmonary disease: GOLD executive summary. *Am J Respir Crit Care Med,* Vol.176, No.6, pp. 532-555

Ribas, J., Díaz, O., Barberà, J.A., Mateu, M., Canalís, E., Jover, L., et al. (1998). Invasive exercise testing in the evaluation of patients at high-risk for lung resection. *Eur Respir J,* Vol.12, No.6, pp. 1429-1435

Richter Larsen, K., Svendsen, U.G., Milman, N., Brenøe, J., Petersen, B.N. (1997). Exercise testing in the preoperative evaluation of patients with bronchogenic carcinoma. *Eur Respir J,* Vol.10, No.7, pp. 1559-1565

Schipper, P.H., Meyers, B.F., Battafarano, R.J., Guthrie, T.J., Patterson, G.A., Cooper, J.D. (2004). Outcomes after resection of giant emphysematous bullae. *Ann Thorac Surg,* Vol.78, No.3, pp. 976-982; discussion 976-982

Sciurba, F.C., Rogers, R.M,, Keenan, R.J., Slivka, W.A., Gorcsan, J. 3rd., Ferson, P.F., et al. (1996). Improvement in pulmonary function and elastic recoil after lung-reduction surgery for diffuse emphysema. *N Engl J Med,* Vol.334, No.17, pp. 1095-1099

Sekine, Y., Iwata, T., Chiyo, M., Yasufuku, K., Motohashi, S., Yoshida, S., et al. (2003). Minimal alteration of pulmonary function after lobectomy in lung cancer patients with chronic obstructive pulmonary disease. *Ann Thorac Surg,* Vol.76, No.2, pp. 356-361; discussion 362

Soriano, J.B., Visick, G.T., Muellerova, H., Payvandi, N., Hansell, A.L. (2005). Patterns of comorbidities in newly diagnosed COPD and asthma in primary care. *Chest,* Vol.128, No.4: 2099-2107

Tashkin, D.P., Celli, B., Senn, S., Burkhart, D., Kesten, S., Menjoge, S., et al. (2008). A 4-year trial of tiotropium in chronic obstructive pulmonary disease. *N Engl J Med,* Vol.359 No.15, pp. 1543-1554

Thomas, J.A. & McIntosh, J.M. (1994). Are incentive spirometry, intermittent positive pressure breathing, and deep breathing exercises effective in the prevention of postoperative pulmonary complications after upper abdominal surgery? A systematic overview and meta-analysis. *Phys Ther,* Vol.74, No.1, pp. 3-10; discussion 10-16

Van Leuven, M., Clayman, J.A., Snow, N. (1999). Bronchial obstruction after upper lobectomy: kinked bronchus relieved by stenting. *Ann Thorac Surg,* Vol.68, No.1, pp. 235-237

Vestbo, J., Anderson, J.A., Calverley, P.M., Celli, B., Ferguson, G.T., Jenkins, C., et al. (2009). Adherence to inhaled therapy, mortality and hospital admission in COPD. *Thorax,* Vol.64, No.11, pp. 939-943

Wernly, J.A., DeMeester, .TR., Kirchner, .PT., Myerowitz, P.D., Oxford, D.E., Golomb, H.M. (1980). Clinical value of quantitative ventilation-perfusion lung scans in the surgical management of bronchogenic carcinoma. *J Thorac Cardiovasc Surg,* Vol.80, No.4, pp. 535-543

Win, T., Jackson, A., Sharples, L., Groves, A.M., Wells, F.C., Ritchie, A.J., et al. (2005). Cardiopulmonary exercise tests and lung cancer surgical outcome. *Chest,* Vol.127, No.4, pp. 1159-1165

Wu, M.T., Pan, H.B., Chiang, A.A., Hsu, H.K., Chang, H.C., Peng, N.J., et al. (2002). Prediction of postoperative lung function in patients with lung cancer: comparison of quantitative CT with perfusion scintigraphy. *AJR Am J Roentgenol,* Vol.178, No.3, pp. 667-672

Wyser, C., Stulz, P., Solèr, M., Tamm, M., Müller-Brand, J., Habicht, J., et al. (1999). Prospective evaluation of an algorithm for the functional assessment of lung resection candidates. *Am J Respir Crit Care Med,* Vol.159, No.5 Pt 1, pp. 1450-1456

Young, R.P., Hopkins, R.J., Christmas, T., Black, P.N., Metcalf, P., Gamble, G.D. (2009). COPD prevalence is increased in lung cancer, independent of age, sex and smoking history. *Eur Respir J,* Vol.34, No.2, pp. 380-386

Zeiher, B.G., Gross, T.J., Kern, J.A,, Lanza, L.A., Peterson, M.W. (1995). Predicting postoperative pulmonary function in patients undergoing lung resection. *Chest,* Vol.108, No.1, pp. 68-72

17

Patients' Survival Expectations Before Localized Prostate Cancer Treatment by Treatment Status

Ravinder Mohan, Hind Beydoun, Myra L. Barnes-Ely, LaShonda Lee, John W. Davis, Raymond Lance and Paul Schellhammer
Department of Family and Community Medicine, Eastern Virginia Medical School, Norfolk, Virginia, USA

1. Introduction

Although around 80% of men aged 80 years and older and 15% to 30% of men aged 50 years and older have microscopic undiagnosed prostate cancer found at autopsy, only 3% men die because of prostate cancer.[1] Increasing prostate-specific antigen (PSA) screening at younger ages has increased overdiagnosis[2] and overtreatment[3] of localized prostate cancer (LPC). More than 90% of US patients currently diagnosed with prostate cancer have LPC and approximately 94% of patients with LPC choose treatment.[4] Based on data from leading studies, a model had recently projected only a 0% to 2% 15-year mortality from low-grade (Gleason score <7) screen-detected LPC in men aged 55 to 74 years if they chose observation instead oftreatment.[5] By consensus, urologists and radiation oncologists recommend treatment for LPC if a patient has a further 10-year life expectancy [6] (the10-year rule[7]) regardless of cancer grade, even though no randomized trials have shown that treatment can improve survival in patients in whom the cancer was screen-detected. National guidelines by the American Cancer Society and the National Comprehensive Cancer Network (NCCN) also recommend treatment for most patients.[8] However, in the review by Zeliadt et al,[9] different studies had found that patients rate the sexual, urinary, and bowel side effects of treatment to be just as important as the potential benefit in survival; that if risks and benefits of treatment were explained with-out bias, 75% of patients chose a lower radiation dose despite a lower predicted survival; that 90% of physicians but fewer than 20% of patients ranked the effect of treatment on survival as one of their top 4 concerns; and that patients who chose treatment believed that treatment was guaranteed to improve survival. At a median of 6 years after treatment, health-related quality of life (HRQOL) of treated patients was worse than that of controlpatients.[10] Many patients regretted that they chosetreatment.[11]

To our knowledge, no studies of patient-physician communication have examined patients' anticipated survival benefit of treatment. Without data from randomized trials in screen-detected patients, it is difficult to counsel patients regarding their survival with and without treatment. Even with the use of multi-factorial models, accuracy of predicted survival is 75% or lower.[12] Physicians are also poor at estimating baseline co-morbidity adjusted life expectancy (CALE), which is critical in making an informed decision.[13] Thus, patients may accept a treatment recommendation not knowing what their baseline CALE is, how much the newly diagnosed cancer could reduce it, or how effectively treatment could minimize that reduction. Current over-treatment of LPC might be because patients do not understand the pros and cons of treatment.

In this study we surveyed newly diagnosed patients about their anticipation of survival with and without treatment. By estimating their baseline CALE without considering the newly diagnosed cancer, we calculated their perceived decrease in longevity with observation (PDLO), and their perceived increase in longevity with treatment (PILT) for the cancer.

2. Methods

We surveyed patients who had been newly diagnosed with LPC (stages T1a to T2c) in the preceding 6 months, had met with their urologist after the diagnosis, were scheduled to receive treatment or observation, and had not yet been treated with surgery or radiation. Patients with dementia, or those who could not read, write, or understand English, were excluded. All patients were recruited from a large, private urology practice in Norfolk, Virginia. Staff at this practice systematically contacted patients newly diagnosed with LPC between March 2005 and November 2007 regarding their interest in participation in a self-administered mailed survey. Two concomitant pretreatment self-administered surveys were used. The first survey asked patients about expectations of survival with and without treatment, co-morbid diseases, mood, social support, satisfaction with life, health, and education by physicians about treatment options. A list of health-related words in a closed envelope was mailed with the survey. Patients were requested to open the envelope and read these words on the telephone to a research assistant. This was done to estimate patient health literacy by using a brief version of the Rapid Estimation of Health Literacy in Medicine scale.[14] Patients were given a $10 stipend for completing this survey. A second pretreatment survey was a part of a longitudinal follow-up by urologists to evaluate generic HRQOL, prostate cancer related symptoms, and fear of cancer recurrence. The study methods were reviewed and approved by an Institutional Review Board.

3. Measures

The Charlson Comorbidity Index (CCI) is a validated measure of co-morbidity. We used a patient self-reported CCI scale that asked about the presence and severity of 12 chronic conditions; the Prostate Cancer Outcomes Study used this CCI version.[15] Score categories are 0, 1, 2, and 3 or more diseases.

The NCCN practice guidelines had recommended, for the first time in 2007,[8] that the health adjusted life expectancy of LPC patients can be estimated by weighting age-based life expectancy by 1.5 for patients in the highest health quartile, using no weighting for patients in the middle 2 health quartiles, and weighting by 0.5 for patients in the lowest health quartile. We used co-morbidity scores as surrogate markers of health status because co-morbidity is the main determinant of life expectancy in older patients, [16] and the most important prognostic factor for patients with LPC who are <75 years old is the co-morbidity score. [17] We categorized patients into health quartiles by using their CCI score (0 disease score = highest health quartile; 1 or 2 disease score = middle 2 health quartiles; 3 or higher disease score = lowest health quartile). Our basis of equating a 1 or 2 disease score with the middle 2 health quartiles was that almost half (49%) of the 3173 patients newly diagnosed with LPC in a Prostate Cancer Outcomes Study15 had a disease score of 1 or 2, and almost half (55.5%) of our patients had a disease score of 1 or 2. Both studies used the same version and scoring of the CCI. Patients were placed in 4 CALE categories: <5 years, 5 to 10 years, 10 to 20 years, and 20 years. These 4 categories were scored, respectively, from 1 to 4.

Patients were asked the following 2 questions: "How long do you expect you will live *without* any treatment for prostate cancer?" (Q1) and "How long do you expect you will live after treatment for prostate cancer?" (Q2). The possible responses to both questions were grouped into 4 categories (similar to the CALE categories): <5 years, 5 to 10 years, 10 to 20 years, and >20 years. These 4 categories were also scored from 1 to 4, respectively. Based on Q1, Q2, and CALE scores, we calculated the patient's PDLO (which is CALE category score minus Q1 category score) and the patient's PILT (which is Q2 category score minus Q1 category score). A PDLO of 10 or more years is at least a 2-category difference between the CALE category and the Q1 category; this is only possible if the CALE was >20 years and the Q1 response was 5 to 10 years or if the CALE was 10 to 20 years and the Q1 response was <5 years. Similarly, a PILT of 10 or more years indicates that the response to Q2 was 10 years or more than the response to Q1. We conducted ordinal logistic regression analyses to identify the main socio-demographic, health, and cancer characteristics that could predict PDLO and PILT of 10 or more years.

The following validated self-administered scales were used. (1) The Short-Form 36 (SF-36, version 2) measures generic HRQOL; we calculated physical component summary and mental component summary scores from SF-36 data.[18] (2) The Prostate Cancer Index measures urinary, sexual, and bowel symptoms and how much they bother the patient.[19] (3) The Duke Activity Status Index[20] measures functional capacity in metabolic equivalents; this scale asks patients whether they could perform 12 activities which have different levels of exertion. (4) The Hospital Anxiety and Depression Scale measures the presence and severity of anxiety and depression.[21] (5) The Fear of Cancer Recurrence Scale measures the fear of possible cancer recurrence.[22] (6) The Medical Outcomes Study Social Support Survey measures social support in an overall score that includes multidimensional sub-scores. [23] (7) The Delighted-Terrible Seven Faces Scale[24] was used to measure patient satisfaction with life, health, and with education given by physicians about treatment options for LPC. (8) The Rapid Estimation of Health Literacy in Medicine scale, discussed earlier, measures health literacy; this was the only scale administered by telephone.[14]

4. Statistical analyses

Frequencies and relative frequencies were used to describe categorical variables. Continuous variables were described using the mean, median, and SD. Chi-square tests, Fisher's exact test, and independent sample *t* tests were used to examine bivariate associations. Unadjusted and adjusted odds ratios (ORs) and their 95% CIs were estimated using ordinal logistic regression analysis. Socio-demographic and health factors that were found to be associated with PDLO and PILT in the bivariate analysis at an alpha level of 0.20 were kept in the multivariate models. All analyses were performed using SAS software (version 9.1, SAS Institute, Inc., Cary, NC).

5. Results

Surveys were mailed to 430 patients newly diagnosed with LPC, but 69 patients had already started treatment by the time the patients received the surveys, 3 patients never received the surveys, and 2 patients were found to be ineligible to participate because their cancer was not localized to the prostate. Of the 356 remaining patients, 104 patients did not return the survey because they were "not interested" in participating and 68 patients who did not return the surveys did not give a reason for not participating or could not be contacted. One hundred eighty-four of 356 patients (survey response rate of 52%) completed and returned the first pretreatment survey; 23 of these 184 patients (12.5%) patients chose observation. Table 1 shows a demographic comparison of patients who chose treatment or observation. Mean patient age was 61.5 years, and most patients reported college education and a family income of >$50,000.

Overall		Treatment	Observation	
Characteristic	(n [%])	(n [%])	(n [%])	P‡
Age (years)	n = 184	n = 161	n = 23	
<60	71 (38.6)	68 (42.2)	3 (13.0)	
60–70	91 (49.5)	81 (50.3)	10 (43.5)	
>70	22 (11.9)	12 (7.5)	10 (43.5)	<.0001
Mean +/- SD	61.5 +/- 7.9	60.6 +/- 7.6	68.2 +/- 5.9	<.0001
Race	n = 184	n = 161	n = 23	
African American	26 (14.1)	26 (16.2)	0 (0.0)	
White	158 (85.9)	135 (83.9)	23 (100)	.05§
Education	n = 180	n = 157	n = 23	
<High school	7 (3.9)	7 (4.5)	0 (0.0)	
High school	65 (36.1)	56 (35.7)	9 (39.1)	
College	108 (60.0)	94 (59.9)	14 (60.9)	.58
Health literacy	n = 173	n = 150	n = 23	
Below 6th grade	1 (0.6)	1 (0.7)	0 (0.0)	
6th-9th grade	16 (9.3)	15 (10.0)	1 (4.4)	
>9th grade	156 (90.2)	134 (89.3)	22 (95.7)	.63
Family income	n = 179	n = 156	n = 23	
Low (>$50,000)	57 (31.8)	50 (32.0)	7 (30.4)	
High (=>$50,000)	122 (68.2)	106 (67.9)	16 (69.6)	.88

*Treatment patients had either surgery or radiotherapy.
†Observation patients had neither surgery nor radiotherapy.
‡Unless otherwise specified, statistical significance is for chi-square test (categorical variables) or independent samples t test (continuous variables).
§Fischer's exact test.

Table 1. Comparison of Socio-demographic Characteristics of Patients with Localized Prostate Cancer who Chose Treatment* and Observation†

Table 2 shows a comparison of patients who chose treatment or observation by cancer grade, PSA, life expectancy by age, and co-morbidity scores. Mean Gleason grade was 6.6. Table 2 also includes a comparison of these patient groups by SF-36 scores (Physical Component and Mental Component Scores), as well as the urinary, sexual, and bowel function scores of the 144 of 184 patients who had also returned the second pretreatment survey. Table 3 shows a comparison of patients who chose treatment or observation by CALE, anxiety and depression, function capacity, social support, and satisfaction. Mean CALE was 22.9 years. Table 4 shows the baseline CALE for the 184 patients and the responses of 170 of the 184 patients who had answered questions about their perceived life expectancy without treatment (Q1) and with treatment (Q2) of the cancer. Without treatment, perceived life expectancy was <5 years in 15.2%, 5 to 10 years in 48.8%, 11 to 19 years in 33.5% and 20 or more years in 2.4% of the patients. With treatment, it was <5 years in 0.6%, 5 to 10 years in 6.5%, 11 to 19 years in 30.0%, and 20 or more years in 62.9% of the patients. By contrast, baseline CALE was <5 years in 0.5%, 5 to 10 years in 2.2%, 11 to 19 years in 36.4%, and 20 or more years in 60.9%. A total of 170 patients had data on CALE, Q1, and Q2. As compared with CALE, 65 (38.2%) of these 170 patients expected their survival to decrease by 10 or more years without treatment. As compared with their perceived survival without treatment, 81 (47.6%) of 170 patients expected their survival to increase by 10 or more years with treatment. Of the 108 patients with a baseline CALE of >20 years, only 2 (1.9%) expected to live beyond 20 years without treatment whereas 84 (77.8%) expected to live beyond 20 years with treatment (data not shown). Neither of these perceptions was significantly related to whether the patients chose treatment or observation. However, to a statistically insignificant extent, patients who chose treatment were more likely than observation patients to expect a 10 or more years reduction in survival without treatment (50% vs. 33.3%, _2 test; *P* = .26) and a 10 or more year increase in survival with treatment (39.9% vs. 16.7%, Fisher's exact test; *P* =.13).

Overall		Treatment	Observation	
Factors	(n [%])	(n [%])	(n [%])	P*
Gleason Grade	n = 184	n = 161	N = 23	
2–4	0 (0.0)	0 (0.0)	0 (0.0)	
5–6	103 (55.9)	84 (52.1)	19 (82.6)	
7	62 (33.7)	60 (37.3)	2 (8.7)	
8–10	19 (10.3)	17 (10.6)	2 (8.7)	0.02
Mean +/- SD	6.6 +/- 0.7	6.6 +/- 0.7	6.2 +/- 0.7	0.02
Prostate-specific antigen	n = 183	n = 161	n = 23	
=<10	159 (86.9)	139 (86.3)	21 (91.3)	
>10	24 (13.1)	22 (13.7)	2 (8.7)	0.74
Mean +/- SD	6.7 +/- 5.3	6.8 +/- 5.5	5.6 +/- 3.4	0.14
Life expectancy by age (years)	n = 183	n = 160	N = 23	
<10	4 (2.2)	2 (1.3)	2 (8.7)	
10–20	104 (56.8)	86 (53.8)	18 (78.3)	
>=20	75 (40.9)	72 (45.0)	3 (13.0)	0.002*
Comorbidity score	n = 184	n = 161	N = 23	

0	74 (40.2)	66 (40.9)	8 (34.8)	
1	75 (40.8)	67 (41.6)	8 (34.8)	
2	27 (14.7)	23 (14.3)	4 (17.4)	
>=3	8 (4.4)	5 (3.1)	3 (13.0)	0.16
Mean +/- SD	0.9 +/- 1.0	0.83 +/- 0.96	1.26 +/- 1.5	0.18
Short Form-36 subscales				
Physical component summary	n = 142	n = 134	n = 8	
Mean +/- SD	54.5 +/- 7.6	54.5 +/- 7.2	52.6 +/- 12.3	0.66
Mental component summary	n = 142	n = 134	n = 8	
Mean+/- SD	44.1 +/-6.8	43.9 +/- 6.9	46.4 +/- 4.5	0.29
Prostate cancer index				
Urinary	n = 141	n = 132	n = 9	
Mean +/- SD	90.2 +/- 16.9	90.1 +/- 17.4	91.3 +/- 9.3	0.83
Bowel	n = 142	n = 133	n = 9	
Mean +/- SD	88.8 +/- 12.5	88.5 +/- 12.8	92.9 +/- 4.5	0.03
Sexual	n = 137	n = 128	n = 9	
Mean +/- SD	57.7 +/- 29.9	57.8 +/-30.4	55.4 +/- 23.8	0.82
Urinary Bother	n = 144	n = 135	n = 9	
Mean +/- SD	86.1 +/- 23.0	85.9 +/- 23.4	88.9 +/- 18.2	0.71
Bowel Bother	n = 144	n = 135	n = 9	
Mean +/- SD	92.5 +/- 17.5	92.0 +/- 17.9	100 +/- 0.0	<0.0001
Sexual Bother	n = 142	n = 133	n = 9	
Mean +/- SD	65.8 +/- 36.8	65.4 +/- 36.8	72.2 +/- 38.4	0.59
Fear of cancer recurrence	n = 141	n = 133	n = 8	
Mean +/- SD	10.7 +/- 3.8	10.7 +/- 3.7	10.9 +/- 4.5	0.92

Table 2. Comparison of Patients who Chose Treatment and Observation by Prostate Cancer-Related and Health Factors

Overall		Treatment	Observation	
Characteristic	(n [%]	(n [%]* **	(n [%]† ***	P‡ *
Comorbidity-adjusted life expectancy				
All ages	184 (100)	161 (100)	23 (100)	
<5 years	1 (0.5)	0 (0)	1 (4.3)	
5–10 years	4 (2.2)	2 (1.2)	2 (8.7)	
11–19 years	67 (36.4)	52 (32.3)	15 (65.2)	
>=20 years	112 (60.9)	107 (66.5)	5 (21.7)	<.0001
Mean +/- SD	22.9 +/- 7.6	23.9 +/- 7.3	<	<.0001
Anxiety score	n = 183	n = 160	n = 23	

None/normal (0–7)	145 (79.2)	123 (76.9)	22 (95.7)	
Mild anxiety (8–10)	23 (12.6)	23 (14.4)	0 (0.0)	
Moderate anxiety (11–14)	12 (6.6)	11 (6.9)	1 (4.4)	
Clinical (15–21)	3 (1.6)	3 (1.9)	0 (0.0)	.18
Mean +/- SD	5.1 +/- 3.5	5.4 +/- 3.5	2.8 +/- 2.9	.0008
Depression score	n = 178	n = 156	n = 22	
None/normal (0–7)	172 (96.6)	150 (96.2)	22 (100)	
Mild depression (8–10)	4 (2.3)	4 (2.6)	0 (0.0)	
Moderate (11–14)	1 (0.6)	1 (0.6)	0 (0.0)	
Clinical (15–21)	1 (0.6)	1 (0.6)	0 (0.0)	.83
Mean +/- SD	1.7 +/- 2.3	1.7 +/- 2.4	1.4 +/- 1.7	.49
Functional capacity	n = 184	n = 160	n = 23	
Mild activities (<3 METs)	1 (0.5)	1 (0.6)	0 (0.0)	
Moderate activities (3–6 METs)	20 (10.9)	15 (9.3)	5 (21.7)	
Vigorous activities (>=6 METs)	163 (88.6)	145 (90.1)	18 (78.3)	.19
Social support	n = 183	n = 160	n = 23	
<50	7 (3.8)	6 (3.8)	1 (4.4)	
50–75	33 (18.0)	29 (18.1)	4 (17.4)	
75–100	143 (78.1)	125 (78.1)	18 (78.3)	.98
Satisfaction with Life	n = 178	n = 156	n = 22	
Delighted or highly satisfied	138 (77.5)	121 (77.6)	17 (77.3)	
Satisfied or lower	40 (22.5)	35 (22.4)	5 (22.7)	.97
Mean +/- SD	6.0 +/- 0.9	5.9 +/- 0.9	6.1 +/- 1.0	.64
Satisfaction with health	n = 178	n = 156	n = 22	
Delighted or highly satisfied	85 (47.8)	72 (46.1)	13 (59.1)	
Satisfied or lower	93 (52.3)	84 (53.9)	9 (40.9)	.26
Mean +/- SD	5.0 +/- 1.3	5.0 +/- 1.3	5.4 +/- 1.4	.19
Satisfaction with education by physician in treatment choices	n = 178	n = 156	n = 22	
Delighted or highly satisfied	141 (79.2)	126 (80.8)	15 (68.2)	
Satisfied or lower	37 (20.8)	30 (19.2)	7 (31.8)	.17
Mean +/- SD	6.1 +/- 0.9	6.1 +/- 0.9	5.9 +/- 1.1	.1

*Treatment patients had either surgery or radiotherapy.
†Observation patients had neither surgery nor radiotherapy.
‡Unless otherwise specified, statistical significance is for chi-square test (categorical variables) or independent samples t test (continuous variables).
MET, metabolic equivalent.

Table 3. Distribution of Men by Prostate Cancer-Related and Health Characteristics

Expected Survival (years)	Baseline CALE Score	Q1	Q2
	(n = 184)	(n = 170)	(n = 170)
<5	1 (0.5)	26 (15.2)	1 (0.6)
5–10	4 (2.2)	83 (48.8)	11 (6.5)
11–19	67 (36.4)	57 (33.5)	51 (30.0)
>=20	112 (60.9)	4 (2.4)	107 (62.9)

Data provided as n (%).
CALE, co-morbidity adjusted life expectancy; Q1, How long do you expect you will live without any treatment for prostate cancer?; Q2, How long do you expect you will live after the treatment of your choice for prostate cancer?

Table 4. Distribution of Men with Localized Prostate Cancer by Calculated Co-morbidity Adjusted Life Expectancy

Tables 5 and 6 present ordinal logistic regression models for PDLO and PILT. Age, CALE, depression, and anxiety scores predicted both PDLO and PILT. Furthermore, PSA level predicted PDLO, whereas social support predicted PILT.

	Unadjusted Effects				Adjusted Effects (OR 95% CI)
	PDLO =<0*	PDLO = 1†	PDLO =>2‡	OR (95% CI)	
Age	25	62	83	1.08 (1.04–1.13)	1.01 (0.92–1.10)
PSA level	25	62	82	0.94 (0.88–1.00)	0.93 (0.86–1.00)
CALE	25	62	83	0.92 (0.88–0.96)	0.93 (0.84–1.02)
Anxiety score	25	62	83	0.88 (0.81–0.96)	0.96 (0.85–1.08)
Depression score	25	58	82	0.79 (0.67–0.93)	0.85 (0.69–1.04)

*A (PDLO) =<0 (reference group) indicates that CALE and self-reported survival expectation without treatment are within the same range or CALE is less.
†A (PDLO) = 1 suggests that CALE exceeds self-reported survival expectation without treatment by one response category.
‡A (PDLO) >=2 suggests that CALE exceeds self-reported survival expectation without treatment by at least 2 response categories (ie.,
about 10 years). All covariates in the ordinal logistic regression model are defined as continuous variables.
PDLO, perceived decrease in longevity with observation (categorized); PSA, prostate-specific antigen; CALE, comorbidity adjusted life expectancy; OR, odds ratio.

Table 5. Ordinal Logistic Regression Modeling for Perceived Decrease in Longevity with Observation (PDLO) among Men with Localized Prostate Cancer

	Unadjusted Effects				Adjusted Effects (OR 95% CI)
	PILT =<0*	PILT = 1†	PILT =>2‡	OR (95% CI)	
Age	18	87	65	1.08 (1.04–1.13)	1.09 (0.99–1.19)
CALE	18	87	65	0.93 (0.89–0.97)	1.02 (0.93–1.12)
Anxiety Score	18	87	65	0.89 (0.82–0.98)	0.91 (0.81–1.02)
Depression score	18	83	64	0.93 (0.82–1.05)	1.06 (0.89–1.26)
Social Support	18	87	65	1.01 (0.99–1.03)	1.00 (0.98–1.02)

*PILT <=0 (reference group) indicates that CALE and self-reported survival expectation with treatment are within the same range or CALE is less.
†A (PILT) = 1 suggests that CALE exceeds self-reported survival expectation with treatment by one response category.
‡A (PILT) >=2 suggests that CALE exceeds self-reported survival expectation with treatment by at least 2 response categories (ie.,
about 10 years). All covariates in the ordinal logistic regression model are defined as continuous variables.
PILT, perceived increase in longevity with treatment (categorized); CALE, comorbidity adjusted life expectancy; OR, odds ratio.

Table 6. Ordinal Logistic Regression Modeling for Perceived Increase in Longevity with Treatment (PILT) among Men with Localized Prostate Cancer

6. Discussion

Prostate cancer is the most common solid cancer in men. Younger patients make up a fast growing population that is being screen-detected and treated for low-risk LPC.[25] To our knowledge, this is the first study to report the perceptions of newly diagnosed patients about how the cancer or its treatment could affect their survival. The mean age of our patients (61.5 years) was similar to the range of 58 to 64 years of US patients currently undergoing radical prostatectomy.[26] The mean Gleason grade was 6.6 in our patients, similar to other series in which almost half of screen-detected cancers were "insignificant."[27] By choosing treatment, these low-risk patients had accepted the treatment side effects in exchange for longer anticipated survival. Our questions were designed to find how much longer these patients expected to live by choosing treatment. These expectations were evaluated after the patients had discussed their treatment options with their urologists. Despite their mean baseline CALE of 22.9 years, without treatment, 26 of 170 patients expected to live <5 years and only 4 expected to live >20 years; with treatment, only 1 expected to live <5 years and 107 patients expected to live >20 years.

What should these patients really be expecting? Nearly 86% of all patients diagnosed through PSA screening are not expected to die because of prostate cancer.[28] The Connecticut Tumor Registry found that almost 20% of patients with Gleason grade 6 or higher who chose observation died as a result of LPC during a period of 20 years.[29] However, all the Registry's patients had been clinically diagnosed; in contrast, patients diagnosed with screen-detected LPC are expected to have a longer survival because of a gain in lead time. Patients in another commonly cited natural history study[30] were also not diagnosed by PSA screening. A review[31] found that only one randomized, high-quality trial[32] could find a survival benefit of treatment, but in this trial 95% of patients had cancer that was clinically palpable (and not detected by PSA screening), putting this cohort in an intermediate- to high-risk category. A study of 44,630 men found a survival benefit of treatment, [33] but only 2.1% of the patient sample had died of prostate cancer. If adjusted for lead time provided by screening and also for the impairment of HRQOL that follows treatment, treatment was projected to enhance quality-adjusted survival by only 0.5 year. [34]

Overtreatment would be expected if patients believe that treatment will lead to a much longer survival. Many studies have found that nearly every patient initially wants eradication of the cancer. [9] In qualitative studies, some patients accepted side effects for any gain in survival but they were convinced that treatment would improve survival.[9] Assuming that tumors would grow exponentially, urologists at the Mayo Clinic were also of the opinion that only 0.3% and 14.5% of screen-detected LPCs were "clinically insignificant."[35] Patient anxiety caused by the new diagnosis of cancer and the consensus advice of specialists that LPC patients with a CALE of >10 years should choose treatment or be offered treatment6 will lead to high treatment rates. In 70% to 90% of patients, a treatment plan is usually made in a single visit to the urologist after a positive biopsy.[36]

The mean Gleason grade of our patients was 6.6, and in 87% of patients the mean PSA was <10, both of which are low-risk categories but for which national guidelines recommend either observation or treatment.[8] Only 12.5% of patients in our study chose observation. Specialists frequently recommend treatment even in low-risk patients because over 10 to 15 years the cancer may progress.[29] To manage this risk, a strategy of active surveillance with deferred initial treatment[28] is being increasingly recommended for patients at lower risk, ie, with cancers of Gleason grade <7, cancer stages T1c to T2a, and PSA <10. Almost half of patients with screen-detected cancer possess such characteristics. [27] In conjunction with specialists, primary care physicians (PCPs) can follow patients who choose this strategy. PCPs may also offer more balanced advice because they might be more knowledgeable about the patient's preferences, co-morbidities, and baseline CALE.[37] Patients with LPC may also want to review educational materials with their PCP. The American Cancer Society website was recommended because its content, accuracy, balance, and readability was rated the highest among 44 patient education materials about LPC.[38]

Overtreatment can also be reduced with decreased screening, and several studies have shown that fewer patients want PSA screening if they are counseled before screening.[39] Enthusiasm for routine screening is high among specialists who treat LPC. In a random nationwide survey, 43% of 559 radiation oncologists recommended routine PSA screening in average-risk patients older than 80.[6] Primary care physicians who frequently order PSA testing without much discussion about risks and benefits of testing cited reasons of lack of time, competing demands, limited patient health literacy, and fear of liability.[40] Prescreening counseling is difficult because it is unclear what and how much discussion should occur. As yet, we cannot say that screening or treatment can improve survival. The deleterious effects of treatment on urinary, bowel, and sexual dysfunction are better known; however, their frequencies and severities after different treatment techniques have been reported in more than 800 publications,[41] vary greatly, and are difficult to balance. We can also share with patients that there is a small risk of immediate morbidity and mortality associated with prostate biopsy and cancer treatment; that a new anxiety results from a positive PSA test, whether or not it is followed by a negative biopsy; and that we cannot compare the risk of death caused by co-morbid diseases with that of death caused by cancer without knowing the grade and stage of the cancer. However, patients must also know that, even if diagnosed with cancer, no randomized controlled trial has shown that treatment can or cannot improve survival in patients with screen-detected cancer. Interestingly, a study found that more African American patients wanted PSA screening after the use of a decision aid, [39] presumably because of the appreciation of the higher risk in African American patients.

In our patients, age, CALE, depression, and anxiety were the most important predictors of PDLO or PILT. Though PSA level also influenced PDLO, PILT was related to social support. PDLO and PILT were not related to other factors such as race; income; education; health literacy; physical and mental summary SF-36 scores; urinary, bowel, and sexual symptoms; choice of treatment or observation; fear of cancer recurrence; functional capacity; and satisfaction with life, health, or with education by physicians in cancer treatment options. Although the association of PDLO and PILT with continuous depression scores was statistically significant, the importance of this finding is unclear given that 96.6% patients had a depression score of <7, which indicates no depression.

Our findings may be difficult to generalize because our study sample was small. However, the differences we found between CALE and patient expectations of survival with and without treatment were large. Also, the mean age[26] and mean cancer grade[27] of patients newly diagnosed with LPC in large series and in our patients were similar. Our patients were treated by urologists in a private practice and more than 80% of urologists in the United States are in private practice.[42] Our method of equating CCI scores with NCCN recommended health quartiles to estimate CALE is new and has not been previously validated. We used this method because we could not find any other validated method to estimate long-term health-adjusted life expectancy in individual ambulatory patients. Finally, we lost accuracy in the estimation of PDLO and PILT by asking patients to predict their survival in ordinal intervals rather than in a discrete number of years. We used ordinal intervals because it might be easier for patients to predict their survival this way, and the intervals allowed an estimation of PDLO and PILT of more than or less than 10 years. We have also published these findings earlier. [43]

We had also studied whether our patients had adequate Knowledge, Understanding and Judgment (KUJ) of their treatment options by using a KUJ 18-item questionnaire that we have developed; we found that although the vast majority of our patients were educated, had good health literacy and had higher income, over half of the patients incorrectly answered over half of the questions on the KUJ scale. These findings have been published separately.[44] Additionally, we had studied whether our patients had chosen treatment or observation in accordance with current NCCN guidelines and we had found that a majority had chosen over-treatment, i.e., they had chosen treatment even though for their clinical situation the NCCN had recommended observation as an equal alternative. These findings were published recently, [45] and had demonstrated that with the use of our method to estimate CALE it becomes feasible to use NCCN guidelines in decision-making in individual patients. Based on our research and NCCN guidelines, in August 2011 we have published a comprehensive and easy-to-understand approach in the journal *American Family Physician* (AFP)[46] which can be used by newly-diagnosed patients and their physicians in quickly reaching an evidence-based and guideline-driven treatment choice. Decision-making is very hard especially for low-risk patients, traditionally primary care physicians are not involved in this process, and over 70% to 80% patients choose a treatment or observation in the first visit to the urologist after a positive biopsy. Although newer guidelines now recommend against PSA screening,[47] this recommendation carries the risk of increasing mortality due to prostate cancer and prostate cancer is already the second most common cause of cancer death in American men. The algorithm and tools provided in our publication in AFP can empower primary care physicians in counseling newly-diagnosed patients and reduce the risk of over-treatment by convincing low-risk patients to choose active surveillance. With this safeguard, patients and physicians can choose screening for prostate cancer with less hesitation.

7. Conclusion

In patients with newly diagnosed LPC, in whom the mean cancer grade was <7 and in whom education, income, and health literacy was intermediate to high, almost 38% of our patients had expectations of a reduction in survival of 10 or more years if they chose observation, and 48.8% patients expected an improvement in survival of 10 or more years through choosing treatment. These expectations are highly unrealistic because no study has shown that the cancer or its treatment can affect survival by even 1 year, especially in screen-detected patients with a cancer Gleason grade of <7.

8. Acknowledgements

This article has been reproduced by permission of the American Board of Family Medicine. We thank Mr. Brian Main, Department of Urology, Eastern Virginia Medical School, for help with data entry and analysis.

9. References

[1] Taichman RS, Loberg RD, Mehra R, Pienta KJ. The evolving biology and treatment of prostate cancer. J Clin Invest 2007;117:2351-61.

[2] Etzioni R, Penson D, Legler JM, et al. Overdiagnosis due to prostate-specific antigen screening: lessons from US prostate cancer incidence trends. J Natl Cancer Inst 2002;94:981-90.

[3] Miller DC, Gruber SB, Hollenbeck BK, Montie JE, Wei JT. Incidence of initial local therapy among men with lower-risk prostate cancer in the United States. J Natl Cancer Inst 2006;98:1134-41.

[4] Harlan SR, Cooperberg MR, Elkin EP, et al. Time trends and characteristics of men choosing watchful waiting for initial treatment of localized prostate cancer: results from CaPSURE. J Urol 2003;170:1804-7.

[5] Parker C, Muston D, Melia J, Moss S, Dearnely D. A model of the natural history of screen-detected prostate cancer, and the effect of radical treatment on overall survival. Br J Cancer 2006;94:1361- 8.

[6] Fowler FJ, Collins MM, Albertsen PC, Zeitman A, Elliott DB, Barry MJ. Comparison of recommendations by urologists and radiation oncologists for treatment of localized prostate cancer. JAMA 2000; 283:3217.

[7] Krahn MD, Bremner KE, Asaria J, et al. The ten year rule revisited: accuracy of clinicians' estimates of life expectancy in patients with localized prostate cancer. Urology 2002;60:258-63.

[8] National Comprehensive Cancer Network. NCCN Clinical Practice Guidelines in Oncology: prostate cancer. Available from http://www.nccn.org/professionals/physician_gls/PDF/prostate.pdf. Accessed, 25 January 2009.

[9] Zeliadt SB, Ramsey SD, Penson DF, et al. Why do men choose one treatment over another? A review of patient decision making for localized prostate cancer. Cancer 2006;106:1865–74.

[10] Miller DC, Sanda MG, Dunn RL, et al. Long-term outcomes among localized prostate cancer survivors: health-related quality-of-life changes after radical prostatectomy, external radiation, and brachytherapy. J Clin Oncol 2005;23:2772- 80.

[11] Hu JC, Kwan L, Saigal CS, Litwin MS. Regret in men treated for localized prostate cancer. J Urol 2003;169:2279–83.

[12] Walz J, Gallina A, Saad F, et al. A nomogram predicting 10-year life expectancy in candidates for radical prostatectomy or radiotherapy for prostate cancer. J Clin Oncol 2007;25:3576–81.

[13] Wilson JRM, Clarke MG, Ewings P, Graham JD, MacDonagh R. The assessment of patient life expectancy: how accurate are urologists and oncologists? BJU Int 2005;95:794–8.

[14] Bass PF, Wilson JF, Griffith CH. A shortened instrument for literacy screening. J Gen Intern Med 2003;18:1036–8.

[15] Hoffman RM, Stone SM, Espey D, Potosky A. Differences between men with screening-detected versus clinically diagnosed prostate cancers in the USA. BMC Cancer 2005;5:27.

[16] Walter LC, Covinsky KE. Cancer screening in elderly patients: a framework for individualized decision making. JAMA 2001;285:2750–6.

[17] Post PN, Hansen BE, Kil PJM, Coebergh JWW. The independent prognostic value of comorbidity among men aged _75 years with localized prostate cancer: a population-based study. BJU Int 2001;87:821–6.

[18] Ware JE, Kosinki M. SF-36 Physical and Mental Health Summary Scales: a manual for users of version 1, 2nd ed. Lincoln (RI): QualityMetric, Inc.; 2005.

[19] Litwin M, Hays RD, Fink A, Ganz PA, Leake B, Brooke RH. The UCLA Prostate Cancer Index: development, reliability, and validity of a health-related quality of life measure. Med Care 1998;36:1002–12.

[20] Hlatky MA, Boineau RE, Higginbotham MB, et al. A brief self-administered questionnaire to determine functional capacity (The Duke Activity Status Index). Am J Cardiol 1989;64:651- 4.

[21] Zigmond AS, Snaith RP. The Hospital Anxiety and Depression scale. Acta Psychiatr Scand 1983;67:361–70.

[22] Mehta SS, Lubeck DP, Pasta DJ, Litwin M. Fear of cancer recurrence in patients undergoing definitive treatment for prostate cancer: results from CaPSURE. J Urol 2003;170:1931–3.

[23] Sherbourne CD, Stewart AL. The MOS Social Support Survey. Soc Sci Med 1991;32:705–14.

[24] Bowling A. Measuring health: a review of quality of life measurement scales, 2nd ed. Buckingham (UK): Open University Press; 1997.

[25] Cooperberg MR, Lubeck DP, Meng MV, Mehta SS, Caroll PR. The changing face of low-risk prostate cancer: trends in clinical presentation and primary management. J Clin Oncol 2004;22:2141–9.

[26] Jang TL, Yossepowitch O, Bianco FJ, Scardino PT. Low risk prostate cancer in men under age 65: the case for definitive treatment. Urol Oncol 2007;25: 510–4.

[27] Draisma G, Boer R, Otto SJ, et al. Lead times and over detection due to prostate-specific antigen screening: estimates from the European Randomized Study of Screening for Prostate Cancer. J Natl Cancer Inst 2003;95:868 –78.

[28] Klotz L. Active surveillance for prostate cancer: for whom? J Clin Oncol 2005;23:8165–9.

[29] Albertsen PC, Hanley JA, Fine J. 20-year outcomes following conservative management of clinically localized prostate cancer. JAMA 2005;293:2095–101.

[30] Johansson JE, Andren O, Andersson SO, et al. Natural history of early, localized prostate cancer. JAMA 2004;291:2713–9.
[31] Alibhai SM, Klotz LH. A systematic review of randomized trials in localized prostate cancer. Can J Urol 2004;11:2110 –7.
[32] Bill-Axelson A, Holmberg L, Ruutu M, et al. Radical prostatectomy versus watchful waiting in early prostate cancer. N Engl J Med 2005;352:1977–84.
[33] Wong YN, Mitra N, Hudes G, et al. Survival associated with treatment vs observation of localized prostate cancer in elderly men. JAMA 2006;296: 2683–93.
[34] Bhatnagar V, Stewart ST, Bonney WW, Kaplan RM. Treatment options for localized prostate cancer: quality-adjusted life years and the effects of leadtime. Urology 2004;63:103–9.
[35] Dugan JA, Bostwick DG, Myers RP, Qian J, Bregstralh EJ, Oesterling JE. The definition and preoperative prediction of clinically insignificant prostate cancer. JAMA 1996;275:288 –94.
[36] Cohen H, Britten N. Who decides about prostate cancer treatment? A qualitative study. Fam Pract 2003;20:724 –9.
[37] Mohan R. Family physicians could help in predicting life expectancy without prostate cancer. J Clin Oncol 2008;26:690 –1.
[38] Fagerlin A, Rovner D, Stableford S, Jentoft C, Wei JT, Holmes-Rovner M. Patient education materials about the treatment of early stage prostate cancer: a critical review. Ann Intern Med 2004;140:721– 8.
[39] Volk RJ, Hawley ST, Kneuper S, et al. Trials of decision aids for prostate cancer screening: a systematic review. Am J Prev Med 2007;33:428 –34.
[40] Guerra CE, Jacobs SE, Holmes JH, Shea JA. Are physicians discussing prostate cancer screening with their patients and why or why not? A pilot study. J Gen Intern Med 2007;22:901–7.
[41] Visser A, van Andel G. Psychosocial and educational aspects in prostate cancer patients. Patient Educ Couns 2003;49:203– 6.
[42] American Urological Association. Member profile. October 2008. Available from http://www.auanet.org/content/about-us/members/membersprofile. pdf. Accessed 28 January 2009.
[43] Mohan R, Beydoun H, Barnes-Ely ML, Lee L, Davis JW, Lance R, Schellhammer P. Patients' survival expectations before localized prostate cancer treatment by treatment status. J Am Board Fam Med. 2009 May-Jun;22(3):247-56.
[44] Beydoun HA, Mohan R, Beydoun MA, Davis J, Lance R, Schellhammer P. Development of a scale to assess patient misperceptions about treatment choices for localized prostate cancer. British Journal of Urology International, 2010 Feb 11. [Epub ahead of print]. Available at: http://www3.interscience.wiley.com/cgi-bin/fulltext/123280002/PDFSTART
[45] Mohan R, Beydoun H, Davis J, Lance R, Schellhammer P. Feasibility of using guidelines to choose treatment for prostate cancer. Can J Urol. 17:4975-84, 2010. Abstract available at: http://www.ncbi.nlm.nih.gov/pubmed/20156376
[46] Mohan R, Schellhammer P. Treatment options in Localized Prostate Cancer. American Family Physician, August 15th, 2011. 84(4):413-20.
[47] Chou R, Croswell JM, Dana T, Bougatsos C, Blazina I, Fu R, Gleitsmann K, Koenig HC, Lam C, Maltz A, Rugge JB, Lin K.Screening for Prostate Cancer: A Review of the Evidence for the U.S. Preventive Services Task Force. Ann Intern Med. 2011 Oct 7. [Epub ahead of print]